2004
YEAR BOOK OF
ONCOLOGY®

The 2004 Year Book Series

Year Book of Allergy, Asthma, and Clinical Immunology™: Drs Rosenwasser, Boguniewicz, Milgrom, Routes, and Spahn

Year Book of Anesthesiology and Pain Management™: Drs Chestnut, Abram, Black, Lang, Roizen, Trankina, and Wood

Year Book of Cardiology®: Drs Gersh, Cheitlin, Graham, Kaplan, Sundt, and Waldo

Year Book of Critical Care Medicine®: Drs Dellinger, Parrillo, Balk, Bekes, Dries, and Roberts

Year Book of Dentistry®: Drs Zakariasen, Boghosian, Burgess, Hatcher, Horswell, McIntyre, and Zakariasen

Year Book of Dermatology and Dermatologic Surgery™: Drs Thiers and Lang

Year Book of Diagnostic Radiology®: Drs Osborn, Birdwell, Dalinka, Gardiner, Groskin, Levy, Maynard, and Oestreich

Year Book of Emergency Medicine®: Drs Burdick, Cone, Cydulka, Hamilton, Handly, and Quintana

Year Book of Endocrinology®: Drs Mazzaferri, Becker, Kannan, Kennedy, Kreisberg, Meikle, Molitch, Osei, Poehlman, and Rogol

Year Book of Family Practice®: Drs Bowman, Apgar, Dexter, Miser, Neill, and Scherger

Year Book of Gastroenterology™: Drs Lichtenstein, Dempsey, Ginsberg, Katzka, Kochman, Morris, Nunes, Reddy, Rosato, and Stein

Year Book of Hand Surgery®: Drs Berger and Ladd

Year Book of Medicine®: Drs Barkin, Frishman, Klahr, Loehrer, Mazzaferri, Phillips, Pillinger, and Snydman

Year Book of Neonatal and Perinatal Medicine®: Drs Fanaroff, Maisels, and Stevenson

Year Book of Neurology and Neurosurgery®: Drs Gibbs and Verma

Year Book of Nuclear Medicine®: Drs Coleman, Blaufox, Royal, Strauss, and Zubal

Year Book of Obstetrics, Gynecology, and Women's Health®: Drs Mishell, Kirschbaum, and Miller

Year Book of Oncology®: Drs Loehrer, Arceci, Glatstein, Gordon, Morrow, Schiller, and Thigpen

Year Book of Ophthalmology®: Drs Rapuano, Cohen, Eagle, Grossman, Myers, Nelson, Penne, Regillo, Sergott, Shields, and Tipperman

Year Book of Orthopedics®: Drs Morrey, Beauchamp, Peterson, Swiontkowski, Trigg, and Yaszemski

Year Book of Otolaryngology-Head and Neck Surgery®: Drs Paparella, Keefe, and Otto

Year Book of Pathology and Laboratory Medicine®: Drs Raab, Grzybicki, Bejarano, Bissell, and Stanley

Year Book of Pediatrics®: Dr Stockman

Year Book of Plastic and Aesthetic Surgery™: Drs Miller, Bartlett, Garner, McKinney, Ruberg, Salisbury, and Smith

Year Book of Psychiatry and Applied Mental Health®: Drs Talbott, Ballenger, Frances, Jensen, Markowitz, Meltzer, and Simpson

Year Book of Pulmonary Disease®: Drs Phillips, Barker, Blanchard, Dunlap, Lewis, and Maurer

Year Book of Rheumatology, Arthritis, and Musculoskeletal Disease™: Drs Panush, Hadler, Hellmann, Hochberg, Lahita, and Seibold

Year Book of Sports Medicine®: Drs Shephard, Alexander, Cantu, Nieman, Sanborn, and Shrier

Year Book of Surgery®: Drs Copeland, Bland, Cerfolio, Daly, Eberlein, Howard, Luce, Mozingo, and Seeger

Year Book of Urology®: Drs Andriole and Coplen

Year Book of Vascular Surgery®: Dr Moneta

2004

The Year Book of ONCOLOGY®

Editor-in-Chief

Patrick J. Loehrer, Sr, MD

Bruce Kenneth Wiseman Professor of Medicine; Director, Division of Hematology-Oncology; and Associate Director for Clinical Research, Indiana University Cancer Center and Indiana University School of Medicine, Indianapolis, Indiana

Mosby

Mosby
Dedicated to Publishing Excellence

Vice President, Continuity Publishing: Timothy M. Griswold
Publisher: Barton Dudlick
Developmental Editor: Shana Murph
Senior Manager, Continuity Production: Idelle L. Winer
Senior Issue Manager: Pat Costigan
Composition Specialist: Betty Dockins
Senior Illustrations and Permissions Coordinator: Chidi M. Nwaseki

2004 EDITION

Printed in the United States of America
Composition by Thomas Technology Solutions, Inc
Printing/binding by Sheridan Books, Inc.

Editorial Office:
Elsevier
300 East
170 South Independence Mall West
Philadelphia, PA 19106-3399

International Standard Serial Number: 1040-1741
International Standard Book Number: 0-323-02087-9

Associate Editors

Table of Contents

Journals Represented

Mosby and its editors survey approximately 500 journals for its abstract and commentary publications. From these journals, the Editors select the articles to be abstracted. Journals represented in this YEAR BOOK are listed below.

American Journal of Clinical Oncology
American Journal of Clinical Pathology
American Journal of Human Genetics
American Journal of Obstetrics and Gynecology
American Journal of Pathology
American Journal of Public Health
American Journal of Roentgenology
American Journal of Surgery
Annals of Internal Medicine
Annals of Surgical Oncology
Annals of Thoracic Surgery
Archives of Surgery
Bone Marrow Transplantation
Breast Journal
British Journal of Cancer
British Medical Journal
Cancer
Cancer Cell
Cancer Epidemiology, Biomarkers and Prevention
Cancer Research
Clinical Cancer Research
Clinical Infectious Diseases
European Journal of Cancer
European Journal of Nuclear Medicine
Gynecologic Oncology
Head and Neck
Human Reproduction
International Journal of Cancer
International Journal of Gynecological Cancer
International Journal of Radiation, Oncology, Biology, and Physics
Journal of Applied Physiology
Journal of Clinical Endocrinology and Metabolism
Journal of Clinical Investigation
Journal of Clinical Oncology
Journal of Computer Assisted Tomography
Journal of Pediatric Hematology/Oncology
Journal of Pediatric Surgery
Journal of Thoracic and Cardiovascular Surgery
Journal of Urology
Journal of the American Medical Association
Journal of the National Cancer Institute
Lancet
Mayo Clinic Proceedings
Molecular Cancer Therapeutics
New England Journal of Medicine
Oncology
Plastic and Reconstructive Surgery

Proceedings of the National Academy of Sciences
Radiology
Radiotherapy and Oncology
Surgery
World Journal of Surgery

Standard Abbreviations

The following terms are abbreviated in this edition: acquired immunodeficiency syndrome (AIDS), cardiopulmonary resuscitation (CPR), central nervous system (CNS), cerebrospinal fluid (CSF), computed tomography (CT), deoxyribonucleic acid (DNA), electrocardiography (ECG), health maintenance organization (HMO), human immunodeficiency virus (HIV), intensive care unit (ICU), intramuscular (IM), intravenous (IV), magnetic resonance (MR) imaging (MRI), ribonucleic acid (RNA), ultrasound (US), and ultraviolet (UV).

Note

The Year Book of Oncology is a literature survey service providing abstracts of articles published in the professional literature. Every effort is made to assure the accuracy of the information presented in these pages. Neither the editors nor the publisher of the Year Book of Oncology can be responsible for errors in the original materials. The editors' comments are their own opinions. Mention of specific products within this publication does not constitute endorsement.

To facilitate the use of the Year Book of Oncology as a reference tool, all illustrations and tables included in this publication are now identified as they appear in the original article. This change is meant to help the reader recognize that any illustration or table appearing in the Year Book of Oncology may be only one of many in the original article. For this reason, figure and table numbers will often appear to be out of sequence within the Year Book of Oncology.

Introduction

Each year, the field of oncology continues to grow. An improved understanding of the mechanisms of malignant process has led to novel therapies. Clinical research trials have helped define the role of traditional approaches for the treatment of patients with cancer and those at risk of developing cancer. On behalf of the co-editors who have reviewed thousands of articles and selected these few, we wish you happy readings.

Patrick J. Loehrer, Sr, MD
Editor-in-Chief

1 Prevention

A Randomized Trial of Aspirin to Prevent Colorectal Adenomas

Baron JA, Cole BF, Sandler RS, et al (Dartmouth-Hitchcock Med Ctr, Lebanon, NH; Dartmouth Med School, Hanover, NH; Univ of North Carolina, Chapel Hill; et al)

N Engl J Med 348:891-899, 2003 1–1

Introduction.—Epidemiologic studies, experimental studies in animals, and randomized trials in patients at risk for the development of colorectal adenomas provide evidence of the anticarcinogenic effects of nonsteroidal anti-inflammatory drugs (NSAIDs). A group of patients with a recent history of colorectal adenomas participated in a randomized, double-blind trial to determine the anti-neoplastic effect of aspirin in the large bowel.

Methods.—The study group included 1121 patients, 372 assigned to placebo, 377 to 81 mg of aspirin, and 372 to 325 mg of aspirin daily. All patients underwent a complete colonoscopy within 3 months of recruitment and had no known remaining colorectal polyps. Excluded were individuals with a history of familial colorectal cancer syndrome, invasive large-bowel cancer, or malabsorption syndromes. At follow-up, patients were advised to avoid aspirin and other NSAIDs; acetaminophen was distributed for treatment of minor pain and fever. A complete surveillance colonoscopy was performed 34 to 40 months after the qualifying examination.

Results.—Follow-up data were available for 1084 randomly assigned patients (96.7%). Reports of compliance were excellent and similar in the aspirin and placebo groups. A majority of patients avoided nonprotocol use of aspirin and other NSAIDs. Six hundred seventy patients had a total of 1812 polyps. At least 1 colorectal adenoma was diagnosed in 47.1% of patients in the placebo group, 38.3% of patients in the 81-mg aspirin group, and 45.1% in the 325-mg aspirin group. Colorectal cancer was diagnosed in 1, 2, and 3 patients, respectively, in these 3 treatment groups. The risks of death and serious bleeding were similar among groups. For advanced neoplasms, the relative risks (as compared with the placebo group) were 0.59 in the 81-mg aspirin group and 0.83 in the 325-mg group.

Conclusion.—Aspirin, taken daily at a low dose (81 mg), had a moderate effect in reducing the risk of recurrent adenoma among patients with a recent history of adenoma. The risk reduction was greater for advanced lesions than for all lesions combined, suggesting that the effects of aspirin may be more important in later stages of the adenoma-carcinoma sequence.

► Aspirin remains one of the most effective drugs in use today for a variety of disease entities. This is a large prospective randomized trial that documents the use of low doses of aspirin as a chemopreventive agent. Would all patients benefit from aspirin? Clearly, no, but perhaps with better molecular markers, we may be able to target those that might. (See Abstract 1–2).

P. J. Loehrer, Sr, MD

Pronounced Reduction in Adenoma Recurrence Associated With Aspirin Use and a Polymorphism in the Ornithine Decarboxylase Gene

Martinez ME, O'Brien TG, Fultz KE, et al (Univ of Arizona, Tucson; Lankenau Inst for Med Research, Wynnewood, Pa)

Proc Natl Acad Sci U S A 100:7859-7864, 2003 1–2

Background.—In most cases of sporadic colon adenoma, mutations in the adenomatous polyposis coli gene (*APC*) and defects in *APC*-dependent signaling are observed. The expression of several genes, such as the *c-myc* oncogene and its antagonist, *Mad1*, are influenced by *APC*. Ornithine decarboxylase (ODC), a transcriptional target of *c-myc*, modifies *APC*-dependent

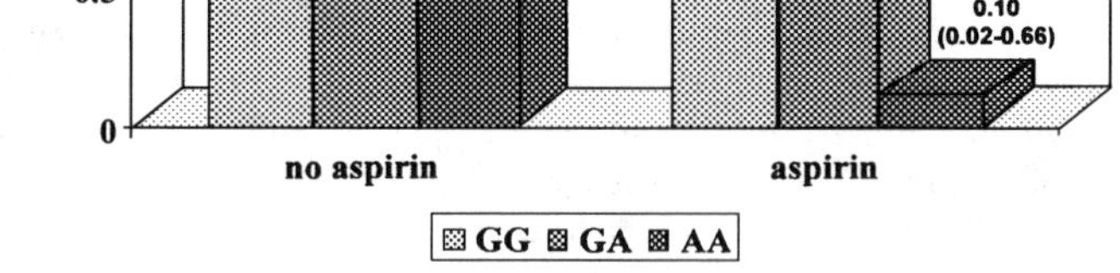

FIGURE 1.—Odds ratios for adenoma recurrence as a function of *ODC* genotype and aspirin use. Results of logistic regression models that control for age, sex, and number of colonoscopies are shown (95% confidence intervals). Individuals homozygous for the G allele and who reported no aspirin use are the reference (*Ref*) group. The number of individuals who recurred over the total in each group among nonaspirin users are 137/266 (51.5%), 100/182 (55%), and 13/31 (41.9%) for GG, AG, and AA variants, respectively; the corresponding figures among aspirin users are 55/116 (47.4%), 34/82 (41.5%), and 2/11 (18.2%). (Courtesy of Martinez ME, O'Brien TG, Fultz KE, et al: Pronounced reduction in adenoma recurrence associated with aspirin use and a polymorphism in the ornithine decarboxylase gene. *Proc Natl Acad Sci USA* 100:7859-7864, 2003.

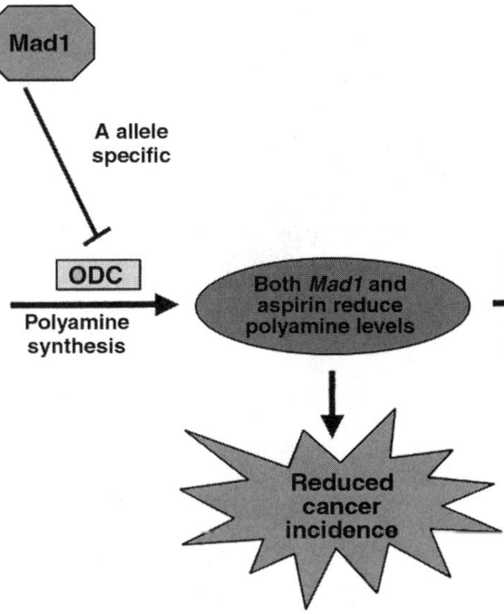

FIGURE 5.—Model depicting actions of *ODC* polymorphism and aspirin on polyamine metabolism, and the consequences for adenoma recurrence. Before acquisition of somatic *APC* mutations, colonic cells in individuals with the minor A allele would have reduced polyamine synthesis from selective suppression of *ODC* promoter activity by *Mad1*. Aspirin would act, in an *ODC* allele–independent manner, to reduce further polyamine levels by activating the transcription of SSAT, thereby increasing polyamine catabolism and export. Cancer risk would be directly related to colonic mucosal polyamine contents, being decreased by decreased polyamine levels. (Courtesy of Martinez ME, O'Brien TG, Fultz KE, et al: Pronounced reduction in adenoma recurrence associated with aspirin use and a polymorphism in the ornithine decarboxylase gene. *Proc Natl Acad Sci USA* 100:7859-7864, 2003. Copyright 2003 National Academy of Sciences U.S.A.)

tumorigenesis. Intron 1 of the human *ODC* gene, which lies between 2 myc-binding domains, contains a single-nucleotide polymorphism. This region has been shown to affect *ODC* transcription. However, there are no data on the association of this polymorphism with colorectal neoplasia risk in human beings. In this colon cancer prevention trial, the relation between *ODC* polymorphism and the risk of adenoma recurrence were investigated.

Methods.—Six hundred eighty-eight patients participating in the adenoma recurrence study were included in the current analysis. In addition, experimental studies conducted in cell culture models were conducted to clarify the epidemiologic findings.

Findings.—Patients homozygous for the minor *ODC* Z allele who reported taking aspirin were approximately 0.1 times as likely as nonaspirin users homozygous for the major G allele to have a recurrence of adenoma (Fig 1). In the human colon cancer–derived cell line HT29, *Mad1* selectively suppressed the activity of the ODC promoter containing the A allele, but not the G allele. The use of 10 μmol/L aspirin or more did not influence *ODC* allele-specific promoter activity, yet it did activate polyamine catabolism and reduced polyamine content in Ht29 cells.

Conclusions.—The ODC polymorphism and aspirin appear to independently decrease the risk of adenoma recurrence. They act, respectively, by suppressing synthesis and activating catabolism of colonic mucosal polyamines (Fig 5). These data also support the hypothesis that the *ODC* polymorphism is a genetic marker for colon cancer risk. The combination of *ODC* inhibitors and aspirin (or other nonsteroidal anti-inflammatory drugs) should be used as a strategy for preventing colon cancer.

▶ This article supports a subgroup who may benefit from aspirin ingestion. Ornithine decarboxylase is the first enzyme involved in polyamine synthesis and is associated with polyp formation. When the variant A allele of the *ODC* gene is homozygous, it is associated with a significantly lower incidence of adenomatous polyp formation. This may be an important pathway to select patients who may benefit from aspirin. This is a nice companion article to Abstract 1–1.

P. J. Loehrer, Sr, MD

Systematic Review of the Effectiveness of Stage Based Interventions to Promote Smoking Cessation

Riemsma RP, Pattenden J, Bridle C, et al (Univ of York, England; Univ of the West of England, Bristol; Univ of Aberdeen, Scotland)

BMJ 326:1175-1177, 2003 1–3

Background.—In 1997, more than 11 million adults in the United Kingdom were regular smokers. In the ensuing 5 years, the proportion of smokers in the population has stabilized or may even be increasing; more recent data indicate that about 25% of 15-year-olds are regular smokers. The risk of disease is reduced after smoking cessation, and several cessation methods are used: pharmacologic methods (nicotine replacement therapy or antidepressants), hypnotherapy, and exercise-based interventions. Behavioral approaches include stage-based interventions, which propose that interventions that account for the current stage of the individual will be more effective and efficient than "one size fits all" interventions. These stage-based models are widely used, yet there is limited evidence of the effectiveness of this approach. The effectiveness of stage-based interventions in effecting positive change in smoking behavior was evaluated.

Methods.—This systematic review used 35 electronic databases, catalogs, and Internet resources. Bibliographies of references were scanned for relevant publications, and authors were contacted where necessary.

Results.—A total of 23 randomized controlled trials were reviewed, including 2 that reported details of an economic evaluation. Eight trials reported effects supportive of stage-based interventions, 3 trials reported mixed results, and 12 trials found no statistically significant difference between a stage-based intervention and a non–stage-based intervention or no intervention. A stage-based intervention was compared with a non–stage-based intervention in 11 trials, and 1 trial reported statistically significant effects for the stage-based intervention. Two studies reported mixed effects, and 8 reported no statistically significant differences between groups. The methodologic quality of the trials was inconsistent, and few of the studies reported any validation of the instrument used to assess participants' stage of change.

Conclusions.—The overall findings of this systematic review indicate that there is limited evidence in support of the effectiveness of stage-based interventions in altering smoking behavior.

► A popular method for smoking cessation in the United Kingdom is "stage-based intervention," in which individuals are separated into 5 stages (precontemplation, contemplation, preparation, action, and maintenance). Progression through the stages is sequential, and interventions are stage-specific. Stage of change needs to be reassessed frequently, as individuals can relapse to an earlier stage or progress to a later 1, and interventions adapt in response to the individual's movement through the stages of change.

Despite the fact that this model is commonly practiced and taught in the United Kingdom, there has been relatively little evidence that this approach is effective. Unfortunately, this systematic review did not find any evidence to support this model system over non–stage-based or no interventions in changing smoking behavior. The authors do admit that the methodologic quality of the reviewed trials was mixed, and only 2 of the 23 trials used a previously validated instrument. This review illustrates the need for more rigorous intervention studies that address the effectiveness of different cessation strategies.

J. H. Schiller, MD

A Controlled Trial of a Human Papillomavirus Type 16 Vaccine

Koutsky LA, for the Proof of Principle Study Investigators (Univ of Washington, Seattle; et al)

N Engl J Med 347:1645-1651, 2002 1–4

Background.—Approximately 20% of adults acquire human papillomavirus type 16 (HPV-16) infections, most of which are benign. In some patients, however, infection progresses to anogenital cancer. Therefore, a vaccine that decreases the incidence of HPV-16 infection may have an important impact on public health.

Methods.—A total of 2392 women (aged 16-23 years) were included in a randomized double-blind study. The women were assigned to 3 doses of placebo or HPV-16 viruslike-particle vaccine, 40 μg, at baseline and at months 2 and 6. Genital samples were obtained periodically. The median follow-up period was 17.4 months after completing the vaccination regimen.

Findings.—The incidence of persistent HPV-16 infection per 100 person years at risk was 3.8 in the placebo group and 0 in the vaccinated group. All 9 women with HPV-16–related cervical intraepithelial neoplasia had been given placebo.

Conclusions.—This HPV-16 vaccine decreases the incidence of HPV-16 infection and HPV-16–related cervical intraepithelial neoplasia. Immunizing HPV-16–negative women may ultimately decrease the incidence of cervical cancer.

▶ This double-blind placebo-controlled study by Koutsky et al evaluated the efficacy of a vaccine against HPV-16 in preventing persistent HPV-16 infection in women between the ages of 16 and 23 years. The data suggest a significant reduction in the rate of persistent infection and raise the possibility of future reduction in the incidence of cervical carcinoma by the use of an HPV vaccine. This may represent an exciting breakthrough in the control of cervical carcinoma.

J. T. Thigpen, MD

Incidence of Cancer and Mortality Following α-Tocopherol and β-Carotene Supplementation: A Postintervention Follow-up

Virtamo J, for the ATBC Study Group (Natl Public Health Inst, Helsinki; et al)
JAMA 290:476-485, 2003 1–5

Objective.—Epidemiologic data have linked low intake of antioxidants to an increased cancer risk. Results of the Alpha-Tocopherol, Beta-Carotene Cancer Prevention (ATBC) Study found a significant reduction in the incidence of prostate cancer among subjects receiving α-tocopherol supplementation but a significant increase in lung cancer and total mortality among those receiving β-carotene. Additional follow-up was performed to clarify the effects of these antioxidants on cancer risk and mortality rate.

Methods.—The postintervention follow-up study included 25,563 Finnish men who participated in the ATBC study. Cancer incidence and cause-specific death were analyzed on the basis of 6-year follow-up data and total mortality rate on the basis of 8-year follow-up data. In the study, more than 29,000 male smokers aged 50 to 69 years were randomly assigned to receive α-tocopherol, β-carotene, both antioxidants, or placebo for 5 to 8 years. Outcomes were assessed by using national cancer and death registry data, with confirmation of all cases of cancer.

Results.—The increase in lung cancer incidence among men receiving β-carotene was nonsignificant on posttrial follow-up: relative risk was 1.06 (95% confidence interval, 0.94 to 1.20). There was also no significant reduction in prostate cancer incidence among men receiving β-carotene: relative risk was 0.88 (95% confidence interval, 0.76 to 1.03). There were no late preventive effects on other types of cancers and no difference in relative mortality risk. The excess risk observed for patients assigned to β-carotene resolved within 4 to 6 years and was mainly attributed to cardiovascular diseases.

Conclusions.—Both the positive and negative effects of antioxidant supplementation reported in the ATBC Study disappear with longer follow-up. Neither α-tocopherol nor β-carotene is effective in preventing cancer. The results still suggest that β-carotene supplementation may be harmful to smokers—total mortality rate is 8% higher among men assigned to β-carotene compared with placebo.

► This is a follow-up from an important prevention trial. With time the results have been muted a bit, but smokers should still avoid β-carotene. We need to be vigilant in advising our patients regarding potential risks of supplemental treatments. Data like this help.

P. J. Loehrer, Sr, MD

2 Breast Cancer

Bilateral Synchronous Breast Cancer: A Population-Based Study of Characteristics, Method of Detection, and Survival

Polednak AP (Dept of Public Health, Hartford, Conn)

Surgery 133:383-389, 2003 2–1

Background.—Bilateral synchronous breast cancer (BSBC) has a reported incidence of 1% to 3%. However, data from population-based cancer registries regarding the clinical and prognostic features of BSBC are limited. The frequency, method of detection, patient and tumor characteristics, and survival for BSBC were defined among all newly diagnosed breast cancer patients in a defined population.

Methods.—The study population included all women with BSBC (cancers in both breasts diagnosed within 3 months of each other) and all women with unilateral breast cancer diagnosed between 1995 and 1999 and reported to the population-based Connecticut Tumor Registry (CTR), which is part of the National Cancer Institute's Surveillance, Epidemiology, and End Results (SEER) Program. The estimated completeness of reporting of cancer cases to SEER registries is approximately 98%, and the quality of SEER coding is generally excellent. Data were obtained on the method of detection of BSBC, and clinical characteristics and survival (through 2000) were compared between BSBC and unilateral breast cancer.

Findings.—BSBC occurred in 300 (1.9%) of the 15,542 patients reported to the CTR during the study period. BSBC was most often detected by mammography of both breasts (35%) or contralateral mammography after detection of a palpable first cancer (18%). There was no difference between BSBC patients and those with unilateral disease in terms of age or stage at diagnosis. However, lobular histology was significantly more frequent in BSBC patients, and the use of total mastectomy (vs less extensive surgery) was more common in BSBC patients than in patients with unilateral disease. Among the BSBC patients, those with cancers detected by breast examination or symptoms had a higher risk of death than those whose BSBC was detected by mammography.

Conclusions.—Bilateral synchronous breast cancer is uncommon. These cancers differ from unilateral cancer with respect to histologic subtype and patient survival. The findings of this study underscore the opportunity for detection of contralateral cancers at an early stage.

▶ The incidence of bilateral breast carcinoma is of interest since many women with a unilateral cancer diagnosis inquire about prophylactic mastectomy of the contralateral breast. The incidence of metachronous cancer in the opposite breast is quite low, affecting slightly less than 1% of women per year.[1] This study uses data from the Connecticut SEER site to determine the incidence of bilateral synchronous breast cancer. Only 1.9% of women had bilateral cancer. The impact of histologic tumor type is of particular interest since there is much concern about the bilaterality of lobular cancer. In this series, lobular cancer was significantly more common in the bilateral cancer group, accounting for 21% of cases compared with 15% in the unilateral group. However, lobular carcinoma in situ was included in this assessment, potentially inflating this statistic. One finding of interest in this study was the increased use of mastectomy in patients with bilateral cancer. Whether this was due to physician advice or patient preference cannot be determined from this report. Bilateral breast-conserving therapy is feasible, and the presence of synchronous cancer does not represent a contraindication to its use. The major message of this study is that the majority of cancers are not bilateral, and a histologic diagnosis of unilateral lobular cancer is not an indication for a bilateral mastectomy.

M. Morrow, MD

Reference

1. Nakhlis F, Morrow M: Prophylactic mastectomy and oophorectomy. *In* Morrow M, Jordan VC, eds: *Managing Breast Cancer Risk*, BC Decker, Hamilton, Ontario, 2003, p 241-258.

Diffusion-Weighted Half-Fourier Single-Shot Turbo Spin Echo Imaging in Breast Tumors: Differentiation of Invasive Ductal Carcinoma From Fibroadenoma

Kinoshita T, Yashiro N, Ihara N, et al (Kameda Med Ctr, Chiba, Japan)
J Comput Assist Tomogr 26:1042-1046, 2002 2–2

Introduction.—Diffusion-weighted (DW) MRI is the most useful clinical tool for diagnosis of cerebral ischemia and stroke. The clinical application of DW-MRI in the breast has been limited; DW echo planar imaging is associated with susceptibility and chemical shift artifacts. Alternative DW echo planar imaging is being considered, including DW half-Fourier single-shot turbo spin echo (HASTE) imaging; it is not affected by such artifacts. The usefulness of DW-HASTE imaging in differentiating invasive ductal carcinoma from fibroadenoma was examined.

Methods.—Between January 2000 and March 2002, 22 women with invasive ductal carcinoma and fibroadenoma (16 and 6 patients, respectively) underwent DW-HASTE imaging. Images were obtained by using diffusion-sensitizing gradients of 0 to 700 mm²/s. The apparent diffusion coefficient (ADC) was determined.

Results.—The DW-HASTE imaging was not influenced by susceptibility or chemical shift artifacts typically present in DW echo planar imaging (Fig 1). The DW-HASTE imaging was linked with low tumor detectability (62%). The difference in mean ADC of invasive ductal carcinoma (1.216×10^{-3} mm²/s) and fibroadenoma (1.495×10^{-3} mm²/s) was significant ($P < .01$).

Conclusion.—ADC measurement using DW-HASTE imaging is useful in the differentiation of invasive ductal carcinoma from fibroadenoma. At

FIGURE 1

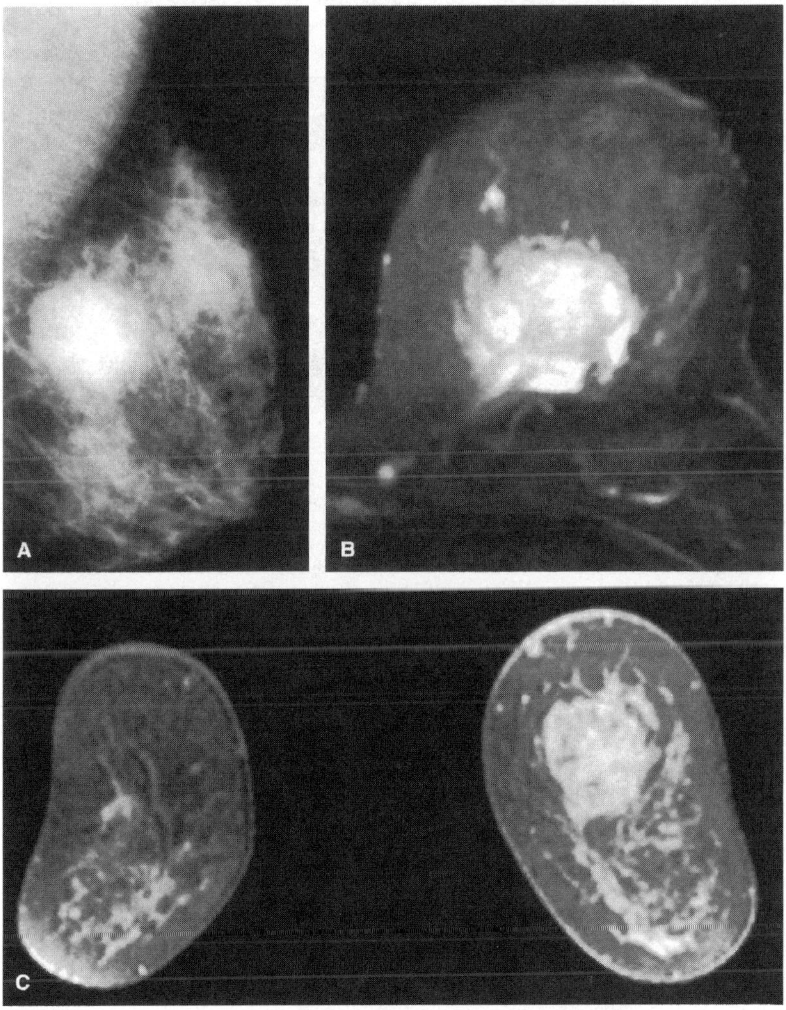

(*Continued*)

FIGURE 1 (cont.)

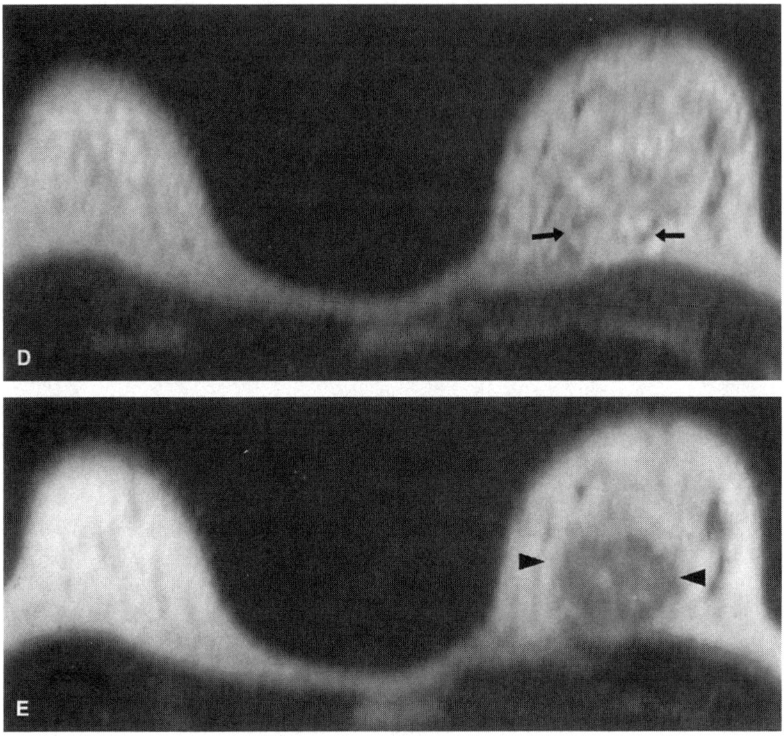

FIGURE 1.—Invasive ductal carcinoma in a 48-year-old woman. **A**, Mediolateral oblique mammogram showed a dense mass with a partial ill-defined margin. **B**, Axial short T1 inversion recovery demonstrated an inhomogeneous hyperintensity mass with an irregular margin. **C**, In a coronal contrast-enhanced 3-dimensional fast long-angle shot image, the mass demonstrated inhomogeneous enhancement with rim enhancement. **D**, A diffusion-weighted half-Fourier single-short turbo spin echo (DS-HASTE) image with a b value of 0 shows a high-intensity mass (*arrows*). **E**, In a DW-HASTE image with a b value of 700 mm^2/s, the signal intensity of the mass is decreased (*arrowheads*). The apparent diffusion coefficient of the invasive ductal carcinoma indicates 1.2×10^{-3} mm^2/s. The DW-HASTE images do not demonstrate image distortion caused by susceptibility and chemical shift. (Courtesy of Kinoshita T, Yashiro N, Ihara N, et al: Diffusion-weighted half-fourier single-shot turbo spin echo imaging in breast tumors: Differentiation of invasive ductal carcinoma from fibroadenoma. *J Comput Assist Tomogr* 26:1042-1046, 2002.)

present, DW-HASTE has low detectability and needs technologic improvement.

► This report from Japan looks at an MR technology called diffusion weighted half-Fourier single-shot turbo spin echo imaging (DW-HASTE). The advantage of this technique is that it is much less susceptible to chemical shift artifacts in the imaging process for MR. The authors report a small series of patients with breast abnormalities in which the DW-HASTE imaging was able to reliably distinguish between invasive ductal carcinoma and fibroadenoma. The numbers are small and it is not a particularly sensitive technique for detection per se. On the other hand, if a lesion is detected and then needs further evaluation, this will prove to be useful, assuming, of course, that it is confirmed by others.

E. Glatstein, MD

Preoperative Assessment of Breast Cancer: Sonography Versus MR Imaging

Hlawatsch A, Teifke A, Schmidt M, et al (Johannes Gutenberg Univ Hosp, Mainz, Germany)

AJR 179:1493-1501, 2003 2–3

Introduction.—Complete tumor removal is essential in patients treated with breast-conserving surgery to prevent recurrence. Thus, precise preoperative information concerning the size of the tumor and the presence and location of multifocal lesions is necessary. The diagnostic value of whole-breast sonography and MRI as adjunct to mammography was examined, along with whether MR imaging should be routinely used in the preoperative evaluation of patients with suspected breast cancer.

Methods.—One hundred four women (mean age, 60 years; range, 34-84 years) in whom breast malignancy was highly suspected underwent preoperative mammography, sonography, and dynamic MRI. All suspicious lesions underwent histologic correlation. The diagnostic relevance of sonographic and MRI was compared with the diagnostic value of clinical examination and mammography alone.

Results.—Twenty-seven tumors demonstrated multifocal or multicentric invasive growth on pathologic examination. Of these, 27 (48%) were correctly diagnosed by mammography alone, 63% with mammography and sonography combined, and 81% with MRI. Nine index tumors were not visible on mammography and were identified on sonography. The use of sonography was beneficial in 13 patients; there were 2 false-positive findings. The use of MRI was beneficial in 7 patients for whom treatment was changed (larger resections or mastectomies in 5 and contralateral resections in 2 patients); there were 8 false-positive findings that prompted unnecessary

TABLE 2.—Patients Evaluated for Breast Cancer Whose Treatment Changed as a Result of Findings of Combined Imaging Techniques

Imaging Method Combination (vs Method on Which Initial Treatment Decision Was Based)	Additional Resection for Tumor		Unnecessary Additional Biopsy or Resection	
	No.	%	No.	%
Combination of mammography and sonography (vs mammography only)	13[a]	13	2	2
Combination of mammography, sonography, and MR imaging (vs combination of mammography and sonography only)	7	7	8	8

*Includes 9 cases of mammographically occult index tumors detected on sonography.

(Courtesy of Hlawatsch A, Teifke A, Schmidt M, et al: Preoperative assessment of breast cancer: Sonography versus MR imaging. *AJR* 179:1493-1501, 2003. Reprinted with permission from the American Journal of Roentgenology.)

contralateral biopsies or larger ipsilateral resections (Table 2). A total of 93% of the cohort had no advantage from MRI. Relevant additional data were significantly more common in patients with dense breasts.

Conclusion.—MRI is most sensitive in identification of small tumors. Yet, it is probably unnecessary in most patients for whom a combination of mammography and whole-breast sonography is used. It is recommended that additional MRI be restricted to problematic cases in women with dense breast parenchyma.

▶ The role of whole breast US and MRI in the preoperative evaluation of the breast cancer patient is controversial. Modern studies of breast-conserving therapy report local control rates of greater than 90% in patients selected for breast conservation with diagnostic mammography. While there is no doubt that both whole-breast US and MRI identify some tumors that are not seen mammographically, the majority of those tumor foci appear to be controlled with radiation. Thus, the routine use of additional imaging techniques raises the disturbing possibility that patients may be subjected to unnecessary mastectomies or cosmetically deforming wide resections due to the detection of subclinical disease that would be treated with radiation. Both MRI and whole breast US are sensitive, but nonspecific, tests. As illustrated in this study, the number of unnecessary biopsies or resections resulting from MRI findings equaled the number of resections that showed cancer. The outcome of US in this study was excellent, but other studies examining the use of whole-breast US have demonstrated a high incidence of biopsies for benign findings.[1,2]

Until the use of whole-breast US and MRI is shown to decrease the incidence of local failure in patients undergoing breast-conserving surgery, these examinations should not be part of the routine preoperative evaluation but should be reserved for problem solving.

M. Morrow, MD

References

1. Golshan M, Fung BB, Wolfman J, et al: The effect of ipsilateral whole breast ultrasound in the surgical management of breast carcinoma. *Am J Surg* 186:391-396, 2003.
2. Gordan PB, Goldenberg SL: Malignant breast masses detected only by ultrasound. A retrospective review. *Cancer* 76:626-630, 1995.

Ultrasonographically-Guided Fine-Needle Aspiration of Axillary Lymph Nodes: Role in Breast Cancer Management

Sapino A, Cassoni P, Zanon E, et al (Univ of Turin, Italy; San Giovanni Hosp, Turin, Italy)

Br J Cancer 88:702-706, 2003 2–4

Background.—Various sophisticated imaging procedures have been proposed for staging of the axillary lymph nodes in breast cancer, but none has been successful enough to replace histologic examination. Whether sonography of axillary lymph nodes followed by fine-needle aspiration cytology (FNAC) of lymph nodes with suspicious findings on sonography is useful in the preoperative treatment of breast cancer patients was evaluated.

Methods.—Axillary sonography was performed in 298 patients with breast cancer (267 with invasive carcinoma and 31 with ductal carcinoma in situ [DCIS]). Ninety-five patients had suspicious nodes on sonography and underwent FNAC of those nodes. Smears were examined by routine cytologic staining. Cases in which the diagnosis was uncertain were stained with a combination of anticytokeratin and antiepithelial membrane antigen antibodies.

Findings.—Of the 95 FNAC procedures, 85 were informative. In 49 cases, lymph nodes were positive for metastases; in 36 cases lymph nodes were negative. Thus, in 49 (18%) of 267 patients with invasive breast cancer, sonography of axillary nodes and FNAC of nodes suspicious on sonography permitted preoperative confirmation of metastatic lymph nodes in the axilla. These patients could continue directly to axillary dissection. Six (16%) of the 36 patients with negative lymph nodes on FNAC were ultimately found to have lymph node metastases. Ultrasonographically guided FNAC presurgically identified 49 (55%) of 88 cases of metastatic lymph nodes. Of the 203 cases in which lymph node findings on sonography were not suspicious and FNAC was not performed, 28 (16%) subsequently proved to be lymph node positive on histologic examination.

Conclusions.—The use of sonographic examination of axillary lymph nodes should be performed in all patients with breast cancer, with FNAC supported by immunocytochemistry performed only on sonographically suspicious lymph nodes. This presurgical protocol is reliable for the screening of patients with lymph node metastases who should proceed directly to axillary dissection or adjuvant chemotherapy and avoid sentinel lymph node biopsy.

► US-guided fine-needle aspiration of axillary lymph nodes could be described as a procedure looking for an indication. Sapino et al make the argument that US-guided aspiration should be routinely employed for staging in all breast cancer patients. This is based on a study of 267 invasive cancer patients. Of these, 95 had nodes described as "suspicious" by US, and fine needle aspiration cytology diagnosed carcinoma in 49. There were 36 patients with a negative aspiration who had a sentinel node biopsy or an axillary dissection; 6 of those were found to have node metastases. The authors report these cases as false-negative results. However, of the 172 patients with normal axillary US, 28 also had nodal metastases, an additional false-negative group. A negative US or a negative needle aspiration is clearly not adequate to exclude the presence of axillary disease. The apparent benefit of the procedure is for the 49 patients who were diagnosed with nodal metastases, allowing them to avoid sentinel node biopsy before axillary dissection. The authors assert that axillary US with needle aspiration is more cost effective than sentinel node biopsy, but no data are provided to support the claim. The US and aspiration procedure is most useful for detecting larger nodal metastases. These metastases are most likely to be identified with a frozen section of the sentinel node, allowing axillary dissection to be performed at the same setting. In this circumstance, the cost savings from avoiding sentinel node biopsy are likely to be minimal. The primary benefit of this procedure seems to be better stratification of patients in trials of neoadjuvant therapy. Off trial it is the status of the nodes after the initial chemotherapy that determines the need for more therapy, not their status before any treatment at all. Based on this report, I would still conclude that US-guided needle aspiration is a procedure looking for an indication in the primary staging of breast cancer.

M. Morrow, MD

Stereotactic 11-Gauge Vacuum-Assisted Breast Biopsy: A Validation Study

Pfarl G, Helbich TH, Riedl CC, et al (Univ of Vienna; Mem Sloan-Kettering Cancer Ctr, New York)

AJR 179:1503-1507, 2002 2–5

Background.—Stereotactic biopsy has been increasingly used for the histologic diagnosis of breast lesions. Several studies in the 1990s found a false-negative rate of 3% to 8% for stereotactic 14-gauge automated core biopsy. Stereotactic 11-gauge vacuum-assisted biopsy technology is now available and has several advantages in comparison with automated core biopsy, including better calcification retrieval, fewer histologic underestimates, and a lower rate of rebiopsy. The false-negative rate of stereotactic 11-gauge vacuum-assisted biopsy was determined in a validation study of lesions that were subsequently surgically excised.

Methods.—A retrospective review was conducted of 318 lesions that underwent stereotactic 11-gauge vacuum-assisted biopsy and subsequent surgical excision. A false-negative result was defined as a pathologically proved cancer in which stereotactic biopsy yielded benign results without atypia. Medical records, imaging studies, and histologic findings were reviewed.

Results.—The false-negative rate for stereotactic 11-gauge vacuum-assisted biopsy was 3.3% of pathologically proved cancers. False-negative findings occurred in 3.5% of malignant calcification lesions versus 3% of malignant masses. Among the 7 false-negative findings were 5 Breast Imaging Reporting and Data System (BI-RADS) category 5 lesions that yielded benign results at biopsy, one BI-RADS category 4 mass that yielded benign breast tissue, and one BI-RADS category 4 cluster of calcifications in which no calcifications were retrieved. The false-negative rate was 10% for radiologists who performed 15 or fewer previous stereotactic vacuum-assisted biopsy procedures compared with 0.6% for radiologists who performed more than 15 previous stereotactic vacuum-assisted biopsy procedures (Table 3).

Conclusions.—The false-negative rate for stereotactic 11-gauge vacuum-assisted biopsy was 3.3%, which declined to 0.6% with experience. All the false-negative findings could be identified prospectively because of failure to sample calcifications or imaging-histologic discordance.

TABLE 3.—Validation Studies of Stereotactic Biopsy

Investigator	Year	No. of Patients	Needle	No. Malignant	No. (%)* False-Negative
Parker et al. [1]	1990	102	Variable automated†	16	1 (6.3)
Parker et al. [2]	1991	102	14-gauge automated	23	1 (4.3)
Dowlatshahi et al. [3]	1991	250	20-gauge automated	76	19 (25.0)‡
Dronkers [4]	1992	53	18-gauge automated	45	2 (4.4)§
Elvecrog et al. [5]	1993	100	14-gauge automated	35‖	1 (2.9)
Gisvold et al. [6]	1994	160	14-gauge automated	64¶	5 (7.8)
Helbich et al. [7]	1997	210	Variable automated**	98	3 (3.1)
Helbich et al. [8]	1998	66	Variable automated††	30	0 (0)
This study	2002	318	11-gauge vacuum-assisted	214	7 (3.3)

*Proportion of pathologically proven cancers in which the stereotactic biopsy histology was benign without atypia.

†Gauge was 18 in 65 lesions, 16 in nine lesions, and 14 in 29 lesions.

‡In an additional 11 (14.5%) of 76 cancers, stereotactic biopsy material was "insufficient for diagnosis." Every lesion in this study underwent fine-needle aspiration biopsy before core biopsy.

§In an additional two (4.4%) of 45 cancers, stereotactic biopsy was "nondiagnostic," with "no representative material obtained" because of "insufficient sampling."

‖Excludes one case of lobular carcinoma in situ.

¶Excludes three cases of lobular carcinoma in situ.

**16-gauge needle in 21 lesions and 14-gauge needle in 189 lesions. Guidance was stereotaxis in 149 (with the patient prone in 82 cases, sitting in 67) lesions and sonography in 61 lesions. All false-negative findings occurred in biopsies performed under stereotactic guidance (sitting in two, prone in one).

††Six passes were performed for each lesion, two with 14-gauge, two with 16-gauge, and two with 18-gauge needles, in random order. Although no false-negative diagnoses were obtained with 14-gauge needle, 16-gauge needle gave false-negative results in two (6.7%) of 30 cancers, and 18-gauge needle gave false-negative results in two (6.7%) of 30 cancers.

(Courtesy of Pfarl G, Helbich TH, Riedl CC, et al: Stereotactic 11-gauge vacuum-assisted breast biopsy: A validation study. *AJR* 179:1503-1507, 2002. Reprinted with permission from the *American Journal of Roentgenology*.)

► Stereotactic biopsy was introduced in the early 1990s and is now widely available. Since the initial validation studies reported in the 1990s, considerable clinical experience has been gained, and well-defined criteria for surgical excision after stereotactic biopsy have been developed.[1] Larger 11-gauge vacuum-assisted biopsy devices have been developed that result in sampling of large amounts of tissue.

In spite of this, significant numbers of women continue to undergo needle localization and surgical excision for the diagnosis of mammographically detected abnormalities. The overwhelming majority of mammographically detected abnormalities are benign. For the woman with a benign lesion, stereotactic biopsy is clearly less morbid and less expensive than a surgical excision.[2] For the woman with an invasive malignancy, a preoperative diagnosis allows the breast and axillary surgery to be performed as a single procedure. Even for the woman who requires mastectomy, a core biopsy diagnosis avoids a skin incision that may interfere with a skin-sparing mastectomy.[3]

The article by Pfarl et al is unusual because it is a modern series, using the vacuum-assisted biopsy device, in which surgical confirmation of the diagnosis was performed for virtually all patients. The study demonstrates an acceptably low false-negative rate of 3.3%, but more importantly, all false-negative cases were identified using standard criteria of lack of concordance of mammographic appearance and pathologic diagnosis, or absence of calcification in the specimen. The study also confirms that even with large vacuum-assisted biopsy devices, a core diagnosis of atypical ductal hyperplasia is an indication for complete excision. In this report, 35% of these patients had carcinoma.

Similarly, a significant number of cases diagnosed as intraductal carcinoma by core biopsy (12% in this study) contained invasive carcinoma, a factor that should be considered when planning local therapy. In spite of these relatively minor drawbacks, it is clear that image-guided core biopsy is the diagnostic procedure of choice for mammographic abnormalities.

M. Morrow, MD

References

1. Bassett L, Winchester DP, Caplan RB, et al: Stereotactic core-needle biopsy of the breast: A report of the Joint Task Force of the American College of Radiology, American College of Surgeons, and College of the American Pathologists. *CA Cancer J Clin* 47:171-190, 1997.
2. Lee CH, Egglin TK, Philpotts L, et al: Cost-effectiveness of stereotactic core needle biopsy: Analysis by means of mammographic findings. *Radiology* 202:849-854, 1997.
3. Morrow M, Venta L, Stinson T, et al: Prospective comparison of stereotactic core biopsy and surgical excision as diagnostic procedures for breast carcinoma. *Ann Surg* 233:537-541, 2001.

Fourteen-Gauge Needle Core Biopsy of Mammographically Evident Radial Scars: Is Excision Necessary?

Cawson JN, Malara F, Kavanagh A, et al (Univ of Melbourne, Fitzroy, Victoria, Australia; Latrobe Univ, Melbourne, Victoria, Australia; Peter MacCallum Cancer Inst, East Melbourne, Victoria, Australia)

Cancer 97:345-351, 2003 2–6

Background.—Radial scars are benign lesions that can mimic breast carcinoma on mammography and are usually managed by excisional biopsy. An experience with using stereotactic needle core biopsy (SNCB) to sample such lesions was reported. In addition, the sensitivity of SNCB in the diagnosis of radial scar and any associated carcinoma was determined.

Methods.—This prospective study examined a consecutive series of 75 mammographically detected radial scars from a population-based screening program between 1993 and 2000. The histologic findings of the core biopsy sample were compared with those of the gold standard of excisional biopsy in patients who underwent lesion sampling by SNCB followed by surgical biopsy.

Findings.—A total of 75 radial scars were detected on mammography; 12 were surgically excised before core biopsy, and 63 were sampled by core biopsy, with SNCB used for 55 patients (87%) and sonographically guided needle core biopsy (UNCB) for 8 patients (13%). One patient who underwent SNCB did not undergo a follow-up excisional biopsy. Preoperative core biopsy led to the diagnosis of radial scars in 51 of 62 patients who underwent excision (82% sensitivity; 95% confidence interval [CI], 70%-91%). The SNCB technique identified 46 of 54 radial scars sampled (85%; 95% CI, 73%-93%), and UNCB identified 5 of 8 radial scars sampled (63%; 95% CI, 24%-91%). Of the 54 patients who underwent SNCB and excision, 4 patients had coexistent ductal carcinoma in situ (DCIS) at the time of excision. SNCB identified DCIS in 1 of these patients and identified atypical ductal hyperplasia (ADH) in the remaining 3 patients. Overall, 5 of 75 radial scars were associated with DCIS (7%), and there were no invasive carcinomas. Coexisting ADH was found at surgical excision in 42 of 74 radial scars (57%; 95% CI, 45%-68%), and ADH had been identified in 21 of 29 radial scars sampled preoperatively by SNCB (72%; 95% CI, 53%-87%).

Conclusions.—The sensitivity of SNCB for the identification of radial scars was 85%. In 4 patients with associated DCIS, SNCB showed either ADH or DCIS, both of which required excision. These findings suggest that cases of SNCB-proven radial scars among a screened population can be managed safely with mammographic follow-up, as long as the lesions are not associated with DCIS, ADH, or lobular carcinoma in situ. Spiculated abnormalities with discordant SNCB findings require surgical biopsy.

► The early experience with needle core biopsy indicated that lack of concordance between imaging and pathology findings, atypical hyperplasia, and a diagnosis of radial scar were indications for surgical excsion.[1] As experience with core biopsy has increased and improvements in technique such as the use of larger needles and more extensive sampling have occurred, these indications for surgery are being reevaluated. Radial scar is an infrequent diagnosis, seen in only 0.09% of screened cases in this study. The strength of this study is that all radial scars in a population-based screening program were examined, and only 1 patient did not have a surgical excision. Only 5 of the 75 radial scars (7%) were associated with malignancies. All of these cases had intraductal carcinoma or atypical hyperplasia identified on core biopsy. This study suggests that when radial scar without associated atypia is identified by core, routine surgical excision is not necessary.

M. Morrow, MD

Reference

1. Bassett L, Winchester DP, Copan RB, et al: Stereotactic core-needle biopsy of the breast. A report of the joint task force of the American College of Radiology, American College of Surgeons, and College of American Pathologists. *CA Cancer J Clin*, 47:171-189, 1997.

Twenty-Year Results of the Naples GUN Randomized Trial: Predictive Factors of Adjuvant Tamoxifen Efficacy in Early Breast Cancer

De Placido S, De Laurentiis M, Carlomagno C, et al (Università 'Federico II," Napoli, Italy; II Università, Napoli, Italy; Istituto Nazionale per lo Studio e la Cura dei Tumori "Pascale," Napoli, Italy)

Clin Cancer Res 9:1039-1046, 2003 2–7

Background.—Tamoxifen is a mainstay of breast cancer treatment, and its use as adjuvant therapy after local-regional treatment of early breast cancer is supported by numerous trials and a meta-analysis of all randomized trials throughout the world. However, tamoxifen is not without toxic effects. Factors with the potential for predicting the efficacy of tamoxifen in patients with early breast cancer were evaluated.

Methods.—A total of 433 patients were enrolled in the Gruppo Universitario Natoletano (GUN) randomized trial from 1978 to 1983, with 206 patients assigned to tamoxifen and 227 patients designated as control subjects. In both groups, premenopausal patients with axillary lymph node involvement also received 9 cycles of CMF therapy. Eight biologic markers were retrospectively assayed for most patients, including estrogen, progesterone, prolactin receptors (PrlRs), microvessel count (MVC), S-phase fraction, tumor ploidy, epidermal growth factor receptor (EGFR), and HER2. A multivariate analysis of the interactions of tamoxifen and covariates was performed to determine whether these variables were predictive of the efficacy of tamoxifen. Estimates of the effect of tamoxifen were expressed as hazard ratio (HR) of death of tamoxifen over no-tamoxifen patients with 95% confidence intervals (CIs).

Results.—PrlRs, MVC, S-phase fraction, ploidy, and EGFR were not predictive of tamoxifen efficacy at a median follow-up of 15 years. However, HER2 was found to have an overall significant predictive effect, with an HR of 0.59 (95% CI, 0.40-0.87) in HER2-negative patients versus an HR of 1.09 (95% CI, 0.63-1.87) in HER2-positive patients. The predictive effect of HER2 was also observed in the subgroup of patients with steroid receptor–positive tumors.

Conclusions.—S-phase, ploidy, EGFR, PRLrs, and microvessel count are not predictive of tamoxifen efficacy. These findings are supportive of the view that patients with tumors overexpressing HER2 may not benefit from adjuvant tamoxifen therapy.

Elevated Serum HER-2/*neu* Level Predicts Decreased Response to Hormone Therapy in Metastatic Breast Cancer

Lipton A, Ali SM, Leitzel K, et al (Penn State Milton S Hershey Med Ctr, Hershey, Pa; Veterans Affairs Med Ctr, Lebanon, Pa; Novartis Pharmaceutical Corp, East Hanover, NJ; et al)

J Clin Oncol 20:1467-1472, 2002 2–8

Background.—HER-2/*neu* overexpression in metastatic breast cancer has been linked with a reduced response rate to first-line hormone therapy in estrogen receptor–positive (ER^+) disease. However, this finding has not been consistent. In this study, a large group of patients with ER^+ or ER status unknown metastatic breast cancer was evaluated for the presence of elevated serum levels of HER-2/*neu* to see if HER-2/*neu* level or ER status affected the response to hormone therapy.

Methods.—The 719 patients (age range, 35-92 years) had been randomly assigned to receive second-line hormone therapy involving megestrol acetate or an aromatase inhibitor. Serum levels of HER-2/*neu* were evaluated with an enzyme-linked immunosorbent assay specific for the extracellular domain of the protein; serum levels higher than 15 ng/mL were considered elevated. End points of the study were response rate and duration, time to progression (TTP) (ie, time to objective disease progression or death), time to treatment failure (TTF) (ie, time to earliest occurrence of progression, death, or withdrawal from randomized trial treatment), and survival.

Results.—Elevated serum levels of HER-2/*neu* were noted in 219 patients; 500 patients had values within normal range. For patients with elevated serum HER-2/*neu* values, the response rate was 23%, whereas that for patients with normal levels was 45% ($P < .0001$). The median TTP was 90 days for patients with elevated serum HER-2/*neu* levels and 180 days for patients with normal levels. The median TTF when serum levels were elevated was 93 days and 175 days when serum levels were normal ($P < .0001$). The duration of clinical response was shorter among those with elevated serum HER-2/*neu* levels than among those with normal levels. At the last follow-up, 475 patients had died; median survival time was much shorter among patients with elevated serum HER-2/*neu* levels than in those whose levels were normal (17.2 vs 29.6 months, $P < .0001$). The results were similar when the analysis was restricted to only the 591 patients for whom hormone receptor status was known to be positive.

Conclusions.—Hormone therapy is likely to be less successful for patients with ER^+ metastatic breast cancer who also have elevated serum levels of HER-2/*neu*. Such patients will also have a shorter duration of response and a shorter survival than patients who have normal serum levels of HER-2/*neu*.

► These 2 trials assess the value of hormonal therapy in patients with breast cancers that overexpress HER-2/*neu*. Both show evidence that hormonal therapy is not as effective in those patients who overexpress the oncogene. Patients overexpressing HER-2/*neu* had significantly worse results than those who were nonoverexpressors of HER-2/*neu*. These observations raise significant questions about the role of hormonal therapy in overexpressing patients and require further study as to exactly how patients positive for ER and progesterone receptor but also positive for overexpression of HER-2/*neu* ought to be managed.

J. T. Thigpen, MD

Endocrine Responsiveness and Tailoring Adjuvant Therapy for Postmenopausal Lymph Node-Negative Breast Cancer: A Randomized Trial

Castiglione-Gertsch M, for the International Breast Cancer Study Group (IBCSG Coordinating Ctr and Inselspital, Bern, Switzerland; et al)

J Natl Cancer Inst 94:1054-1065, 2002 2–9

Background.—Between 1992 and 1996, more than 43% of the women having surgery for nonmetastatic invasive breast cancer in the United States were aged 50 years or older and had negative lymph nodes. Relapses and death are substantially reduced when tamoxifen is taken for at least 5 years by such women. For postmenopausal women with lymph node–positive disease, chemotherapy combined with tamoxifen has been shown to improve the results as compared with tamoxifen alone. The role of adjuvant chemotherapy before tamoxifen treatment for patients with lymph node–negative disease was assessed in a randomized controlled trial.

Methods.—The 1669 patients were stratified by estrogen receptor (ER) status (382 had ER-negative and 1217 had ER-positive tumors, with 70 of unknown ER status) and were randomly assigned to receive (1) three 28-day courses of classic adjuvant CMF chemotherapy and then tamoxifen, 20 mg/d orally for 57 months; or (2) only tamoxifen at the same dose for 60

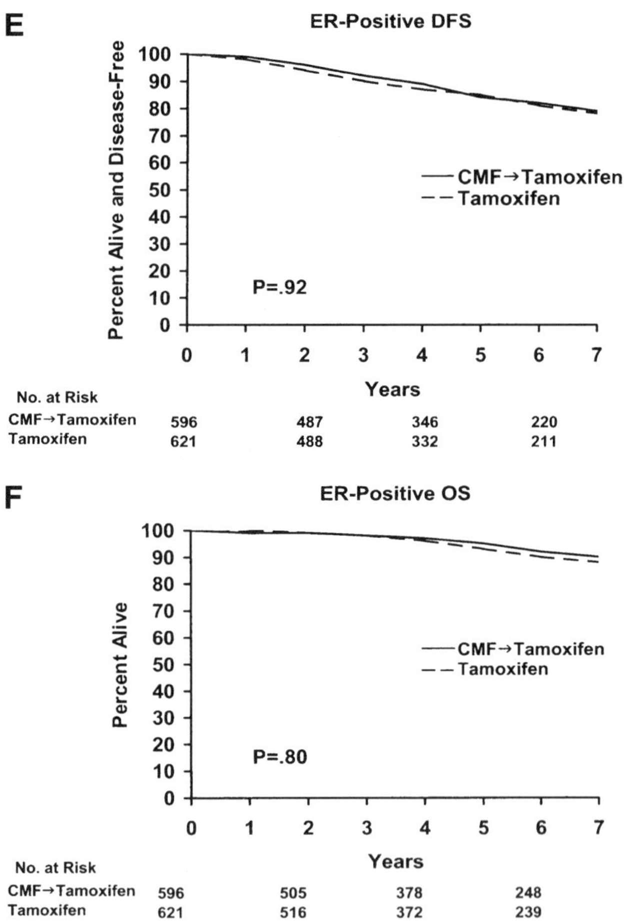

FIGURE 2.—Kaplan-Meier plots of disease-free survival (*DFS*) (E) and overall survival (*OS*) (F) for 1217 postmenopausal women with lymph node–negative, estrogen receptor (*ER*)-positive breast cancer according to randomized treatment group at a median follow-up of 71 months. E, $P = .92$ for DFS for the two treatment groups. F $P = .80$ for OS for the two treatment groups. All statistical tests were two-sided. (Courtesy of Castiglione-Gertsch M, for the International Breast Cancer Study Group: Endocrine responsiveness and tailoring adjuvant therapy for postmenopausal lymph node-negative breast cancer: A randomized trial. *J Natl Cancer Inst* 94:1054-1065, 2002. By permission of Oxford University Press.)

months. The chemotherapy consisted of oral cyclophosphamide, 100 mg/m^2 on days 1 to 14; IV methotrexate, 40 mg/m^2 on days 1 and 8; and IV 5-fluorouracil, 600 mg/m^2 on days 1 and 8. Follow-up extended for a median of 71 months.

Results.—Patients who received 3 courses of CMF followed by tamoxifen had better disease-free survival (DFS) than those who only received tamoxifen, and overall survival (OS) was also trending toward better results for the combination therapy. Among ER-negative patients, the group receiving chemotherapy plus tamoxifen had a statistically significantly better DFS of 84% at 5 years versus 69% for the ER-negative women receiving tamoxifen only; their OS was also statistically significantly better (89% vs 81%). ER-positive women did not show this difference in DFS or OS (Fig 2, E and F). Only patients with ER-negative tumors of 1 cm or less or with grade 1 tumors did not have statistically significantly better DFS with CMF, whereas CMF did not improve DFS for any of the patients with ER-positive tumors. Prognostically significant factors for ER-negative cases were treatment, tumor size, and tumor grade; those for ER-positive cases were age and tumor grade.

Conclusions.—Substantial benefit was documented for postmenopausal women with lymph node–negative, endocrine-nonresponsive breast cancer when treatment included adjuvant chemotherapy. The use of adjuvant chemotherapy for patients with similar tumors that are endocrine responsive did not provide this benefit; tamoxifen alone for at least 5 years produced similar outcomes.

► In recent years, it has become increasingly clear that for the patient with hormone receptor–positive breast cancer, endocrine therapy rather than chemotherapy provides the major therapeutic benefit. The amount of additional benefit obtained from adding chemotherapy to tamoxifen in the treatment of ER-positive, node-negative postmenopausal women remains the subject of debate. In this study, no benefit for the addition of 3 cycles of CMF to tamoxifen was observed in ER-positive patients. Patients at higher risk of relapse on the basis of grade or tumor size were not found to benefit from the additional chemotherapy. A companion quality-of-life analysis showed that patients receiving CMF scored significantly worse than those receiving tamoxifen alone on an overall subjective health rating and on all reported quality-of-life measures except hot flash severity. These differences were confined to the first 12 months after treatment. The findings of this study are consistent with those of the National Surgical Adjuvant Breast and Bowel Project (NSABP) B-20 trial,[1] which also examined the benefit of adding chemotherapy to tamoxifen in women with receptor-positive, node-negative disease. No significant benefit was observed for patients older than 60 years. These studies emphasize that in this population, the benefits of chemotherapy are minimal, and the rationale for its use must be carefully considered for each individual patient. Improvements in survival with more effective endocrine therapy, such as those observed in the Arimidex and Tamoxifen: Alone or in Combination (ATAC) trial comparing anastrozole to tamoxifen, are more likely to provide benefit to this subset of women.

M. Morrow, MD

Reference

1. Fisher B, Dignan J, Wolmark N, et al: Tamoxifen and chemotherapy for lymph node negative, estrogen receptor positive breast cancer. *J Natl Cancer Inst* 89:1673-1682, 1997.

Randomized Trial of Dose-Dense Versus Conventionally Scheduled and Sequential Versus Concurrent Combination Chemotherapy as Postoperative Adjuvant Treatment of Node-Positive Primary Breast Cancer: First Report of Intergroup Trial C9741/Cancer and Leukemia Group B Trial 9741

Citron ML, Berry DA, Cirrincione C, et al (ProHEALTH Care Associates LLP, Lake Success, NY; Mem Sloan-Kettering Cancer Ctr, New York; Univ of Texas, Houston; et al)

J Clin Oncol 21:1431-1439, 2003 2–10

Background.—Dose-escalation approaches have met with little success in improving responses to adjuvant chemotherapy for primary operable breast cancer. Dose-density approaches seek to minimize residual tumor burden by giving chemotherapy drugs with a shorter interval between treatments. The effects of dose-dense versus conventional neoadjuvant chemotherapy, and of a sequential versus a concurrent schedule of administration, for women with node-positive primary breast cancer were compared.

Methods.—The randomized trial enrolled 2005 women with T0 to T3, N1 to N2, M0 primary adenocarcinoma of the breast in a 2 × 2 factorial design. Group I was given sequential therapy with 4 doses of doxorubicin, then 4 doses of paclitaxel, then 4 doses of cyclophosphamide, with doses given every 3 weeks. Group II received sequential doxorubicin, paclitaxel, and cyclophosphamide, given every 2 weeks with filgrastim. Patients in group III received concurrent doxorubicin and cyclophosphamide followed by paclitaxel every 3 weeks, and those in group IV received concurrent doxorubicin and cyclophosphamide followed by paclitaxel every 2 weeks with filgrastim. Disease-free survival, overall survival, and toxicity were compared among groups.

Findings.—At a planned analysis performed at a median 36 months' follow-up, 315 relapses or deaths had occurred compared with 515 expected treatment failures. Dose-dense chemotherapy was associated with significant improvement in the primary end point of disease-free survival (risk ratio [RR], 0.74; $P = .01$) as well as in overall survival (RR, 0.69; $P = .013$). Patients receiving dose-dense therapy (ie, that given every 2 weeks) had a 4-year disease-free survival rate of 82% (95% confidence interval [CI], 80.7%-83.3%) compared with 75% (95% CI, 73.7%-76.2%) in the conventional groups. Treatment sequence was not correlated with disease-free or overall survival; no interaction was found between dose density and treatment sequence. Grade 4 granulocytopenia was more common with the 3-week than the dose-dense regimen (33% vs 6%; $P < .0001$), and grade 3 to

4 emesis was more common in the concurrent regimens than in the sequential regimens (7% vs 3%; $P = .0002$).

Conclusions.—For women receiving postoperative neoadjuvant chemotherapy for node-positive breast cancer, dose-dense combination chemotherapy improves outcome over that obtained with a conventional dose schedule in terms of both disease-free and overall survival. Outcomes were similar for sequential versus concurrent chemotherapy.

▶ This phase III randomized trial of the Cancer and Leukemia Group B evaluated the concepts of sequential versus concurrent chemotherapy and of dose density. The significant finding in the trial is that dose density (shortening the interval between chemotherapy cycles rather than escalating the dose per cycle) appears to confer a statistically significant, albeit small, absolute progression-free and overall survival advantage. The dose-dense approach requires the use of growth factors and is logistically more difficult. The questions that remain include: (1) Does the advantage for dose density apply to all patients or only to a high-risk subset? (2) Are the increased logistical difficulty and cost justified by the gain?

J. T. Thigpen, MD

Improved Outcomes From Adding Sequential Paclitaxel but Not From Escalating Doxorubicin Dose in an Adjuvant Chemotherapy Regimen for Patients With Node-Positive Primary Breast Cancer

Henderson IC, Berry DA, Demetri GD, et al (Univ of California, San Francisco; Cancer and Leukemia Group B (CALGB) Statistical Ctr, Durham, NC; Wake Forest Univ, Winston-Salem, NC; et al)

J Clin Oncol 21:976-983, 2003 2–11

Background.—Adjuvant systemic therapy with a combination of cyclophosphamide, methotrexate, and fluorouracil (CMF) reduces the annual odds of recurrence and early death in patients with breast cancer by 24% (±SD 3%) and 14% (±4%), respectively. In trials in which an anthracycline (doxorubicin or epirubicin) was added to cyclophosphamide, the anthracycline regimens resulted in a reduction in annual odds of 12% (±1%) and 11% (±5%) in recurrence or death, respectively, compared with CMF. Whether increasing the dose of doxorubicin in or adding paclitaxel to a standard adjuvant chemotherapy regimen in patients with breast cancer would increase the time to recurrence and survival was investigated.

Methods.—A total of 3121 women with operable breast cancer and involved lymph nodes were randomly assigned to adjuvant chemotherapy with a combination of cyclophosphamide (C), 600 mg/m^2, with 1 of 3 doses of doxorubicin (A), 60, 75, or 90 mg/m^2, for 4 cycles. This regimen was followed by either no additional therapy or 4 cycles of paclitaxel at 175 mg/m^2. Tamoxifen was given to 94% of patients with hormone receptor–positive tumors.

Results.—There was no evidence of a dose effect for doxorubicin: the 5-year disease-free survival was 69%, 66%, and 67% for patients who received 60, 75, and 90 mg/m^2, respectively. The hazard reductions from the addition of paclitaxel to CA therapy were 17% for recurrence and 18% for death. The disease-free survival at 5 years was 65% (±1%) and 70% (±1%) for CA alone or CA plus paclitaxel, respectively. Overall survival at 5 years was 77% (±1%) and 80% (±1%) for CA alone or CA plus paclitaxel, respectively. An unplanned subset analysis showed that the hazard ratio of CA plus paclitaxel versus CA alone was 0.72 for those with estrogen receptor–negative tumors and just 0.91 for patients with estrogen receptor–positive tumors, with nearly all these patients receiving adjuvant tamoxifen. The addition of 4 cycles of paclitaxel resulted in generally modest additional toxicity.

Conclusions.—In patients with early breast cancer, the addition of 4 cycles of paclitaxel after a standard course of cyclophosphamide and doxorubicin improves both disease-free and overall survival.

► This phase III randomized study of the Cancer and Leukemia Group B evaluates the importance of the dose intensity of an anthracycline and the value of the addition of sequential paclitaxel as a part of adjuvant therapy for patients with node-positive breast carcinoma. Patients were randomized to receive doxorubicin at a dose of either 60 mg/m^2, 75 mg/m^2, or 90 mg/m^2 in combination with cyclophosphamide and then were rerandomized to receive either no further chemotherapy or 4 cycles of paclitaxel after the completion of 4 cycles of doxorubicin/cyclophosphamide. The study showed no advantage for the higher doses of doxorubicin, a result similar to a prior study that showed no advantage to escalation of the cyclophosphamide dose in the doxorubicin/cyclophosphamide combination. Those patients who received 4 cycles of paclitaxel after completion of the doublet, however, did demonstrate a superior progression-free and overall survival. It would appear that the addition of 4 cycles of paclitaxel improves the results of adjuvant therapy in patients with node-positive breast carcinoma. Two questions remain: (1) Is the benefit observed confined to a specific subset of patients (e.g., those who are HER2/*neu* overexpressors)? (2) Does the absolute 3% improvement in overall survival justify the increased toxicity of the added paclitaxel?

J. T. Thigpen, MD

Conventional Adjuvant Chemotherapy With or Without High-Dose Chemotherapy and Autologous Stem-Cell Transplantation in High-Risk Breast Cancer

Tallman MS, Gray R, Robert NJ, et al (Northwestern Univ, Chicago; Dana-Farber Cancer Inst, Boston; Inova Fairfax Hosp, Falls Church, Va; et al)
N Engl J Med 349:17-26, 2003 2–12

Background.—Women with primary breast cancer and 10 or more involved ipsilateral axillary lymph nodes are at high risk of recurrence. Adjuvant chemotherapy improves 5-year disease-free survival in these patients to 20% to 50%, depending on the regimen. Some trials have suggested high-dose chemotherapy with autologous hematopoietic stem-cell transplantation can improve 5-year disease-free survival to approximately 65% to 70% in patients at high risk of recurrence. Whether adding high-dose chemotherapy with autologous stem-cell transplantation to conventional adjuvant chemotherapy improves outcomes in patients with stage II or III breast cancer at high risk of recurrence was examined.

Methods.—The subjects were 511 women (median age, 44 years) with primary breast cancer and 10 or more involved ipsilateral axillary lymph nodes. Patients were randomly assigned in a 1:1 ratio to receive conventional adjuvant chemotherapy (CAF) alone or in combination with high-dose chemotherapy plus autologous hematopoietic stem-cell transplantation. CAF consisted of cyclophosphamide (100 mg/m^2 on days 1-14), doxorubicin (30 mg/m^2 on days 1 and 8), and fluorouracil (500 mg/m^2 on days 1 and 8) every 28 days for 6 cycles. Patients in the high-dose chemotherapy group also received cyclophosphamide (6 gm/m^2) and thiotepta (800 mg/m^2) on days 6, 5, 4, and 3 before autologous bone marrow or peripheral blood stem cells infusion. All patients underwent radiation therapy after the end of chemotherapy, and patients with steroid receptor–positive tumors were given tamoxifen. Patients were followed up for a median of 6.1 years to determine disease-free and overall survival and time to recurrence. Additionally, the incidence of second (nonbreast) cancers and adverse effects were monitored.

Results.—At 6 years, the CAF alone and the combined therapy groups did not differ significantly in disease-free survival (47% vs 49%, respectively), overall survival (62% vs 58%), and time to recurrence (48% vs 55% of patients remained free of recurrence). However, during the study there were many minor protocol violations (eg, failure to document a negative pregnancy test, the receipt of chemotherapy before enrollment). When only the 417 patients who fulfilled the strict eligibility requirements were considered, the addition of high-dose chemotherapy and autologous stem-cell transplantation significantly improved 6-year recurrence-free survival compared with CAF alone (55% vs 45%). Nine patients in the CAF alone group had a second cancer develop compared with 15 patients in the combined therapy group. In particular, 9 patients in the combined therapy group died of transplantation-related complications, and 9 had a myelodysplastic syndrome or acute myeloid leukemia develop.

Conclusion.—In patients with breast cancer and 10 or more involved ipsilateral axillary lymph nodes, adding high-dose chemotherapy and autologous hematopoietic stem-cell transplantation to 6 cycles of standard adjuvant chemotherapy may reduce the risk of relapse. However, this additional treatment does not significantly improve outcomes, but it does carry the risk of transplantation-related morbidity and mortality. Therefore, adjuvant chemotherapy remains the standard of care for patients with primary breast cancer and a high risk of recurrence.

▶ This randomized phase III trial evaluates the value of high-dose chemotherapy with stem-cell support as consolidation therapy in patients who have completed adjuvant chemotherapy for node-positive breast cancer associated with 10 or more positive nodes. The study shows a reduction in the relapse rate without a concomitant improvement in survival. The authors conclude that standard chemotherapy remains the standard of care. This is consistent with the results of other trials of high-dose chemotherapy with stem-cell support in breast cancer.

J. T. Thigpen, MD

High-Dose Chemotherapy With Hematopoietic Stem-Cell Rescue for High-Risk Breast Cancer

Rodenhuis S, for the Netherlands Working Party on Autologous Transplantation in Solid Tumors (The Netherlands Cancer Inst, Amsterdam; et al)

N Engl J Med 349:7-16, 2003 2–13

Background.—Among patients with breast cancer who are at high risk of recurrence, some studies suggest high-dose adjuvant chemotherapy with hematopoietic stem-cell infusion improves progression-free survival compared with conventional adjuvant chemotherapy. Other studies have not supported these claims. A large prospective study was therefore undertaken to investigate the effect of high-dose adjuvant chemotherapy with hematopoietic stem-cell infusion on disease recurrence and survival in patients with stage II or III breast cancer at risk of recurrence.

Methods.—The subjects were 885 women younger than 56 years old who had undergone surgery for breast cancer and who had 4 or more tumor-positive axillary lymph nodes but no distant metastases. Patients were randomly assigned in a 1:1 ratio to receive conventional adjuvant chemotherapy alone or in combination with high-dose chemotherapy plus hematopoietic stem-cell infusion. Conventional adjuvant chemotherapy (FEC) consisted of fluorouracil (500 mg/m^2), epirubicin (90 mg/m^2, and cyclophosphamide (500 mg/m^2) every 3 weeks for 5 cycles. Patients in the high-dose chemotherapy group received FEC for the first 4 cycles. Their fifth cycle was replaced by cyclophosphamide (6 gm/m^2), thiotepta (480 mg/m^2), and carboplatin (1600 mg/m^2) infused over a 4-day period, followed 48 hours later by peripheral blood progenitor cell infusion. All patients underwent radiation therapy after the end of chemotherapy and were given tamoxifen. Patients were followed up for a median of 57 months to determine disease-free and overall survival. Additionally, the incidence of second cancers and adverse effects was monitored.

Results.—At 5 years, the FEC alone and the combined therapy groups did not differ significantly in disease-free survival (59% vs 65%) or overall survival. However, for patients with 10 or more tumor-positive axillary lymph nodes, relapse-free survival was significantly better in the combined therapy group (61% vs 51%). There was no significant correlation between survival and treatment for patients with HER2/neu-positive tumors. For patients with HER2/neu-negative tumors, however, relapse-free survival was significantly better in the combined therapy group (hazard ratio for relapse, 0.66), and overall survival tended to be better, too (P = .07). In particular, in the patients with HER2/neu-negative tumors, combined therapy had significant advantages for patients younger than 40 years old, for premenopausal patients, for patients who underwent mastectomy, for patients with 10 or more tumor-positive axillary lymph nodes, for progesterone receptor–positive tumors, for p53-positive tumors, and for less aggressive (grade I) tumors. Fifteen patients in the FEC alone group had a second cancer develop compared with 21 patients in the combined therapy group. One patient (in the FEC alone group) developed myelodysplasia or leukemia, and 4 patients in the combined therapy group died within 100 days of stem-cell infusion (2 from cardiac causes, 2 from septicemia).

Conclusion.—In patients with breast cancer and 10 or more involved axillary lymph nodes, adding high-dose chemotherapy and hematopoietic stem-cell infusion to 4 cycles of standard adjuvant chemotherapy improves relapse-free survival, although this benefit appears limited to patients with HER2/neu-negative tumors.

► This article constitutes the final report on a randomized trial of high-dose chemotherapy in women with breast cancer. Patients were randomized to receive either standard anthracycline-based therapy or high-dose chemotherapy with stem cell support. Subjects were women with breast cancer with at least 4 positive lymph nodes. Overall survival among the 885 women randomized to the 2 arms was not different, though the studied suggested an improvement in relapse-free survival for the women with 10 or more positive lymph nodes. Subset analysis did demonstrate a modest advantage for women whose tumors were HER-2/*neu* positive, suggesting that a population of biologically aggressive tumors may be better treated with more aggressive therapy. Overall, this negative trial, in terms of overall survival, provided some hints for improvement in outcomes in selective subsets of women with breast cancer at the highest risk of relapse. Although high-dose chemotherapy has given way to more dose-dense adjuvant regimens, it does suggest that stratification of adjuvant therapy based on tumor profiling may be appropriate.

M. S. Gordon, MD

A Gene-Expression Signature as a Predictor of Survival in Breast Cancer

van de Vijver MJ, He YD, van 't Veer LJ, et al (Netherlands Cancer Inst, Amsterdam; Ctr for Biomedical Genetics, Amsterdam; Rosetta Inpharmatics, Kirkland, Wash)

N Engl J Med 347:1999-2009, 2002 2–14

Introduction.—Most clinicians agree that patients with poor prognostic characteristics benefit the most from adjuvant therapy. A more accurate method for prognostication in breast cancer will improve the selection of patients who are appropriate for adjuvant systemic therapy.

Methods.—A microarray analysis was used to examine a previously established 70-gene prognostic profile to classify a series of 295 consecutive

C Lymph-Node–Negative Patients

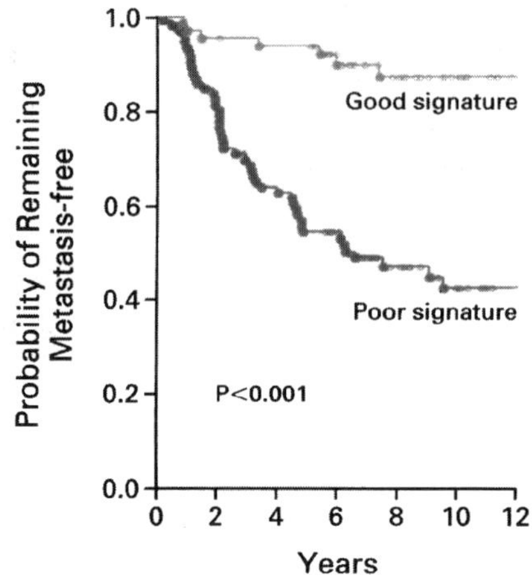

No. at Risk

Good signature	60	57	54	45	31	22	12
Poor signature	91	72	55	41	26	17	9

E Lymph-Node–Positive Patients

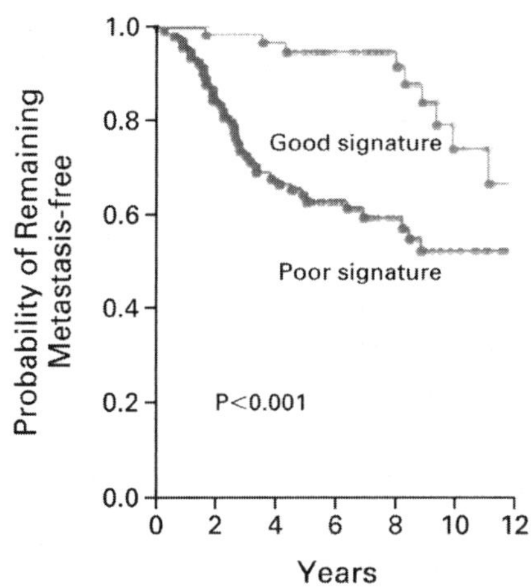

No. at Risk

Good signature	55	54	53	42	28	14	7
Poor signature	89	74	56	43	26	16	8

FIGURE 2.—Kaplan-Meier analysis of the probability that patients would remain free of distant metastases among patients with lymph-node–negative disease (C) and patients with lymph-node–positive disease (E), according to whether they had a good-prognosis or a poor-prognosis signature. The *P* values were calculated with use of the log-rank test. (Reprinted by permission of *The New England Journal of Medicine* from van de Vijver MJ, He YD, van't Veer LJ, et al: A gene-expression signature as a predictor of survival in breast cancer. *N Engl J Med* 347:1999-2009, 2002. Copyright 2002, Massachusetts Medical Society. All rights reserved.)

patients with primary breast cancer as having a gene expression signature that is either linked with a poor or good prognosis. The predictive value of the prognosis profile was examined by both univariate and multivariate analyses.

Results.—Of 295 patients, 180 had a poor prognosis signature and 115 had a good prognosis signature. The mean overall 10-year survival rates were 54.6% and 94.5%, respectively, for those with poor and good prognosis signatures. At 10 years, the probability of remaining free of distant metastases was 50.6% and 80.2% in these groups, respectively. The estimated hazard ratio for distant metastases was 5.1 (95% confidence interval [CI], 2.9-9.0; $P < .001$) for the poor compared with good prognosis signature group. This ratio continued to be significant when the groups were evaluated according to lymph node status (Fig 2). Multivariate Cox regression analysis demonstrated that the prognosis profile was a strong independent factor in predicting disease outcome.

Conclusion.—The gene expression profile examined was a more powerful predictor of outcome of distant disease in young patients with breast cancer than standard systems based on clinical and histologic criteria.

▶ Treatment tailored to an individual patient's risk of relapse is a major unrealized goal of breast cancer therapy. This study of gene expression profiling as a method of predicting outcome validates earlier work by this group,[1] which suggests that a 70-gene panel can be used to identify patients with good and poor outcomes, independent of nodal status. This work has numerous clinical implications. The good-prognosis subset is substantially larger than that identified with criteria suggested by the National Institutes of Health Consensus Conference[2] or the St Gallen Consensus Conference.[3] Most patients in this favorable-prognosis subset have tumors that contain the estrogen receptor, suggesting that the addition of chemotherapy to endocrine treatment may be overtreatment. Conversely, 2 distinct groups within the population of lymph-node–positive patients are identified, offering the possibility of tailoring the intensity of treatment.

However, exciting as this work is, it requires independent validation before being ready for routine clinical use. All clinicians have puzzled over why the patient with a large cancer and 15 positive nodes survives, while a woman with a 1-cm, node-negative tumor develops metastases and dies. It appears that through gene profiling, we may finally begin to understand if not why, at least who.

M. Morrow, MD

References

1. van't Veer LJ, Dai H, van de Vijver MF, et al: Gene expression profiling predicts clinical outcome of breast cancer. *Nature* 415:530-536, 2002.
2. Eifel P, Axelson JA, Costa J, et al: National Institutes of Health Consensus Development Conference Statement: Adjuvant therapy for breast cancer, November 1-3, 2000. *J Natl Cancer Inst* 93:979-989, 2001.

3. Goldhirsch A, Glick JH, Gelber RD, et al: Meeting highlights: International Consensus Panel on the Treatment of Primary Breast Cancer: Seventh International Conference on Adjuvant Therapy of Primary Breast Cancer. *J Clin Oncol* 19:3817-3827, 2001.

Patterns of Recurrence After Sentinel Lymph Node Biopsy for Breast Cancer

Badgwell BD, Povoski SP, Abdessalam SF, et al (Ohio State Univ, Columbus)
Ann Surg Oncol 10:376-380, 2003 2–15

Introduction.—The development and validation of sentinel lymph node biopsy (SLNB) in the staging and treatment of breast cancer has been an important medical advance that has allowed this technique to become a standard of care in many specialty medical centers. The incidence and pattern of disease recurrence after SLNB were examined in patients who underwent SLNB between April 6, 1998, and October 27, 1999.

Methods.—A prospectively maintained breast cancer database was used to identify female patients who had undergone successful SLNB more than 24 months previously. A total of 222 consecutive patients met these criteria. A retrospective medical record review and data analysis were performed to identify variables predictive of recurrence.

Results.—The median follow-up was 32 months (range, 24-43 months). Of 222 patients, 159 (72%) were SLN negative and did not undergo any further axillary treatment. Five (3.1%) patients had recurrence (1 local, 4 distant), with no isolated regional (axillary) recurrences. Sixty-three (28%) patients were SLN positive. They underwent a subsequent axillary lymph node dissection. Six (9.5%) of these patients had recurrence (3 local, 1 regional, 2 distant). Pathologic tumor size ($P < .001$), lymphovascular invasion ($P = .018$) and a positive SLN ($P = .048$) were statistically significantly linked with disease recurrence.

Conclusion.—With a minimum follow-up of 24 months, patients with a negative SLN and no subsequent axillary treatment have a low rate of disease recurrence. These findings support the use of SLNB as the sole axillary procedure in patients who are SLN negative.

► A major unanswered question regarding SLNB is the incidence of isolated axillary recurrence after the procedure. Studies of SLNB followed by axillary dissection demonstrate false-negative rates of 5% to 10%.[1] However, reported rates of axillary recurrence are much lower. In this study of 222 patients, no isolated axillary recurrences were noted. In a review of 1493 patients treated with SLNB alone, only 2 (0.13%) isolated axillary recurrences were reported.[1] In part, the low incidence of axillary recurrence can be explained by the use of breast irradiation, which includes a significant portion of the lower axilla in the breast tangents since the majority of women in these studies were treated with lumpectomy and radiotherapy. In addition, the NSABP B04 trial demonstrated that a significant number of patients with untreated axillary node metastases do not develop clinical evidence of axillary recurrence.[2] The growing body of data on the excellent rates of local control and low morbidity after SLNB support its use as the preferred staging procedure for the clinically node-negative axilla.

M. Morrow, MD

References

1. Grube B, Giuliano AE: Management of the axilla. In Harris JR, Lippman ME, Morrow M, Osborne CK, eds: *Diseases of the breast.* Lippincott, Williams & Wilkins, Philadelphia, 2004. In press.
2. Fisher B, Redmond C, Fisher ER, et al: Ten-year results of a randomized clinical trial comparing radical mastectomy and total mastectomy with or without radiation. *N Engl J Med* 312:674-681, 1985.

The Prognostic Value of Vascular Endothelial Growth Factor in 574 Node-Negative Breast Cancer Patients Who Did Not Receive Adjuvant Systemic Therapy

Manders P, Beex LVAM, Tjan-Heijnen VCG, et al (Univ Med Centre Nijmegen, The Netherlands; Rotterdam Cancer Inst, The Netherlands)

Br J Cancer 87:772-778, 2002 2–16

Introduction.—The growth and metastasizing capacity of solid tumors depend on angiogenesis, for which vascular endothelial growth factor (VEGF) is a mediator. Several trials have demonstrated that in invasive breast cancer, the level of VEGF is highly correlated with the degree of angiogenesis. The prognostic value of VEGF for relapse-free survival (RFS) and overall survival (OS) was examined in patients with node-negative breast cancer who were not treated with adjuvant systemic therapy.

Methods.—The cytosolic levels of VEGF were determined by means of a quantitative enzyme-linked immunosorbent assay to examine tumor samples from 574 patients with node-negative invasive breast cancer. These patients did not undergo adjuvant systemic therapy. Follow-up was a median of 61 months (range, 2-155 months) after primary diagnosis. Correlations were examined with well-known prognostic factors.

Results.—There was a positive correlation between VEGF and age and tumor size (P = .042 and P = .029, respectively). The VEGF level was inversely, yet weakly associated with progesterone receptor levels (r_s = −0.090; P = .035). A high VEGF level (equal to or above the median level of 0.53 ng/mg protein) predicted a decreased RFS and OS in univariate survival rate analysis (for both, P = .005) (Fig 1). Multivariate analysis also showed that VEGF was an independent predictor of poor RFS and OS (P = .045 and P = .029, respectively), in addition to age, tumor size, and progesterone receptor level.

Conclusion.—Cytosolic levels of VEGF in tumor tissue samples are independently indicative of prognosis in patients with node-negative breast cancer who do not undergo adjuvant systemic therapy, implying that VEGF is associated with the natural course of breast cancer progression.

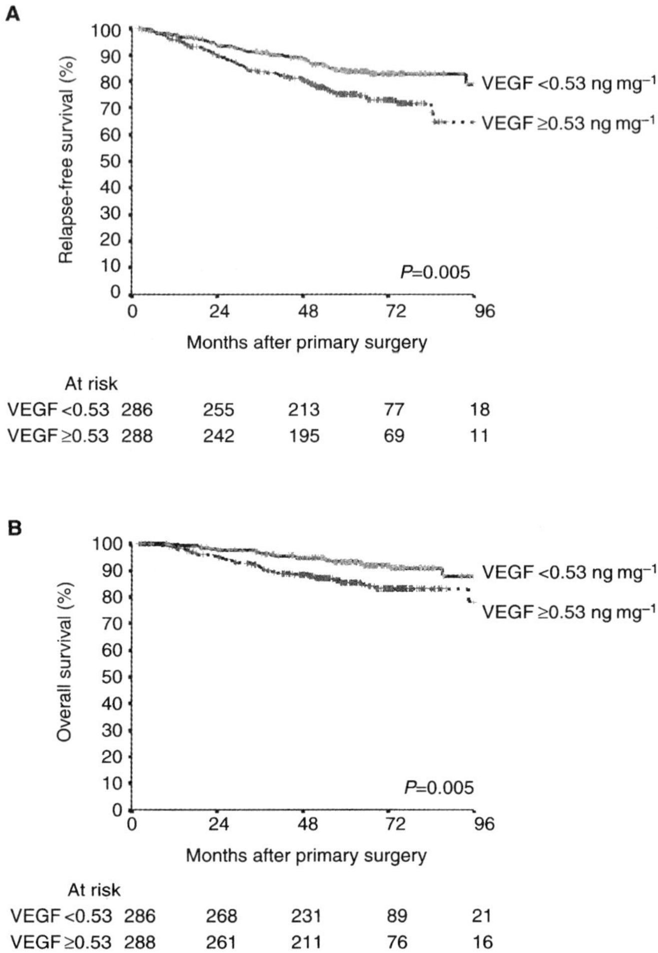

FIGURE 1.—Relapse-free survival (A) and overall survival (B) as a function of vascular endothelial growth factor (*VEGF*) values. For each data set, original VEGF values in the primary breast tumors were divided into 2 groups: less than 0.53 ng/mg protein or 0.53 ng/mg or greater. Events indicate the number of patients at risk in each group. Patients at risk at 0, 24, 48, 72, and 96 months after primary surgery are indicated. (Courtesy of Manders P, Beex LVAM, Tjan-Heijnen VCG, et al: The prognostic value of vascular endothelial growth factor in 574 node-negative breast cancer patients who did not receive adjuvant systemic therapy. *Br J Cancer* 87:772-778, 2002.)

► These Dutch investigators report on 574 patients with node-negative invasive breast cancer. They have evaluated the level of VEGF and conclude that the cytosolic level of VEGF in the tumor tissue samples was independently predictive of prognosis for these patients with node-negative breast cancer who are not treated with adjuvant systemic therapy. The observation they make is interesting. The differences, although statistically significant, are fairly modest, and one has to wonder if there are not other factors that are responsible for the separation of the curves.

E. Glatstein, MD

BRCAPRO Validation, Sensitivity of Genetic Testing of *BRCA1/BRCA2*, and Prevalence of Other Breast Cancer Susceptibility Genes

Berry DA, Iversen ES, Gudbjartsson DF, et al (Baylor College of Medicine, Houston; Duke Univ, Durham, NC; Harvard Univ, Boston; et al)

J Clin Oncol 20:2701-2712, 2002 2–17

Background.—Mutations of the susceptibility genes *BRCA1* and *BRCA2* are more likely to be found in persons who have a family history of breast or ovarian cancer, or both. Genetic testing to detect these mutations is being done much more commonly than in the past. Genetic testing carries both health and cost consequences and requires complex risk assessment. Models to predict the results of genetic testing currently depend on regression or classification approaches wherein certain family characteristics are used. A computer program, BRCAPRO, applies a statistical model to predict the probability of carrying a mutation of these genes based on the person's cancer status and whether first- or second-degree relatives have had breast and ovarian cancer. The limitations and practical application of BRCAPRO and other carrier probability models were explored.

Methods.—The data were gathered from 6 high-risk genetic counseling clinics and applied to persons whose family had a minimum of one member who had been tested for mutations at *BRCA1* and *BRCA2*. BRCAPRO was used to predict genetic predispositions to breast and ovarian cancer, and the predictions were compared with the results of genetic testing. Three hundred one persons were included.

Results.—One hundred twenty-six families were Ashkenazi Jewish (AJ). The average numbers of cases of breast cancer, ovarian cancer, and bilateral breast cancer in the 301 families were 3.0, 0.8, and 0.5, respectively. Seventy-one percent of the probands had 3 or more cases of familial breast or ovarian cancer, placing them at high risk for carrying mutations. Probands who had extensive family histories of these cancers tended to have higher carrier probabilities, but many probands with these histories had low carrier probabilities, and some probands with only a few familial cancers had high probabilities. Thus, genetic risk could not be based solely on family history. The mean carrier probability was 61%: 79% for persons who tested positive and 39% for those who tested negative. There was good correspondence between carrier probabilities and proportions of positive tests, although BRCAPRO tended to underestimate the true proportion of positive tests when the carrier probability was lowest or highest. AJ and non-AJ patients were also evaluated (Fig 2, B). The sensitivity of genetic testing was estimated as 85% or better.

Conclusions.—BRCAPRO proved to be accurate in determining the carrier probability for mutations of the *BRCA1* and *BRCA2* genes. The use of genetic testing for these genes missed an estimated 15% of mutations. Among the persons evaluated, genes indicating a susceptibility to breast cancer other than *BRCA1* and *BRCA2* were found to be rare, nonexistent, or carry low disease penetrance.

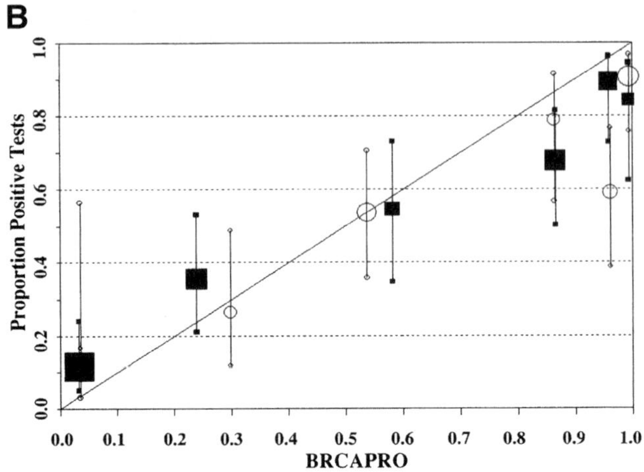

FIGURE 2.—B, Comparison of BRCAPRO carrier probability and results of genetic testing by subgroups of Ashkenazi Jewish (AJ) and not AJ. Each *circle/square* represents a sextile of the data set; each 95% confidence interval is shown by a *vertical line with dotted end points.* (Courtesy of Berry DA, Iversen ES, Gudbjartsson DF, et al: BRCAPRO validation, sensitivity of genetic testing of *BRCA1/BRCA2*, and prevalence of other breast cancer susceptibility genes. *J Clin Oncol* 20[11]:2701-2712, 2002. Reprinted with permission from the American Society of Clinical Oncology.)

► As awareness of genetic predisposition mutations increases among both physicians and patients, clinical questions about which women to refer for genetic counseling and possible testing arise. This is particularly true in the case of women with unilateral breast carcinoma, where the presence of a mutation in *BRCA1* or *2* will significantly change the risk of second primary cancers in the ipsilateral breast as well as the risk of contralateral cancer. This information may affect a woman's choice of operative procedure, but awaiting the results of genetic testing significantly delays surgery and may be a source of anxiety.

This study provides validation for the BRCAPRO model, a computer program which predicts the probability that an individual carries a *BRCA1* or *2* mutation. The model performed well and was most accurate for those with neither extremely high (>70%) or extremely low (<5%) carrier probabilities. These women of intermediate risk are precisely those in whom clinical uncertainty is greatest. This study indicates that this model is a useful tool for counseling patients about the likelihood that genetic testing will provide informative results.

M. Morrow, MD

Concordance Between Local and Central Laboratory HER2 Testing in the Breast Intergroup Trial N9831

Roche PC, Suman VJ, Jenkins RB, et al (Mayo Clinic, Rochester, Minn; Eastern Cooperative Oncology Group, Brookline, Mass; Southwest Oncology Group, San Antonio, Tex; et al)

J Natl Cancer Inst 94:855-857, 2002 2–18

Background.—The efficacy of trastuzumab in patients with metastases prompted an investigation of this agent as an adjuvant therapy in women with primary, operable, node-positive breast carcinoma with strong overexpression of HER2 protein or HER2/neu gene amplification. Concordance between local and central laboratory HER2 testing in this trial was investigated.

Methods.—Eligibility of women enrolled in the study was determined by local laboratory testing. The protocol stipulated verification of HER2 status by central testing with use of the HercepTest immunohistochemistry and the Vysis PathVysion fluorescence in situ hybridization (FISH) assays.

Findings.—Among tumor specimens obtained from the first 119 enrolled patients and centrally tested, 74% were HercepTest 3-positive. Sixty-six per-

TABLE 1.—A, Comparison of Local HER2 Testing Performed for Study Entry Onto N9831 and Central HercepTest*

	Central HercepTest™ Score†				
	0	1+	2+	3+	Total
Local HER2 testing					
IHC‡	8	9	12	81	110
FISH	1	1	0	7	9
Total	9	10	12	88	119

B, Comparison of Local HER2 Testing Performed for Study Entry Onto N9831 and Central FISH

	Central FISH Result§		
	Not Amplified	Amplified	Total
Local HER2 testing			
IHC	37	73	110
FISH	3	6	9
Total	40	79	119

*All specimens originally scored in a local laboratory as either HER2 positive (3+) by immunohistochemistry or the presence of HER2/neu gene amplification by fluorescence in situ hybridization.

†HER2 overexpression was tested with the HercepTest and a DAKO Autostainer in strict accordance with the manufacturer's instructions in the Immunohistochemistry Laboratory (P. C. Roche, Mayo Clinic, Rochester, Minnesota). The stained slides were interpreted and scored on a 0-3+ scale according to the Food and Drug Administration–approved guidelines for HercepTest by the study pathologist.

‡FISH is performed with the PathVysion HER2/neu DNA probe kit following the manufacturer's instructions in the Cytogenetics Laboratory (R. B. Jenkins, Mayo Clinic, Rochester, Minnesota). The stained slides were independently analyzed and interpreted by 2 technicians as described.

Abbreviations: FISH, Fluorescence in situ hybridization; *IHC*, immunohistochemistry.

(Courtesy of Roche PC, Suman VJ, Jenkins RB, et al: Concordance between local and central laboratory HER2 testing in the breast intergroup trial N9831. *J Natl Cancer Inst* 94:855-857, 2002, by permission of Oxford University Press.)

cent were found to have HER2 gene amplification. Only 67% of the specimens submitted by local laboratories as FISH positive were verified by central assays. Central HercepTest and central FISH assays were 92% concordant. The 74% concordance between local and central testing for HER2 status resulted in modifications in the eligibility criteria (Table 1).

Conclusions.—The overall performance of HER2 testing at local laboratories in the initial study sample was disappointing. Levels of discordance with central testing were unacceptably high. The use of FISH by local oncology and pathology practices needs to be evaluated. Further research on interlaboratory agreement is required.

Real-World Performance of HER2 Testing—National Surgical Adjuvant Breast and Bowel Project Experience

Paik S, Bryant J, Tan-Chiu E, et al (Natl Surgical Adjuvant Breast and Bowel Project Operation Ctr, Pittsburgh, Pa; Univ of Pittsburgh, Pa; Univ of Kentucky, Lexington; et al)

J Natl Cancer Inst 94:852-854, 2002 2–19

Background.—Trastuzumab (Herceptin), a monoclonal antibody against HER2 growth factor receptor, is beneficial in patients with metastatic breast cancer with HER2 overexpression. Currently, this therapy combined with polychemotherapy is being tested in several clinical trials. The National Surgical Adjuvant Breast and Bowel Project Protocol B-31 tested the advantage of adding Herceptin to the adjuvant chemotherapy regimen of doxorubicin and cyclophosphamide, followed by paclitaxel, in patients with stage II breast cancer with HER2 overexpression or gene amplification. A snapshot of the quality of HER2 assays performed in laboratories nationwide was presented.

TABLE 1.—Results From a Central Testing Facility Confirming Original IHC Assay Results Submitted by NSABP B-31 Accruing Institutions*

Test Used for Eligibility	Type of Laboratory Used	No. of Negative Cases Detected By the Central Testing Facility	
		HercepTest™†	PathVysion FISH‡
HercepTest™ 3+ (n = 80)	Small-volume§	10 of 52	12 of 52
	Large-volume‖	1 of 28	1 of 28
Other IHC assays (n = 24)¶	Small-volume	11 of 23	9 of 23
	Large-volume	0 of 1	0 of 1

*HercepTest immunohistochemistry is scored on a 3-point scale. For eligibility in NSABP B-31, a positive score of 3+ was required. A negative score was 0-2+.

†PathVysion FISH is scored as either positive or negative for HER2 gene amplification.

‡Small-volume laboratories were arbitrarily determined to perform no more than 99 tests per month.

§Large-volume laboratories were arbitrarily determined to perform at least 100 tests per month.

‖Other IHC assays refers to any immunohistochemistry test that did not use the HercepTest.

Abbreviations: IHC, Immunohistochemistry; *NSABP*, National Surgical Adjuvant Breast and Bowel Project; *FISH*, fluoresnce in situ hybridization.

(Courtesy of Paik S, Bruant J, Tan-Chiu E, et al: Real-world performance of HER2 testing—National Surgical Adjuvant Breast and Bowel Project Experience. *J Natl Cancer Inst* 94:852-854, 2002, by permission of Oxford University Press.)

Methods and Findings.—In the study, 4 cycles of doxorubicin and cyclophosphamide followed by 4 cycles of paclitaxel was compared with the same treatment plus weekly Herceptin for 1 year. Data on the first 104 patients enrolled in the trial were reviewed. Immunohistochemistry (IHC) results were analyzed. Fifty-eight small-volume laboratories contributed a total of 75 cases, and 9 large-volume laboratories contributed 29. Eighteen percent of the community-based assays used to determine the eligibility of patients to participate in the study could not be verified by HercepTestT IHC or fluorescence in situ hybridization (FISH) by a central testing facility (Table 1).

Conclusions.—This analysis found that an appreciable proportion of community-based assay results could not be confirmed by testing in a central facility. Quality control measures in laboratories that use IHC assays needs to be improved, including periodic testing for concordance with FISH.

▶ Trastuzumab (Herceptin) is beneficial only to breast cancer patients whose tumors overexpress the HER2 protein or who have amplification of the HER2 gene. Determination of patient eligibility for treatment requires accurate testing by immunohistochemistry or FISH. These tests are performed at the local hospital level, where methods and quality control measures may vary considerably. Inaccurate determination of HER2 status has the potential to significantly affect the results of clinical trials. In both of these reports (Abstracts 2–18 and 2–19) patients enrolled in cooperative group trials using Herceptin had HER2 testing performed at the local level, with repeat testing done in a central laboratory. Concordance of results was observed in only 74% and 82% of the cases, respectively, in the Breast Intergroup and NSABP studies, and problems were observed with both immunohistochemistry and FISH. In the NSABP study (Abstract 2–19), discrepancies were more frequent in laboratories that performed fewer than 99 tests per month. These results have important implications, not only for the use of Herceptin. Today, many laboratories use immunohistochemistry for prognostic markers. In the future, other targeted therapies may also use immunohistochemistry for patient selection. These reports emphasize the importance of quality control and cross validation studies to ensure that results obtained from central laboratories are reproducible in the community.

M. Morrow, MD

A CHEK2 Genetic Variant Contributing to a Substantial Fraction of Familial Breast Cancer

Vahteristo P, Bartkova J, Eerola H, et al (Helsinki Univ; Inst of Cancer Biology, Copenhagen; Tampere Univ, Finland; et al)

Am J Hum Genet 71:432-438, 2002 2–20

Introduction.—Cell-cycle–checkpoint kinase 2 (CHEK2 [MIM 604373]) (previously known as "CHK2") is a human homologue of budding yeast that phosphorylates p53 and BRCA1 in response to DNA damage. A protein-truncating mutation, 1100delC in exon 10, which eradicates the kinase

TABLE 1.—Frequency of the CHEK2 1100delC Mutation in the Cohorts of Unselected Patients and Patients With Familial Breast Cancer, According to Family History

Cohorts and Subgroups	No. of Subjects	No. With Mutation (%)	OR*	95% CI	*P*
Population controls	1,885	26 (1.4)			
Unselected patients with breast cancer:	1,035	21 (2.0)	1.48	.83-2.65	.182
No family history	677	10 (1.5)			
≥1 Affected first- or second-degree relative	358	11 (3.1)	2.27	1.11-.63	.021
Breast cancer only	318	11 (3.5)	2.56	1.25-5.23	.008
Breast and ovarian cancer	40	0			
Patients with familial breast cancer:	507	28 (5.5)	4.18	2.4-7.2	.0002
By type(s) of cancer:					
Breast cancer only	448	23 (5.1)	3.87	2.19-6.85	<.00005
Breast and ovarian cancer	59	4 (6.8)	5.20	1.75-15.41	.012
By no. of affected relatives:					
Index with 1 affected first-degree relative	291	18 (6.2)	4.70	2.55-8.71	<.00005
≥3 Affected family members†:	216	10 (4.6)	3.50	1.65-7.3	.002
Index with affected first-degree relatives	164	7 (4.3)	3.19	1.36-7.46	.013
Index with affected second-degree relatives only	52	3 (5.8)	4.38	1.28-14.95	.041

*Compared with population control subjects.
†First- or second-degree relatives with breast or ovarian cancer (including the index patient).
Abbreviations: OR, Odds ratio; *CI*, confidence interval.
(Courtesy of Vahteristo P, Bartkova J, Eerola H, et al: A CHEK2 genetic variant contributing to a substantial fraction of familial breast cancer. *Am J Hum Genet* 71:432-438, 2002. Reproduced by permission of The University of Chicago Press.)

function of CHEK2, has been identified in families with Li-Fraumeni syndrome and in patients with a cancer phenotype suggestive of Li-Fraumeni syndrome, including breast cancer. The significance of the CHEK2 genetic variant for breast cancer susceptibility was examined in a large trial involving germline mutation screening of more than 3000 persons. Germline CHEK2 mutation data were compared with analysis of CHEK2 protein expression in breast tumors by using tissue microarrays.

Findings.—The frequency of 1100delC was 2.0% in an unselected population-based series of 1035 patients with breast cancer. This was slightly, yet not significantly ($P = .182$) higher than the 1.4% rate among a population of 1885 controls (Table 1). A significantly increased frequency was identified among the 358 patients with a positive family history (11/358 [3.1%]; odds ratio [OR], 2.27; 95% confidence interval [CI], 1.11-4.63; $P = .021$ compared with population controls). Patients with bilateral breast cancer were 6-fold more likely to be carriers of 1100delC than patients with unilateral cancer (95% CI, 1.87-20.32; $P = .007$). Analysis of the 1100delC variant in an independent set of 507 patients with familial breast cancer and no BRCA1 or BRCA2 mutations verified a significantly increased frequency of 1100delC (28/507 [5.5%]; OR, 4.2; 95% CI, 2.4-7.2; $P = .0002$) compared with controls. A high frequency was also observed in patients with only a single first-degree relative (18/291 [6.2%]). Tissue microarray revealed that breast tumors from patients with 1100delC mutation demonstrated decreased CHEK2 immunostaining.

Conclusion.—It is likely that CHEK2 acts as a low-penetrance tumor suppressor gene in breast cancer, and that it makes a substantial contribution to familial clustering of breast cancer, including families with only 2 affected relatives, which are more common than families that include larger numbers of affected females.

► In spite of the enthusiastism surrounding the identification of BRCA1 and BRCA2 genes, only 5% to 10% of breast cancers can be attributed to mutations in these genes. Multiple laboratories attempting to identify other high-penetrance susceptibility genes have, to date, been unsuccessful. This raises the possibility that most breast cancer, even that which occurs in familial clusters, is caused by a combination of low-penetrance susceptibility genes, or interactions between low-penetrance genes and environmental factors.

In this study, the relationship between CHEK2 mutations and breast cancer in sporadic and familial breast cancer was examined. The incidence of CHEK2 mutations was not significantly elevated in unselected patients compared with controls. However, those with a family history had a significantly higher rate of CHEK2 mutations: 3.1% versus 1.4% in the initial study, and 4.2% in an independent group of patients. The likelihood of a CHEK2 mutation was not related to the number of affected relatives, nor did it correlate with mutations of BRCA1 and BRCA2. While this provides a number of interesting avenues for research, it has little practical clinical application at this time since in families found to have the mutation, a significant number of carriers are unaffected by breast cancer. Until factors interacting with CHEK2 to produce the breast cancer phenotype are identified, testing for this mutation should remain a research procedure.

M. Morrow, MD

High Prevalence of Premalignant Lesions in Prophylactically Removed Breasts From Women at Hereditary Risk for Breast Cancer

Hoogerbrugge N, Bult P, de Widt-Levert LM, et al (Univ Med Ctr Nijmegen, The Netherlands)

J Clin Oncol 21:41-45, 2003 2–21

Background.—Many women with a hereditary predisposition for breast cancer consider prophylactic mastectomy to avoid the extremely high risk of invasive breast carcinoma that is associated with this hereditary predisposition. However, the utility of mastectomy for breast cancer prevention is a matter of debate. Whether women at high hereditary risk for breast cancer have high-risk histopathologic lesions was determined, as well as the variables related to, and predictive for, the presence of such high-risk lesions.

Methods.—This prospective study examined breast specimens from 67 women at extremely high genetic risk of breast cancer, with or without previous breast cancer, who had undergone prophylactic mastectomy. Two thirds of these women were carriers of a *BRCA1* or *BRCA2* mutation. Breast specimens were studied by radiographic and macroscopic examination of 5-mm tissue slices. Histologic analysis involved suspicious lesions and random samples from each quadrant of the breast and the nipple area.

TABLE 2.—Histopathologic Findings and Relevant Risk Indicators of Patients Younger vs Older Than 40 Years

	N = 67 (%)	< 40 Years, n = 37 (%)	≥ 40 Years, n = 30 (%)	P*
Overall presence of high-risk lesions	38 (57)	16 (43)	22 (73)	.01
ALH	25 (37)	8 (22)	17 (57)	.003
ADH	26 (39)	10 (27)	16 (53)	.03
LCIS	17 (25)	4 (11)	13 (43)	.002
DCIS	10 (15)	3 (8)	7 (23)	.08
Oophorectomy before mastectomy	17 (25)	5 (14)	12 (40)	.013
BRCA mutation carrier	44 (66)	29 (78)	15 (50)	.015
Previous breast cancer	26 (39)	7 (19)	19 (63)	.000

Data are presented as n (%).

*Indicates significance of difference between the group older and younger than 40 years.

Abbreviations: ALH, Atypical lobular hyperplasia; *ADH*, atypical ductal hyperplasia; *LCIS*, lobular carcinoma in situ; *DCIS*, ductal carcinoma in situ.

(Courtesy Hoogerbrugge N, Bult P, de Widt-Levert LM, et al: High prevalence of premalignant lesions in prophylactically removed breasts from women at hereditary risk for breast cancer. *J Clin Oncol* 21:41-45, 2003. Reprinted with permission from the American Society of Clinical Oncology.)

Findings.—One or more different types of high-risk histopathologic lesions were present in 57% of the women. One woman had a 4-mm invasive ductal carcinoma with ductal carcinoma in situ. None of these lesions had been detected by palpation or mammography. The presence of high-risk lesions was independently related to age older than 40 years (odds ratio, 6.6; P = .01; Table 2) and to bilateral oophorectomy before prophylactic mastectomy (odds ratio, 0.2; P = .02).

Conclusions.—Many women at high risk of hereditary breast cancer have high-risk histopathologic lesions develop, particularly after age 40 years. These high-risk histopathologic lesions are not detected by surveillance.

► The ductal epithelium of the breast undergoes a series of changes from simple hyperplasia to hyperplasia with atypia to in situ carcinoma that are associated with increasing levels of risk for the development of invasive breast cancer. This study of prophylactic mastectomy specimens in women with genetic risk for the development of breast cancer indicates that a high proportion (57%) of high-risk women have histologic risk lesions that are clinically silent. The likelihood of these lesions increases with increasing age, suggesting a time-dependent element in their development. In addition, the frequency of risk lesions was decreased in women who had undergone oophorectomy, an intervention known to decrease risk in gene mutation carriers. These findings suggest that the identification of high-risk lesions through epithelial sampling techniques such as random fine-needle aspiration or ductal lavage could further stratify risk in women with a genetic predisposition to breast cancer and might influence the timing of chemoprevention or prophylactic surgery. Since this study was limited to women at a high genetic risk for breast cancer development, its application to women at risk on the basis of other factors is uncertain, but worthy of study.

M. Morrow, MD

Twenty-Year Follow-up of a Randomized Trial Comparing Total Mastectomy, Lumpectomy, and Lumpectomy Plus Irradiation for the Treatment of Invasive Breast Cancer

Fisher B, Anderson S, Bryant J, et al (Natl Surgical Adjuvant Breast and Bowel Project, Pittsburgh, Pa; Univ of Pittsburgh, Pa)

N Engl J Med 347:1233-1241, 2002 2–22

Background.—Previous results from the National Surgical Adjuvant Breast and Bowel Project (NSABP) B-06 trial of breast-conserving surgery for women with stage I or II breast cancer have suggested similar survival outcomes for women undergoing total mastectomy, lumpectomy with postoperative breast irradiation, or lumpectomy alone. However, the risk of recurrence in the operated breast was lower in women undergoing lumpectomy plus irradiation than in those undergoing lumpectomy alone. The 20-year results of the B-06 trial were reported.

Methods.—Between 1976 and 1984, a total of 2163 women with stage I or II breast cancer and tumor diameters of 4 cm or less were randomly assigned to undergo total mastectomy, lumpectomy alone, or lumpectomy with postoperative breast irradiation. At follow-up in 2002, complete data

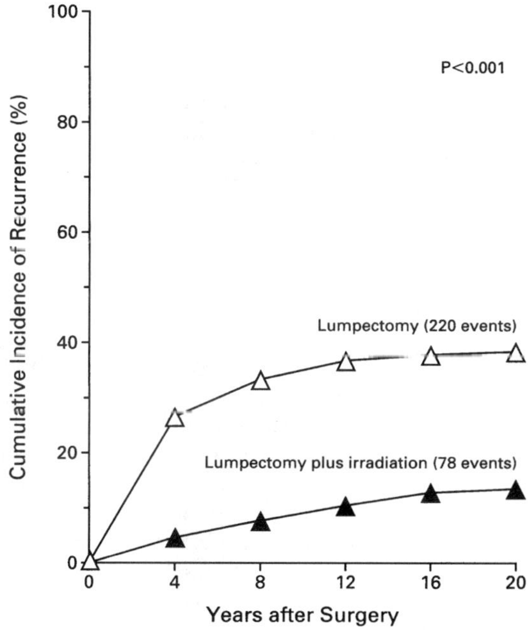

FIGURE 1.—Cumulative incidence of a first recurrence of cancer in the ipsilateral breast during 20 years of follow-up among 570 women treated with lumpectomy alone and 567 treated with lumpectomy plus breast irradiation. The data are for women whose specimens had tumor-free margins. (Reprinted by permission of *The New England Journal of Medicine* from Fisher B, Anderson S, Bryant J, et al: Twenty-year follow-up of a randomized trial comparing total mastectomy, lumpectomy, and lumpectomy plus irradiation for the treatment of invasive breast cancer. *N Engl J Med* 347:1233-1241, 2002. Copyright 2002, Massachusetts Medical Society. All rights reserved.)

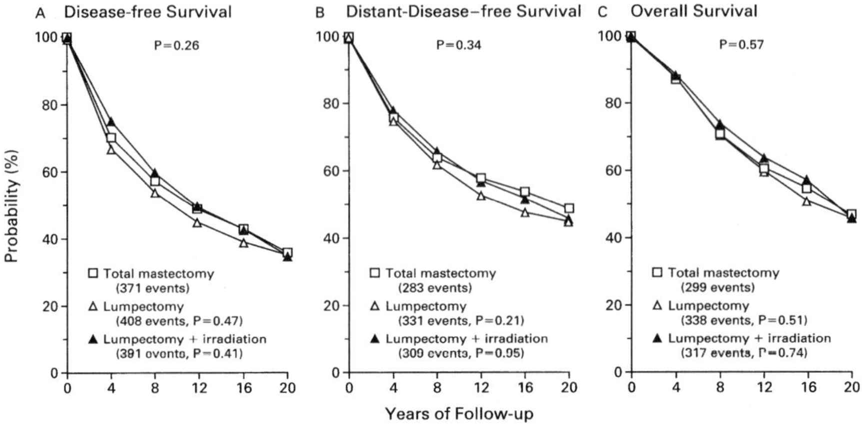

FIGURE 2.—Disease-free survival (A), distant-disease–free survival (B), and overall survival (C) among 589 women treated with total mastectomy, 634 treated with lumpectomy alone, and 628 treated with lumpectomy plus irradiation. In each panel, the *P* value above the curves is for the three-way comparison among the treatment groups; the *P* values below the curves are for the two-way comparisons between lumpectomy alone or with irradiation and total mastectomy. (Reprinted by permission of *The New England Journal of Medicine* from Fisher B, Anderson S, Bryant J, et al: Twenty-year follow-up of a randomized trial comparing total mastectomy, lumpectomy, and lumpectomy plus irradiation for the treatment of invasive breast cancer. *N Engl J Med* 347:1233-1241, 2002. Copyright 2002, Massachusetts Medical Society. All rights reserved.)

including lymph node status were available on 1851 patients. Survival and tumor recurrence rates were compared among the 3 groups.

Results.—The tumor recurrence rate in the ipsilateral breast was 39.2% in the lumpectomy-only group versus 14.3% in the lumpectomy plus irradiation group (Fig 1). All survival outcomes continued to be similar among the 3 groups, including disease-free survival, distant-disease–free survival, and overall survival (Fig 2). Compared with the mastectomy group, hazard ratios for death were nonsignificant in both lumpectomy groups. On analysis of women undergoing lumpectomy who had tumor-free resection margins, the risk of death was not significantly different between those who did and those who did not undergo irradiation. Women receiving radiation had a marginally significant reduction in the risk of death from breast cancer, with some increase in death from other causes.

Conclusions.—The 20-year follow-up data continue to show similar survival rates for women with early stage breast cancer treated with mastectomy or with lumpectomy. For women undergoing lumpectomy, postoperative irradiation is associated with a significant reduction in the risk of tumor recurrence in the ipsilateral breast. As long as the resection margins are tumor free, and the cosmetic results are satisfactory, lumpectomy plus irradiation is an appropriate choice of treatment for breast cancer. The findings underscore the need for long-term follow-up after breast cancer treatment, since many events occur after 5 years.

► The results of the National Surgical Adjuvant Breast and Bowel Project (NSABP) B-06 trial comparing total mastectomy with lumpectomy alone or lumpectomy with breast irradiation have been published before. This 20-year follow-up is important because of the long natural history of breast cancer. No survival benefit for mastectomy is seen. In addition, there is no evidence of an increase in the risk of contralateral breast cancer in the women who received radiotherapy. The incidence of local recurrence after lumpectomy and irradiation is surprisingly low; 14.3% at 20 years, in spite of the fact that women were entered into NSABP B-06 between 1976 and 1984. During this period, the extent of mammographic evaluation before surgery was limited compared with the diagnostic workups done today, and US and MR were not routinely used. The low rate of local recurrence in patients selected by mammography alone should serve as a cautionary note for those who advocate the routine use of other imaging modalities to identify multicentric cancer, which is then considered an indication for mastectomy. Clearly, much of this subclinical disease is controlled by radiotherapy. In contrast, the incidence of local failure without breast irradiation was 39.2%, suggesting that improved imaging techniques might allow identification of a subset of women who require radiation only to the quadrant of the breast in which the primary tumor is located. Finally, this study emphasizes the importance of lifelong surveillance of the breast cancer patient. Eleven percent of all recurrences, including 9% of local recurrences, 7% of regional recurrences, and 13% of distant recurrences, were detected more than 10 years after diagnosis. In addition, 32% of contralateral breast cancer occurred more than 10 years after diagnosis. This study clearly demonstrates that breast conservation with radiotherapy is a safe and effective treatment that allows the majority of women to preserve their breasts, even with long-term follow-up.

M. Morrow, MD

Local Recurrence After Skin-Sparing Mastectomy: Tumor Biology or Surgical Conservatism?

Carlson GW, Styblo TM, Lyles RH, et al (Emory Univ, Atlanta, Ga)

Ann Surg Oncol 10:108-112, 2003 2–23

Introduction.—Skin-sparing mastectomy (SSM), which removes the breast, nipple-areola complex, previous biopsy incisions, and skin overlying superficial tumor (Fig 1), is being used with increasing frequency in patients with breast cancer. This surgical approach preserves the inframammary fold and native skin and greatly enhances the aesthetic results of immediate breast reconstruction. Long-term follow-up of the use of SSM in the treatment of breast cancer is reported to ascertain the impact of local recurrence (LR) on patient survival.

Methods.—A retrospective review was performed in 539 consecutively treated patients (565 cases of breast cancer) who underwent immediate reconstruction after SSM between January 1, 1989, and December 31, 1998. Medical records were examined for demographic, oncologic, and reconstructive data. The American Joint Committee on Cancer pathologic staging was used and revealed breast cancer was stage 0 in 175 (31%) patients, stage I in 135 (23.9%), stage II in 173 (30.6%), stage III in 54 (9.6%), and stage IV

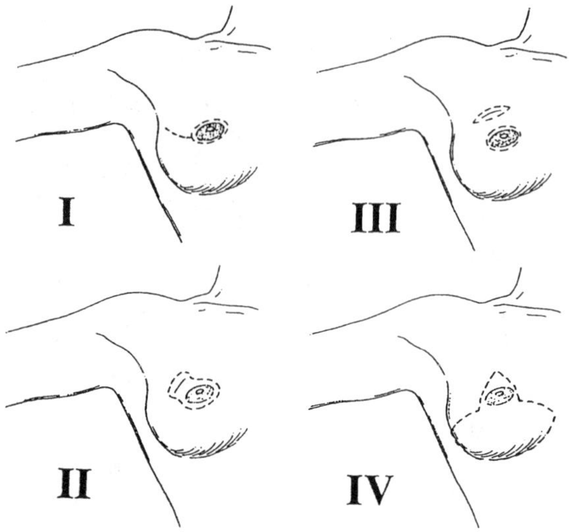

FIGURE 1.—Types of SSM. (Courtesy of Carlson GW, Styblo TM, Lyles RH, et al: Local recurrence after skin-sparing mastectomy: Tumor biology or surgical conservatism? *Ann Surg Oncol* 10:108-112, 2003.)

in 8 patients (1.4%). The disease was recurrent in 20 (3.5%) patients. Follow-up ranged from 23.7 to 86.3 months, with 5 patients lost to follow-up.

Results.—A LR was identified in 31 patients during follow-up, including 5 patients who underwent adjuvant radiation. The distribution of LR, stratified by cancer stage, was stage 0, I, II, III, and recurrent disease in 1, 5, 17, 6, and 2 patients, respectively. The overall incidence of LR was 5.5%. Twenty-four patients (77.4%) had a systemic relapse and 7 (22.6%) remained free of recurrent disease at a mean follow-up of 78.1 months. The cancer stage of patients who remained disease free was stage 0, I, and II, respectively, in 1 (100%), 4 (80%), and 2 (11.8%) patients.

Conclusion.—LR of breast cancer after SSM is not always linked with systemic relapse. Patients with early stage disease may be salvaged by surgical resection and radiotherapy.

► SSM involves removal of the nipple-areolar complex and the surgical biopsy scar, if present. Preservation of the remaining skin decreases the size of the surgical scars and allows more rapid completion of tissue expansion when expanders are used for reconstruction. A recent survey indicates that considerable concern exists that SSM increases the risk of LR after mastectomy.[1] This study is one of many documenting that rates of LR after SSM are similar to those seen after conventional mastectomy. Factors related to poor prognosis, such as the number of involved nodes and tumor size, are predictive of the risk of LR after both SSM and conventional mastectomy. In addition, the majority of LR after mastectomy occurs in the skin or subcutaneous tissue,[2] so the presence of the reconstructed breast mound does not delay detection. The use of SSM optimizes the cosmetic outcome of reconstruction without increasing the risk of cancer recurrence.

M. Morrow, MD

Reference

1. Bleicher RJ, Hansen NM, Giuliano AE: Skin-sparing mastectomy: Specialty bias and world wide lack of consensus. *Cancer* 2316-2321, 2003.
2. Newman LA, Kucrer HM, Hunt KK, et al: Presentation treatment and outcome of local recurrence after skin-sparing mastectomy and immediate breast reconstruction. *Ann Surg Oncol* 5:620-626, 1998.

Compliance With Breast-Conservation Standards for Patients With Early-Stage Breast Carcinoma

White J, Morrow M, Moughan J, et al (Med College of Wisconsin, Milwaukee; Northwestern Univ, Chicago; American College of Radiology, Philadelphia; et al)

Cancer 97:893-904, 2003 2–24

Background.—Several sets of treatment guidelines and practice standards have been developed for use in the management of breast carcinoma. However, few studies have been done as to the penetration and utility of these practice standards. In 1992, several groups—the American College of Surgeons, the American College of Radiology, the College of American Pathologists, and the Society of Surgical Oncology—jointly established standards for breast-conservation therapy (BCT). Whether practice patterns for the treatment of breast carcinoma with BCT were consistent with these standards 2 years after their dissemination was determined, as well as whether compliance varied according to patient and hospital factors associated with the amount of BCT performed.

Methods.—A 72-item questionnaire was developed specifically for this study and circulated to 1400 cancer hospitals with programs accredited by the Commission on Cancer of the American College of Surgeons. Each program was asked to submit reports on the first 25 consecutive patients with stage I and II breast carcinoma who were treated in 1994. Responses were obtained from 842 predominantly community hospitals in the United States, providing a total of 16,643 analyzable patients. The frequency of compliance with 1992 standards was determined for 7097 patients who received BCT. This evaluation included variation in compliance rates by patient age, race, and insurance status and the treating hospital's geographic location and cancer program.

Findings.—Of the 22 standards evaluated in the areas of preoperative mammography (2 standards), labeling of the surgical specimen (3 standards), pathology report content (10 standards), radiation after lumpectomy (6 standards), and systemic therapy for patients with positive lymph nodes (1 standard), treatment adherence was at least 80% for 16 standards. Poor compliance was observed on 6 standards: documentation of size of the abnormality in the mammogram report; labeling of the lumpectomy specimen with the affected quadrant of the breast; spatial orientation of the lumpectomy specimen; and inclusion of lymphatic/vascular invasion, ductal carcinoma in situ, and macroscopic margin assessment in the pathology report. Variation in compliance with a standard was common across the type of hospital cancer program and geographic region (77% for both). Variation was less frequent across the patient variables of age (32%), race (41%), and payer (23%). No pattern of more frequent compliance was noted for variables associated with BCT use.

Conclusions.—Large-scale evaluation of the penetration of treatment standards is feasible. Practice standards seem to be consistent (80% compliance or greater) for patients who underwent lumpectomy, with 73% of 22 treatment standards followed. The standards for which compliance was poor are areas that should be targeted for physician education and reevaluation. Significant differences in adherence to standards on the basis of the hospital's geographic location and the type of cancer program were frequently observed. This observation underscores the importance of adequate dissemination of treatment standards.

▶ The adoption of BCT, consisting of lumpectomy and radiotherapy, has occurred slowly in the United States, in spite of a large body of high-quality scientific data supporting the effectiveness of the procedure. In a somewhat alarming report using Surveillance, Epidemiology, and End Results (SEER) data, Nattinger and colleagues[1] noted that as the use of BCT increased between 1990 and 1995, the use of "inappropriate care" also increased. In an era when quality of care is assuming increasing importance, this is a noteworthy finding.

In this study, White et al examine compliance with a series of standards for BCT in 7097 patients treated in 1994. It is important to recognize that the standards were developed at a time when BCT was a relatively new and infrequently performed procedure. They represent fundamentals of evaluation and care, not sophisticated high-tech guidelines appropriate only for tertiary care centers. For example, the size of the cancer was reported in only 47% of mammogram reports, 12% of patients had a biopsy without a preoperative mammogram, and the surgical specimen was oriented in only 67% of cases. Considerable geographic variation was seen in compliance with standards, as was variation according to hospital type. This variation actually exceeded the variation observed on the bases of patient age, race, or payer. The greatest variation in compliance with standards related to perioperative evaluation (mammography, surgical specimens, pathology report) was seen in community hospitals without comprehensive cancer programs. Two studies of the use of second opinions in breast cancer surgery[2,3] have documented that patients who are candidates for BCT are not being offered the procedure, often after an incomplete initial evaluation. The widespread application of what has been learned through the clinical trials' process remains a problem. The application of high-quality standards and guidelines at the local level is a low-cost way for physicians to ensure that the process of care is appropriate.

M Morrow, MD

References

1. Nattinger AB, Hoffmann RG, Kneusel RT, et al: Relation between appropriateness of primary therapy for early stage breast carcinoma and increased use of breast conserving surgery. *Lancet* 386:1148-1153, 2000.
2. Chang HJ, Vines E, Bertsch H, et al: The impact of a multidisciplinary breast cancer center on recommendations for patient management: The University of Pennsylvania experience. *Cancer* 91:1231-1237, 2001.
3. Clauson J, Hsieh YC, Acharya S, et al: Results of the Lynn Sage Second Opinion Program for the local therapy of breast cancer: Changes in management and determinants of where care is delivered. *Cancer* 95:1185-1190, 2002.

Node-Positive Left-Sided Breast Cancer Patients After Breast-Conserving Surgery: Potential Outcomes of Radiotherapy Modalities and Techniques

Johansson J, Isacsson U, Lindman H, et al (Univ of Uppsala, Sweden)

Radiother Oncol 65:89-98, 2002 2–25

Introduction.—Protons have a finite range of penetration in tissues and an increased dose delivery at the end of the range, properties which can be used to create dose distributions with very low dose to the critical structures outside the target volume. Intensity modulated radiotherapy (IMRT) for photons allows an improved therapeutic ratio and thus dose delivery that is more conformed to the target volume. Protons, IMRT, and conventional external radiotherapy were compared in the treatment of node-positive left-sided breast cancer after breast-conserving surgery to ascertain the possibilities of reducing the risks of cardiac mortality and radiation pneumonitis with preserved mean dose to the planning target volume, so that tumor control probability could be kept at a high level.

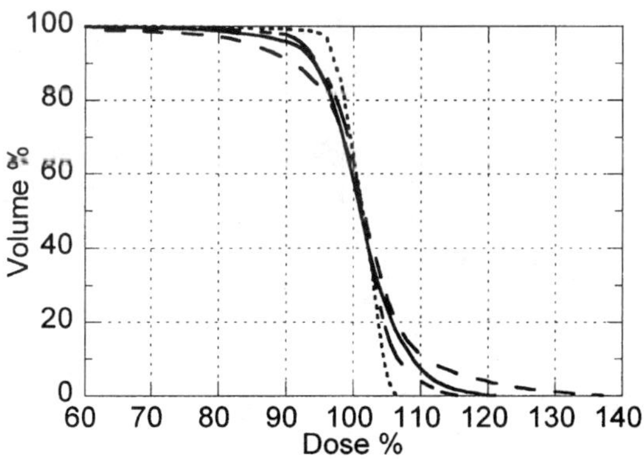

FIGURE 2.—Cumulative dose-volume histograms of the planning target volume for a representative patient. The proton plan is represented by the *dotted line*; the IMRT plan, *solid line*; the patched technique, *broken line*; and the tangential technique, *broken dotted line*. (Reprinted from Johansson J, Isacsson U, Lindman H, et al: Node-positive left-sided breast cancer patients after breast-conserving surgery: Potential outcomes of radiotherapy modalities and techniques. *Radiother Oncol* 65:89-98, 2002. Copyright 2002, with permission from Elsevier Science.)

Methods.—Four different treatment plans were created for 11 consecutive patients with left-sided stage II (International Union Against Cancer stage $T_{1\text{-}2}$ $N_{1\text{-}2}$ M_0) breast cancer (mean age, 59 years) with the use of a 3-dimensional treatment planning system, the Helax-TMS. The 4 were 1 proton plan, 1 IMRT, and 2 conventional plans (tangential and patched). Assessment of the different treatment plans was made by applying the normal tissue complication probability model (NTCP) on the dose distribution in terms of dose-volume histograms (Fig 2). The organs at risk are the spinal cord, the left lung, and the heart. The noncritical normal tissues included the right breast.

Results.—Proton treatment plans provided significantly lower NTCP values for the heart and lung, compared with conventional radiation qualities including IMRT for all 11 women. At a prescribed dose of 50 Gy in the planning target volume, the calculated mean NTCP value for patients dropped, on the average, from 14.7% to 0.6% for the lung (radiation pneumonitis) for the proton plan versus the best plan using conventional radiation qualities. The corresponding figures for the heart (cardiac mortality) fell from 2.1% to 0.5%. The values for cardiac mortality for IMRT, the tangential technique, and the patched technique were 2.2%, 6.7%, and 2.1%, respectively (Fig 3).

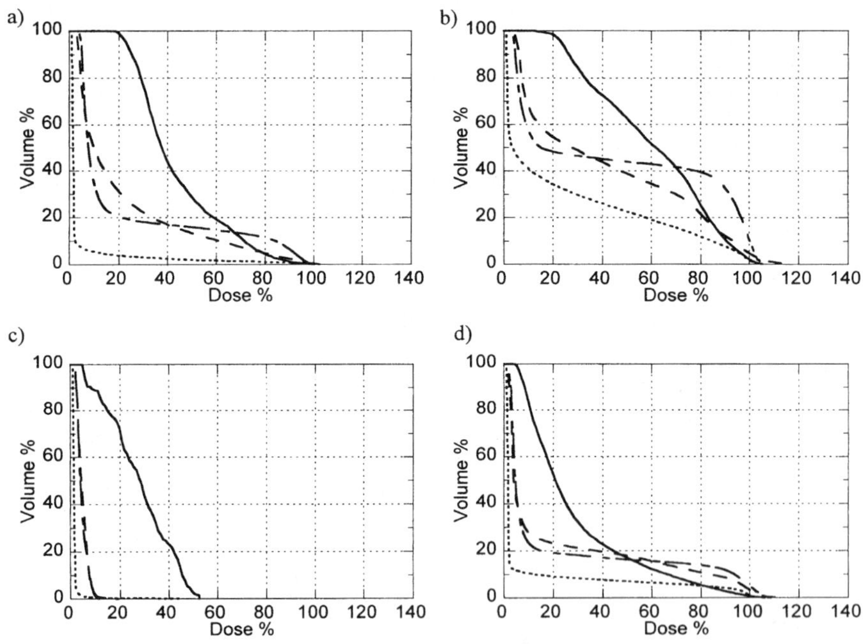

FIGURE 3.—Cumulative dose-volume histograms of a representative patient for (**A**) the left lung, (**B**) the heart, (**C**) the spinal cord, (**D**) the non-target tissue volume for the proton plan (*dotted line*), the IMRT plan (*solid line*), patched technique (*broken line*) and the tangential technique (*broken dotted line*). (Reprinted from Johansson J, Isacsson U, Lindman H, et al: Node-positive left-sided breast cancer patients after breast-conserving surgery: Potential outcomes of radiotherapy modalities and techniques. *Radiother Oncol* 65:89-98, 2002. Copyright 2002, with permission from Elsevier Science.)

Conclusion.—Lower complication risks were observed with protons, compared with treatments that used conventional radiation qualities for the treatment of node-positive left-sided breast cancer after breast-conserving surgery.

► In today's world, there seems to be great concern about morbidities from radiation therapy related to left-sided breast cancer when breast conservation approaches are used. There are concerns about lung and cardiac function in particular.

Much has been touted concerning the impact of IMRT, which effectively divides the target volume into a series of small fields coming from multiple angles so that many fields integrate into a high dose within the tumor volume, but the adjacent lower tissues see a lower dose. It is rarely mentioned, but the price that is paid for multiple fields is that larger volumes of normal tissue see radiation. The dose may be modest but the volume is considerably increased by multiple fields. The concern is that the mutagenecity resulting from radiation therapy is a random event, at least to the best of our knowledge.

As a consequence, this means more cells will see mutagenic doses within the normal tissue volumes being exposed. On the other hand, the doses will be small enough that cells that have been mutated by radiation therapy will probably not be destroyed since the total dose will be small. Once again, the old axiom says that you cannot get something for nothing, or as my mother used to say, "Keep your eye on the donut and not on the hole."

E. Glatstein, MD

Skin-Sparing Mastectomy and Immediate Autologous Tissue Reconstruction After Whole-Breast Irradiation

Disa JJ, Cordeiro PG, Heerdt AH, et al (Mem Sloan-Kettering Cancer Ctr, New York)

Plast Reconstr Surg 111:118-124, 2003 2–26

Background. Long term follow up in patients treated with breast con servation has revealed a local recurrence rate of 3% to 16%. Meta-analyses have reported a generally accepted local recurrence rate of 10% at 10 years for women receiving lumpectomy, axillary dissection, and radiation therapy, compared with 23% local recurrence in patients not receiving adjuvant radiation therapy. Traditionally, local recurrence of breast cancer in the absence of systemic disease has been managed with salvage mastectomy.

In the absence of local or systemic contraindications, these women are candidates for reconstructive surgery. Skin-sparing mastectomy and immediate autologous tissue reconstruction is an accepted method for management of primary breast malignancies that provides exceptional aesthetic results. Skin-sparing mastectomy and autologous tissue reconstruction were evaluated in the previously irradiated breast.

Methods.—This retrospective review evaluated all patients who underwent skin-sparing mastectomy and immediate reconstruction with autologous tissue after failed breast conservation therapy from 1995 to 1999. A total of 11 patients with a mean age of 45 years were included in the study. Indications for initial lumpectomy were ductal carcinoma in situ in 6 patients and infiltrating carcinoma in 5 patients. The mean interval from lumpectomy to salvage mastectomy was 44 months (range, 12 to 169 months).

Results.—The reconstructive techniques used included unipedicled transverse rectus abdominis musculocutaneous (TRAM) flap in 4 patients , free TRAM flap in 4 patients, and latissimus flap with immediate placement of a saline implant in 3 patients. Flap survival was 100% with no early flap complications. Partial-thickness mastectomy flap loss developed in 1 patient and was managed conservatively. There were no cases of full-thickness mastectomy skin loss. The late complications included capsular contracture in 2 patients, fat necrosis in 1 patient, and ventral hernia in 1 patient. There was 1 late death from metastatic disease. The remaining 10 patients showed no evidence of disease at a mean of 48 months, with a range of 30 to 75 months. The aesthetic results were determined to be excellent in 4 patients, good in 5 patients, fair in 1 patient, and poor in 1 patient.

Conclusion.—Skin-sparing mastectomy and immediate autologous tissue reconstruction is a safe and efficacious procedure in patients who have previously undergone whole-breast irradiation. In this series, the pedicled or free TRAM flap provided the best results. Careful selection of patients is the key factor in this technique, with close attention paid to the quality of the irradiated breast skin and the anatomical location of the recurrent disease.

▶ The issues of the interactions of radiation therapy and breast reconstruction continue to be somewhat controversial. This article presents a small number of patients (11) who underwent lumpectomy and radiation therapy and later a salvage mastectomy. As part of the mastectomy, the skin was spared and a TRAM flap was used. In most instances in this small series, the outcome was apparently good.

To the oncologist, the reconstructive procedures are difficult to fit in with our general principles of cancer management. For the reconstructive surgeon, it is important to maximize the tissues that remain for reconstruction. To the oncologist, the usual principle would be to remove everything, including the skin. Given this kind of internal conflict and considering the nature of the surgery, the obvious point is that these patients need to be very carefully selected in terms of low risk of cutaneous involvement.

E. Glatstein, MD

Randomized, Placebo-Controlled Trial of Clodronate in Patients With Primary Operable Breast Cancer

Powles T, Paterson S, Kanis JA, et al (Univ of Sheffield, England; Univ of Calgary, Canada; Central Hosp, Jyväskylä, Finland; et al)

J Clin Oncol 20:3219-3224, 2002 2–27

Background.—Experimental evidence shows that the development of bone metastases from breast cancer is facilitated by the release of substances from tumor cells that activate osteoclasts to cause local osteolysis. The use of nonsteroidal anti-inflammatory drugs or bisphosphonates such as clodronate inhibits tumor-induced osteolysis in vitro and prevents bone destruction and hypercalcemia in vivo. Whether clodronate might reduce the subsequent incidence of bone metastases in patients with primary breast cancer was determined.

Methods.—A total of 1069 patients with operable breast cancer were enrolled in this trial from 1989 to 1995. All the patients received surgery, radiotherapy, chemotherapy, and tamoxifen as needed. The patients were randomly assigned to receive oral clodronate, 1600 mg/d, or a placebo for 2 years beginning within 6 months of primary treatment. The main outcome measures was relapse in bone, analyzed as intention to treat, during the medication period and during the total follow-up period (median, 2007 days). The secondary outcome measures were relapse in other sites, mortality, and toxicity.

Results.—There was a nonsignificant reduction in bone metastases during the total follow-up period for patients receiving clodronate. During the medication period, there was a significant reduction in the occurrence of bone metastases (clodronate, n = 12; placebo, n = 28). The occurrence of nonosseous metastases was similar for both groups, but there was a significant reduction in mortality during the total follow-up period.

Conclusions.—In patients with primary operable breast cancer, clodronate may reduce the incidence of bone metastases. In this trial, the reduction in incidence was only significant during the medication phase. There was a significant reduction in mortality.

► Bone metastases are a frequent occurrence in breast cancer, and a major cause of morbidity. This prospective, randomized trial confirms the findings of Diehl et al[1] that the use of a bisphosphonate, clodronate, in the adjuvant setting reduces the incidence of bone metastases during the time the clodronate is given. No increase in metastases at other sites, and significant prolongation of survival were seen. Another randomized trial has failed to observe a benefit for clodronate.[2] An ongoing National Surgical Adjuvant Breast and Bowel Project Study randomizing 3000 women to 3 years of clodronate or placebo after completion of traditional adjuvant therapy should help provide a definitive answer to this question.

M. Morrow, MD

References

1. Diehl I, Solomayer EF, Costa S, et al: Reduction in new metastases in breast cancer with adjuvant clodronate treatment. *N Engl J Med* 339:357-363, 1998.
2. Saarto T, Blomquist C, Virkkunen P, et al: Adjuvant clodronate treatment does not reduce the frequency of skeletal metastases in node-positive breast cancer patients: 5-year results of a randomized controlled trial. *J Clin Oncol* 19:10-17, 2001.

Axillary Sentinel Lymph Node Biopsy in Patients With Pure Ductal Carcinoma In Situ of the Breast

Intra M, Veronesi P, Mazzarol G, et al (European Inst of Oncology, Milan, Italy; Univ of Milan, Italy; Mem Sloan-Kettering Cancer Ctr, New York)

Arch Surg 138:309-313, 2003 2–28

Background.—Because of the widespread use of mammography, the incidence of pure ductal carcinoma in situ (DCIS) has increased by 15-fold in the past 10 years, so that pure DCIS now accounts for at least 20% of mammographically detected carcinomas and 12% of all newly diagnosed breast cancers. It was hypothesized that a sentinel lymph node (SLN) biopsy should not be considered standard in the treatment of all patients with DCIS of the breast if the lesion is completely excised by radical surgery and there are free margins of resection.

Methods and Findings.—This prospective case series included 223 unselected consecutive patients with pure DCIS who underwent SLN biopsy between January 1998 and December 2001. Metastases in the SLN were detected in only 7 (3.1%) of the patients. Complete axillary dissection was subsequently done in 6 of these 7 patients. Five of the 7 patients had only micrometastases in the SLNs. In the 6 patients who underwent complete axillary dissection, the SLN was the only positive node.

Conclusions.—Because the prevalence of metastases is low, SLN biopsy should not be done routinely in all patients with DCIS. In patients with pure DCIS with complete lesion excision at radical surgery, an SLN biopsy can be avoided. An SLN biopsy may be considered in patients with DCIS who undergo mastectomy because in such patients, an SLN biopsy cannot be done after mastectomy. If the SLN contains only micrometastatic disease, complete axillary dissection may not be necessary.

▶ The low morbidity and high accuracy of SLN biopsy have led some to recommend that it be performed not only for patients with invasive cancer, but for those with DCIS and those undergoing prophylactic mastectomy. As this study by Intra et al demonstrates, the likelihood of axillary nodal disease in patients with an initial diagnosis of DCIS is extremely low. Patients with DCIS diagnosed by core biopsy will be found to have invasive cancer in 10% to 20% of cases. Does it really make sense to perform 80 to 90 unnecessary SLN biopsies to avoid returning the 10 to 20 patients who need the procedure to the operating room?

I agree with Intra et al that the answer to that question is no. A fundamental tenet of the biology of DCIS is that it lacks the capacity to metastasize. Although it is true that sometimes the pathologist fails to identify invasion, this should be fairly infrequent with the small, mammographically detected lesions that make up most of the DCIS that is seen today. The breast cancer–specific survivals of 96% to 99% reported for women with DCIS treated with therapy to the breast alone suggest that this is relatively infrequent. The danger in performing routine SLN biopsy, often with serial sectioning or immunohistochemistry of the node, or both, is well illustrated in this article. Such close scrutiny of the node leads to the identification of single tumor cells, small clusters of cells in the subcapsular sinus, or micrometastases. The prognostic significance of such cells in invasive cancer is uncertain enough that it is the subject of 2 prospective trials. In the patient with DCIS, their meaning is even more unclear, but their identification usually leads to treatment of the patient as if she had invasive breast cancer metastatic to the axillary nodes.

The policy proposed in this article is sensible and one that we have adopted in our practice—performance of SLN biopsy for DCIS only in patients having mastectomies. Patients undergoing mastectomy for DCIS usually have large areas of DCIS, with a higher probability of unsampled invasion. After a mastectomy, the opportunity for SLN biopsy is lost. For the remainder, SLN biopsy is reserved for those who have invasion (including microinvasion) identified after definitive surgical excision.

M. Morrow, MD

Is Axillary Lymph Node Dissection Necessary in Elderly Patients With Breast Carcinoma Who Have a Clinically Uninvolved Axilla?

Martelli G, Miceli R, De Palo G, et al (Istituto Nazionale per lo Studio e la Cura dei Tumori, Milan, Italy; Univ of Milan, Italy)

Cancer 97:1156-1163, 2003 2–29

Background.—Nearly 40% of all breast carcinomas occur in patients aged 70 years or older. However, elderly women are usually excluded from clinical trials in breast carcinoma, primarily because they often have concurrent medical conditions that impose modifications on trial protocols. The optimal primary treatment for older patients is controversial. Axillary dissection in elderly patients with early-stage breast carcinoma without palpable axillary lymph nodes is controversial because of the morbidity associated with the surgery, the reduced life expectancy of the patients, and the efficacy of hormone therapy in the prevention of recurrences and axillary events.

Methods.—A retrospective analysis was conducted of 671 consecutive patients with breast carcinoma who were 70 years or older and who underwent conservative breast surgery with axillary dissection (172 patients) or without axillary dissection (499 patients) (Table 2). Tamoxifen was administered to all patients. The effects of axillary dissection compared with no axillary dissection on breast carcinoma mortality rate and distant metasta-

TABLE 2.—Number of Events by Treatment Group

Event	No AD (n = 499 Patients)	AD (n = 172 Patients)	Total (n = 671 Patients)
	No. of Patients (%)		
First event	208 (41.6)	51 (29.6)	259 (38.5)
Ipsilateral recurrence	24 (4.8)	11 (6.4)	35 (5.2)
Axillary occurrence	27 (5.4)	0 (0.0)	27 (4.0)
Distant metastases	37 (7.4)	15 (8.7)	52 (7.7)
Contralateral breast carcinoma	8 (1.6)	2 (1.2)	10 (1.5)
Second primary malignancy	17 (3.4)	3 (1.7)	20 (3.0)
Deaths from unrelated conditions	95 (19.0)	20 (11.6)	115 (17.1)
Mortality			
Total deaths	163 (32.6)	37 (21.5)	200 (29.8)
Deaths from breast carcinoma	46 (9.2)	14 (8.1)	60 (8.9)
Deaths from other malignancies	11 (2.2)	1 (0.6)	12 (1.8)
Deaths from unrelated conditions	106 (21.2)	22 (12.8)	128 (19.1)

Abbreviations: No AD, No axillary lymph node dissection; *AD*, axillary lymph node dissection.

(Courtesy Martelli G, Miceli R, De Palo G, et al: Is axillary lymph node dissection necessary in elderly patients with breast carcinoma who have a clinically uninvolved axilla? *Cancer* 97:1156-1163, 2003.

ses were analyzed with multiple proportional-hazards regression models. The assignment of patients to axillary treatment was not random, so covariate adjustments were made for baseline variables that influenced the decision to perform axillary dissection and for prognostic factors.

Results.—There was no significant difference apparent between the 2 groups in the crude cumulative incidence curves for breast carcinoma mortality rate and distant metastasis. The crude cumulative incidences of axillary lymph node occurrence at 5 years and 10 years were 4.4% and 5.9%, respectively.

Conclusions.—Elderly patients with breast carcinoma with no evidence of axillary lymph node involvement can be treated effectively with conservative surgery and tamoxifen. Immediate axillary dissection is not necessary in these patients but should be performed in the small proportion of patients who later develop overt axillary lymph node involvement.

► Although there is a lack of consensus regarding the impact of axillary treatment on survival, axillary dissection is recognized as an effective method of maintaining local control in the axilla. Recurrences in the untreated axilla occur at a mean of 2 to 3 years after diagnosis, making axillary management a relevant issue even for elderly women with comorbid conditions.

In this study, Martelli et al report a cumulative incidence of axillary recurrence at 5 and 10 years of 4.4% and 5.9%, respectively, in clinically node-negative women aged 70 years and older treated with tangent field irradiation to the preserved breast and no axillary surgery. Axillary dissection necessitates the use of general anesthesia and has significant long-term morbidity in older women.[1] Since axillary nodal status usually is not the primary determinant of the need for systemic therapy in women aged 70 years and older, this study provides reassurance that it can be omitted with high rates of local control.

These findings may not seem to be relevant in the era of axillary staging with sentinel node biopsy, but it is useful to remember that rates of sentinel node identification in women older than 50 or 60 years are consistently lower than identification rates in their younger counterparts. Before undertaking sentinel node biopsy or axillary dissection in older women, it is useful to ask how the findings will change management to benefit the patient.

M. Morrow, MD

Reference

1. Veronesi U, Paganelli G, Viale G, et al: A randomized comparison of sentinel node biopsy with routine axillary dissection in breast cancer. *N Engl J Med* 349:546-553, 2003.

Chronic Arm Morbidity After Curative Breast Cancer Treatment: Prevalence and Impact on Quality of Life

Kwan W, Jackson J, Weir LM, et al (British Columbia Cancer Agency-Fraser Valley Centre, Surrey, Canada; Vancouver Centre, BC, Canada; Vancouver Island Centre, Victoria, BC, Canada)

J Clin Oncol 20:4242-4248, 2002 2–30

Background.—Shoulder stiffness and pain, lymphedema, and risk of cellulitis—can be difficult problems for breast cancer survivors. Despite the disruptiveness of these complications, they have rarely been studied with modern quality-of-life (QOL) assessments. A sample of breast cancer survivors were surveyed regarding chronic arm morbidity and its effects on quality-of-life (QOL).

Methods.—A random sample of 744 women who had undergone curative treatment for breast cancer at 1 of 2 Canadian cancer centers between 1993 and 1997 were sent a 4-item questionnaire. Sampling was stratified by diagnosis year, axillary treatment, and nodal status. Random samples of respondents who reported or denied arm-related morbidity were invited for further investigation, including assessment of lymphedema. Two QOL instruments were used: the European Organization for Research and Treatment of Cancer QOL Questionnaire C-30 and a questionnaire that specifically addressed everyday arm function.

Results.—The response rate to the initial survey was 63% (467 of 744). Among the respondents, 50% reported arm symptoms. Detailed assessments were carried out in 57 women with arm symptoms and 55 without. Examination revealed lymphedema in 10 of 57 patients with arm symptoms (17.5%) and 4 of 55 asymptomatic patients (7%), for an overall rate of 12.5%. Analysis of treatment variables suggested that axillary dissection and postdissection axillary radiography approximately tripled the risk of lymphedema: associated odds ratios were 3.3 (95% confidence interval [CI], 2.0-5.4) and 3.1 (95% CI, 2.0-4.7), respectively. Both QOL instruments indicated significant impairments in physical functioning, social functioning, cognitive functioning, nausea, and pain for patients with symptoms and patients with lymphedema, regardless of symptom status ($P < .01$). Impairments in arm functioning were reflected in reductions in shoulder abduction and external rotation.

Conclusions.—Even with modern treatment techniques, this retrospective study suggests that 1 of 8 breast cancer survivors has chronic lymphedema. The proportion of women with at least mild shoulder symptoms may be as high as 70%. Axillary dissection and radiation therapy are significant risk factors for lymphedema, which, along with associated symptoms, significantly affects QOL.

Sequelae of Axillary Lymph Node Dissection in Older Women With Stage 1 and 2 Breast Carcinoma

Mandelblatt JS, and the OPTIONS Research Team (Georgetown Univ, Washington, DC; et al)

Cancer 95:2445-2454, 2002 2–31

Background.—The long-term sequelae of axillary dissection among older patients with breast carcinoma have not been well studied. This effects of axillary dissection among a group of patients 67 years old or older are reported.

Methods.—Subjects were 571 women with stage I or II breast cancer from 29 hospitals in 5 geographic areas of the United States between 1995 and 1997. The minimum age limit of 67 years was chosen to allow estimation of preexisting comorbid conditions from 2 years of Medicare claims. Baseline interviews were conducted 3 months after surgery and again at 12 and 24 months after surgery.

Findings.—During follow-up, 60% of women reported arm problems at some time after surgery. The cumulative risk of having arm problems during the 2 years after treatment was 3 times greater among those who had axillary surgery, after adjusting for covariates, than among those who had not had axillary surgery (83% vs 17%, $P = .0001$). At 2 years after surgery, the effects of axillary dissection and arthritis were multiplicative. Arm problems were the main determinant of lower physical ($P = .0001$) and mental functioning ($P = .04$), again after adjustment for other factors. Undergoing axillary surgery did not reduce patients' fears about recurrences; women diagnosed with stage II disease were more worried about recurrence than patients diagnosed with stage I disease ($P < .04$).

Conclusions.—The occurrence of arm problems after axillary dissection has a consistent negative impact on quality of life. Thus, in older women with breast cancer, the risks associated with this procedure may outweigh the potential benefits.

► The long-term sequelae of axillary dissection have often been overlooked since they are rarely life threatening and occur in the outpatient setting. With the switch from mastectomy to breast-conserving surgery, axillary dissection has become the major cause of long-term morbidity after the local therapy of breast cancer. The studies of Kwan et al (Abstract 2–30) and Mandelblatt et al (Abstract 2–31) examine the sequelae of axillary dissection in different populations, using different methodologies, but have similar findings. Between 50% and 60% of patients studied reported arm problems after axillary dissection, and these arm problems were associated with a significant impairment in quality of life. The study of Mandelblatt et al examined the cohort of women aged 67 years and older and observed that in those with arthritis undergoing axillary dissection the effects were multiplicative. These studies both rely on self-reporting of symptoms and may underestimate the actual impairment seen after axillary dissection. A major advantage of sentinel node biopsy is the lower morbidity of the procedure. This was convincingly demonstrated in the randomized trial of Veronesi et al.[1] In this study, the patients were randomized to sentinel node biopsy alone or followed by axillary dissection. A comparison of arm function at 6 months and 2 years demonstrated significantly less pain, better range of motion, fewer sensory changes, and less lymphedema after sentinel node biopsy than axillary dissection at both the time points studied. While there is little doubt that sentinel node biopsy is rapidly becoming the standard technique for managing the node negative axilla,[2] the studies discussed here emphasize the importance of determining whether axillary dissection is necessary after finding metastases in the sentinel node. This will only be accomplished if prospective randomized trials such as the American College of Surgeons Oncology Group Z-11 trial, which addresses this question, are successfully completed.

M. Morrow, MD

References

1. Veronesi U, Paganelli G, Viale G, et al: A randomized comparison of sentinel-node biopsy with routine axillary dissection in breast cancer. *N Engl J Med* 349:546-553, 2003.
2. Edge SB, Niland JC, Bookman MA, et al: Emergence of sentinel node biopsy in breast cancer as standard-of-care in academic comprehensive cancer centers. *J Natl Cancer Inst* 95:1514-1521, 2003.

Completion Axillary Lymph Node Dissection Minimizes the Likelihood of False Negatives for Patients With Invasive Breast Carcinoma and Cytokeratin Positive Only Sentinel Lymph Nodes

Jakub JW, Diaz NM, Ebert MD, et al (H Lee Moffitt Cancer Ctr and Research Inst, Tampa, Fla; Lakeland Regional Cancer Ctr, Fla)
Am J Surg 184:302-306, 2002 2–32

Background.—Regional lymph node status continues to be the strongest prognostic factor for invasive breast cancer. Immunohistochemical staining to identify cancer cells in regional sentinel lymph nodes (SLNs) serves as an indicator of clinical prognosis and reduces false-negative findings. The incidence of metastatic disease was determined in complete axillary lymph node dissection (CALND) specimens from patients with invasive carcinoma after

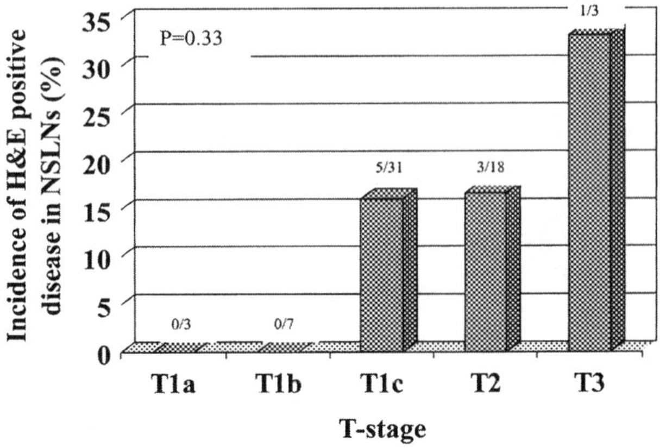

FIGURE 3.—Tumor size as a predictor of non-SLN (*NSLNs*) hematoxylin and eosin (*H & E*) positive metastatic disease in patients with SLNs only positive by cytokeratin immunohistochemical (CK-IHC) staining. (Courtesy of Jakub JW, Diaz NM, Ebert MD, et al: Completion axillary lymph node dissection minimizes the likelihood of false negatives for patients with invasive breast carcinoma and cytokeratin positive only sentinel lymph nodes. *Am J Surg* 184:302-306, 2002. Copyright 2002, with permission from Excerpta Medica Inc.)

an SLN biopsy sample was found to be positive only by immunohistochemical staining for cytokeratin (CK-IHC).

Methods.—All 1380 patients undergoing lymphatic mapping and SLN biopsy for invasive breast cancer at one center between April 1998 and May 2001 were studied. Sections of all SLNs that had negative findings by routine histology were immunostained and analyzed for cytokeratin-positive cells. Routine hematoxylin and eosin (H&E) staining was used to interpret sections of lymph nodes collected by CALND.

Findings.—Metastatic disease was found in at least one SLN by H&E analysis in 409 patients (29.6%), and 78 patients (of 971 with negative findings on H&E) had positive findings only by CK-IHC. Of the 62 patients with CK-IHC–positive SLNs who underwent CALND, 9(14.5%) had metastases in the CALND specimen. All 9 patients had tumors larger than 1 cm (Fig 3).

Conclusions.—In this series, 14.5% of patients with invasive breast cancer and SLNs that were positive only by CK-IHC had H&E-positive lymph nodes on CALND. Thus, CK-IHC should be used to assess SLNs. In addition, CALND should be considered when SLNs are positive by CK-IHC only. The use of this approach would provide an absolute reduction in the number of false-negative findings.

► The identification of the sentinel node(s), defined as the node(s) most likely to contain metastatic disease, allows the pathologist to perform a much more detailed evaluation of the node(s) than is feasible with an axillary specimen containing 20 to 30 nodes. This examination usually takes the form of additional sections of the node and may include immunohistochemical (IHC) staining. The prognostic significance of tumor cells detected by IHC only is subject to debate, and is being addressed in prospective studies by the National Surgical Adjuvant Breast and Bowel Project and American College of Surgeons Oncology Group. In practice, women found to have IHC-positive nodes usually receive systemic therapy as if they had H&E-identified metastases. But, completion axillary dissection is often omitted in this group since the risk of additional nodal metastases is thought to be "low."

In this study, Jakub et al report that 14.5% of 62 patients with metastases in the sentinel node detected only by IHC had additional H&E-identified metastases in nonsentinel nodes after axillary dissection. A total of 78 patients had IHC-only metastases, and even if no additional metastases were present in the 16 patients who did not have a dissection, this is still an 11% rate of additional nodal disease. Metastases were present in 10% of those with IHC involvement of a single sentinel node and 33% of those with multiple IHC-positive nodes, and patients with T1 and T2 tumors did not differ significantly in the risk of additional nodal disease. This study would suggest that if IHC is performed outside a clinical trial, an IHC-positive sentinel node should be considered an indication for completion axillary dissection.

M. Morrow, MD

3 Gynecologic Cancer

International Collaborative Ovarian Neoplasm Trial 1 and Adjuvant ChemoTherapy In Ovarian Neoplasm Trial: Two Parallel Randomized Phase III Trials of Adjuvant Chemotherapy in Patients With Early-Stage Ovarian Carcinoma

Trimbos JB, for the International Collaborative Ovarian Neoplasm 1 (ICON1) and European Organisation for Research and Treatment of Cancer Collaborators–Adjuvant ChemoTherapy In Ovarian Neoplasm (EORTC-ACTION) (Leiden Univ, The Netherlands; et al)

J Natl Cancer Inst 95:105-112, 2003 3–1

Background.—Adjuvant chemotherapy may be a strategy for improving survival in women with early stage ovarian cancer. However, the randomized studies done to date have been too small to adequately address this question. A combined analysis of 2 parallel, randomized clinical trials was presented.

Methods.—The International Collaborative Ovarian Neoplasm 1 (ICON1) trial and the Adjuvant ChemoTherapy in Ovarian Neoplasm (ACTION) trial were included in the analysis. Both compared platinum-based adjuvant chemotherapy with observation postoperatively. A total of 925 patients undergoing surgery for early stage ovarian cancer were enrolled in the studies between 1990 and 2000. The patients were randomly assigned to receive either platinum-based adjuvant chemotherapy or observation until chemotherapy was indicated. The median follow-up was more than 4 years.

Findings.—Two hundred forty-five patients died or had a recurrence during follow-up. At 5 years, the overall survival was 82% in the chemotherapy group and 74% in the observation group. Recurrence-free survival at 5 years was 76% and 65%, respectively.

Conclusions.—Platinum-based adjuvant chemotherapy appears to improve 5-year overall survival and recurrence-free survival in women with early stage ovarian cancer as defined by the inclusion criteria of the ICON1 and ACTION studies. This combined analysis enabled the study of a large number of patients.

Impact of Adjuvant Chemotherapy and Surgical Staging in Early-Stage Ovarian Carcinoma: European Organisation for Research and Treatment of Cancer–Adjuvant ChemoTherapy in Ovarian Neoplasm Trial

Trimbos JB, for the EORTC-ACTION Collaborators (Leiden Univ Med Ctr, The Netherlands; et al)

J Natl Cancer Inst 95:113-125, 2003 3–2

Background.—None of the previously published randomized trials of adjuvant chemotherapy for early stage ovarian cancer have had the statistical power to show a difference in the effect on survival between adjuvant and no adjuvant chemotherapy. Also, previous research has not considered the adequacy of surgical staging. In a prospective, unblinded, randomized phase III study, the efficacy of adjuvant chemotherapy in patients with early stage ovarian cancer was tested, emphasizing the extent of surgical staging.

Methods.—Four hundred forty-eight patients from 40 centers in 9 European countries were enrolled between 1990 and 2000. The patients were randomly assigned to receive adjuvant platinum-based chemotherapy or observation after operation. The median follow-up was 5.5 years

Findings.—The 2 groups did not differ significantly in overall survival. However, recurrence-free survival was significantly better in the adjuvant chemotherapy recipients. Only about one third of patients had had optimal staging. In the observation group, optimal staging correlated with a significant improvement in overall and recurrence-free survival. This correlation was not evident in the adjuvant chemotherapy group. Among patients who had not been staged optimally, adjuvant chemotherapy was associated with significant improvement in overall and recurrence-free survival. Adjuvant chemotherapy appeared to have no benefits among optimally staged patients.

Conclusions.—Adjuvant chemotherapy correlated with significantly improved recurrence-free survival in patients with early stage ovarian cancer. The benefits of adjuvant chemotherapy appeared to be limited to patients who had not been staged optimally.

International Collaborative Ovarian Neoplasm Trial 1: A Randomized Trial of Adjuvant Chemotherapy in Women With Early-Stage Ovarian Cancer

Parmar M, for the International Collaborative Ovarian Neoplasm (ICON1) Collaborators (Medical Research Council Clinical Trials Unit, London)

J Natl Cancer Inst 95:125-132, 2003 3–3

Background.—Establishing whether platinum-based adjuvant chemotherapy improves outcomes in patients with early stage epithelial ovarian cancer is important. The effects of adjuvant chemotherapy on overall and recurrence-free survival were determined in women with early stage epithelial ovarian cancer.

Methods.—In this multicenter, open randomized trial, 84 centers in 5 countries enrolled 477 patients between 1991 and 2000. The patients were randomly assigned to receive either adjuvant chemotherapy immediately after surgery or no adjuvant chemotherapy until indicated clinically.

Findings.—Overall survival was better in women receiving adjuvant chemotherapy than in those who did not, with a hazard ratio of 0.66. The 5-year survival rates were 79% for women receiving adjuvant therapy, compared with 70% for those who did not. In addition, adjuvant chemotherapy increased recurrence-free survival, with 5-year rates of 73% for women receiving adjuvant chemotherapy and 62% for those who did not.

Conclusions.—Platinum-based adjuvant chemotherapy appears to improve survival in patients with early stagy ovarian cancer. Recurrence-free survival is also prolonged in women receiving such adjuvant therapy.

Systematic Review of Adjuvant Therapy for Early Stage (Epithelial) Ovarian Cancer

Winter-Roach B, Hooper L, Kitchener H (St Mary's Hosp, Manchester, England)

Int J Gynecol Cancer 13:395-404, 2003 3–4

Background.—Even women with stage I ovarian cancer have a high incidence of recurrent disease. Adjuvant therapy can be used to reduce recurrence. Unfortunately, many adjuvant chemotherapy trials in this patient group have had insufficient statistical power to demonstrate the efficacy of adjuvant therapy. A systematic review of adjuvant therapy trials was performed to determine whether adjuvant chemotherapy is effective for the treatment of women with early stage ovarian cancer.

Study Design.—A comprehensive search was performed of MEDLINE, Embase, Cancer Lit, and the Central Cochrane database. Only prospective, randomized clinical trials that reported survival in patients with stage I and II epithelial ovarian cancer treated with adjuvant therapy were considered for inclusion. Only studies with formal surgical staging at laparotomy were considered. The primary outcomes were overall and disease-free survival. Meta-analyses were performed for those trials comparing adjuvant chemotherapy versus radiotherapy or adjuvant chemotherapy versus observation.

Findings.—The systematic review identified 15 trials with 3162 total patients for inclusion in the meta-analysis. Two recent trials, ICON 1 and ACTION, dominated this meta-analysis. Early ovarian cancer patients who received adjuvant chemotherapy had significantly better disease-free and overall survival rates than those treated by observation alone. There was no significant difference between adjuvant radiotherapy and chemotherapy in patient outcome.

Conclusions.—Women with early stage ovarian cancer who are adequately staged with well-differentiated disease confined to the ovaries with intact capsule (FIGO stage IA/IB) can be managed by observation alone. All

other women should be offered platinum-based chemotherapy to improve disease-free and overall survival rates.

► Studies of limited-stage ovarian carcinoma (stage I-II) have historically been difficult because of lack of availability of these patients for clinical trials. This situation is beginning to change, and our basis for treatment of these patients is now on a somewhat firmer footing. There has been agreement for 20 years that patients should be divided into those at low risk and those at high risk for recurrence. In the United States at least, the standard of care for patients at high risk for recurrence has long been adjuvant chemotherapy, and more recently adjuvant platinum-based chemotherapy. This approach has been based on staging studies performed in the early 1980s and relatively small clinical trials showing improvement in disease-free survival in those high-risk patients so treated. The ACTION trial (Abstract 3–2) and the ICON1 trial (Abstract 3–3) are each larger than most studies that preceded them. The ACTION trial included 448 patients at high risk for recurrence based on appropriate staging procedures and showed a statistically significant improvement in recurrence-free survival (hazard ratio = 0.63, P = .02) but no significant improvement in overall survival for those patients who received platinum-based adjuvant chemotherapy compared with those who received no further therapy after surgical resection. The ICON1 trial included 477 patients with early stage ovarian carcinoma deemed to require chemotherapy and showed a statistically significant improvement in both recurrence-free (hazard ratio = 0.65, P = .01) and overall (hazard ratio = 0.66, P = .03) survival rates for those patients treated with platinum-based chemotherapy as opposed to those with no further therapy after surgery. A pooled analysis (Abstract 3–1) of the 2 studies was also published and showed, in the population of 925 patients, a statistically significant absolute 11% improvement in recurrence-free (65% to 76%) and 8% improvement overall (74% to 82%) survival at 5 years. These 3 articles report results from the largest studies yet in patients with limited-stage ovarian carcinoma and build a strong case to support the use of adjuvant platinum-based chemotherapy in those patients at high-risk for recurrence.

The fourth of these articles on limited-stage ovarian carcinoma (Abstract 3–4) is a review of all randomized trials conducted over the last 2 decades and provides an excellent overview of the topic. It should be noted that, prior to the ACTION and ICON1 trials, the average size of randomized trials in these patients fell below the 300-patient mark; such trials are underpowered to detect a clinically probable difference with treatment. It should further be noted that, although this overview plus the 3 articles on the ACTION and ICON1 trials provide a basis for the use of adjuvant chemotherapy, a number of unanswered questions remain. These include the optimal regimen, the optimal duration of therapy, and the role of newer agents such as the biologicals. Ongoing trials addressing these questions will hopefully begin to fill in these gaps in our knowledge. For now, based on the best evidence to date, adjuvant therapy should consist of at least 3 cycles of paclitaxel plus carboplatin after complete surgical resection of high-risk stage I to II disease.

J. T. Thigpen, MD

Adjuvant Treatment for Early Ovarian Cancer: A Randomized Phase III Trial of Intraperitoneal ^{32}P or Intravenous Cyclophosphamide and Cisplatin—A Gynecologic Oncology Group Study

Young RC, Brady MF, Nieberg RK, et al (Fox Chase Cancer Ctr, Philadelphia; Roswell Park Cancer Inst, Buffalo, NY; Univ of California, Los Angeles; et al)

J Clin Oncol 21:4350-4355, 2003 3–5

Background.—Clinical trials performed by the Gynecologic Oncology Group (GOG) have defined subsets of patients with early stage ovarian cancer who have good long-term prognosis (stage IA/IB International Federation of Gynecology and Obstetrics [FIGO] classification) without adjuvant therapy. The majority of patients, however, would benefit from appropriate adjuvant therapy to decrease the incidence of recurrence. The 10-year follow-up of a prospective, randomized phase III study comparing ^{32}P to cyclophosphamide-cisplatin (CP) adjuvant therapy for women with early-stage ovarian cancer at high risk for recurrence is described.

Study Design.—Women with high-risk ovarian cancer received a thorough surgical staging. Those who were FIGO stage IA or IB (grade 3) or stage IC or II (any grade) were randomly assigned to receive either a single intraperitoneal dose of ^{32}P (110 patients) or CP every 21 days for 3 cycles (119 patients). There were no significant differences between these 2 groups.

Findings.—The cumulative incidence of recurrence at 10-year follow-up was 35% for patients in the ^{32}P adjuvant therapy group and 28% for those in the CP adjuvant therapy group. Patients in the CP group had a 29% lower recurrence rate and a 17% lower death rate than patients in the ^{32}P group, but these differences were not significant. The 10-year cumulative incidence for all stage I patients was 27% and for all stage II patients was 44%. Patients with ascites had a worse prognosis than patients without ascites. Both regimens were tolerated, yet inadequate distribution and small-bowel perforation problems made ^{32}P adjuvant therapy less acceptable.

Conclusions.—There were no statistical differences in recurrence rates after ^{32}P versus CP adjuvant therapy for patients with early stage ovarian cancer, but survival trends and complication rates made CP the preferred adjuvant therapy for this patient group. Despite this adjuvant chemotherapy, only 65% of stage I patients and 52% of stage II patients can be expected to be alive and disease free at 10 years. Better adjuvant therapy is still needed to treat patients with early ovarian cancer at high risk for recurrence.

▶ This study lends further support to the need for adjuvant chemotherapy for patients with high-risk stage I to II disease. Although there were no statistically significant differences in efficacy between the 2 arms, strong trends favoring the chemotherapy option in terms of progression-free and overall survival, taken together with the statistically significant survival advantage observed in the ICON1/ACTION analysis, establish adjuvant platinum-based chemotherapy as the standard of care for these high-risk patients.

J. T. Thigpen, MD

Phase III Trial of Carboplatin and Paclitaxel Compared With Cisplatin and Paclitaxel in Patients With Optimally Resected Stage III Ovarian Cancer: A Gynecologic Oncology Group Study

Ozols RF, Bundy BN, Greer BE, et al (Fox Chase Cancer Ctr, Philadelphia; Roswell Park Cancer Inst, Buffalo, NY; New York Presbyterian Hosp-Cornell Med Ctr; et al)

J Clin Oncol 21:3194-3200, 2003 3–6

Background.—In the United States, standard therapy for advanced epithelial ovarian cancer is cisplatin plus paclitaxel, on the basis of trials performed by the Gynecologic Oncology Group (GOG). Carboplatin is an analogue of cisplatin with less hematologic toxicity. GOG 158 was designed as a noninferiority study comparing the efficacy and toxicity of carboplatin plus paclitaxel with cisplatin plus paclitaxel for treatment of small-volume stage III ovarian cancer.

Study Design.—The study group consisted of 792 women with stage III epithelial ovarian cancer, no prior therapy, and no residual disease greater than 1.0 cm in diameter after surgery. These women were randomly assigned to receive either cisplatin and paclitaxel or carboplatin and paclitaxel. These 2 groups were similar in terms of prognostic factors. Analysis was by intention to treat. Outcomes included overall survival (OS), progression-free survival (PFS), and adverse effects.

Findings.—Gastrointestinal, renal, and metabolic toxicity and grade 4 leukopenia were significantly more common among patients treated with cisplatin plus paclitaxel. Grade II or more thrombocytopenia was significantly more common among patients treated with carboplatin plus paclitaxel. Neurologic toxicity was similar for both treatments. The median PFS was 19.4 months and OS was 48.7 months for those in the cisplatin arm and 20.7 and 57.4 months, respectively, for those in the carboplatin arm.

Conclusions.—For patients with advanced ovarian cancer, chemotherapy with carboplatin plus paclitaxel was less toxic, easier to administer, and not inferior to chemotherapy with cisplatin plus paclitaxel. Because more than 70% of patients will have recurrence with a median progression time of less than 2 years, more effective therapies are still needed. GOG is currently participating in an international, randomized clinical trial of new 3-drug and sequential combinations. For the present, carboplatin and paclitaxel continue to be the standard therapy for ovarian cancer.

A Randomized Clinical Trial of Cisplatin/Paclitaxel Versus Carboplatin/Paclitaxel as First-Line Treatment of Ovarian Cancer

du Bois A, et al for the Arbeitsgemeinschaft Gynäkologische Onkologie (AGO) Ovarian Cancer Study Group (Dr-Horst-Schmidt-Kliniken, Wiesbaden, Germany; et al)

J Natl Cancer Inst 95:1320-1330, 2003 3–7

Purpose.—OVAR-3, a randomized, phase III, noninferiority trial, was designed to compare the safety and efficacy of cisplatin-paclitaxel (PT) to carboplatin-paclitaxel (TC) in patients with advanced ovarian cancer.

Study Design.—The study group consisted of 798 adult women with FIGO stage IIB to IV ovarian cancer who had undergone radical debulking surgery within the previous 6 weeks. Patients were randomly assigned to receive TC or PT. The primary end point was the proportion of patients without disease progression at 2 years. Secondary end points included toxicity, quality of life (QOL), overall survival (OS), progression-free survival (PFS), and treatment response. Survival curves were calculated with the Kaplan-Meier method and hazard ratios were estimated by the Cox proportional hazards model.

Findings.—In the patients without disease progression, the median PFS and median OS were not significantly different between the 2 treatment groups. TC therapy was associated with greater hematologic toxicity but lower gastrointestinal and neurologic toxicity than PT therapy. The mean global QOL scores were significantly better for the TC patients.

Conclusions.—Therapy with TC was as effective as therapy with PT but was better tolerated and associated with better QOL. The use of carboplatin instead of cisplatin may be better for the patient and should be considered a first-line treatment option for patients with advanced ovarian cancer and for use in clinical trials.

► The current standard chemotherapy regimen for advanced ovarian carcinoma, paclitaxel plus a platinum compound, is based on 2 independent studies (GOG Protocol 111 and a European-Canadian study OV-10) that compared cyclophosphamide/cisplatin to PT and found the PT regimen to be superior in terms of response rate, clinical complete response rate, PFS, and OS. By far the more common regimen used in the United States, however, is TC on the basis of prior studies suggesting that carboplatin had similar activity to that of cisplatin but a more favorable therapeutic index. This is an assumption, however, that is potentially incorrect since it does not account for the fact that paclitaxel and carboplatin clearly interact with each other. This interaction results in a marked decrease in the amount of myelosuppression observed with the combination compared with single-agent carboplatin. Since the mechanism of this bone marrow protection is not clear, it could not be stated with confidence that the interaction did not also protect the tumor.

These concerns led to 2 large trials comparing TC to PT to determine whether the 2 regimens were equivalent. DuBois et al (Abstract 3–7) evaluated the 2 regimens in patients with stages IIB to IV disease and used an area under the curve of 6 for carboplatin. This trial showed no significant difference in efficacy but small trends favoring the cisplatin regimen. Ozols et al (Abstract 3–6) studied the regimens in patients with small-volume residual stage III disease and used an area under the curve of 7.5 for carboplatin. This trial also produced no significant difference in efficacy, but there were strong trends favoring the carboplatin regimen.

Taken together, the 2 trials suggest that the 2 regimens are equivalent (at almost 800 eligible patients, each study had, in round figures, a 90% probability of detecting a 30% difference in survival). The trends, however, raise some interesting concerns about the dose of carboplatin. If in fact the interaction between carboplatin and paclitaxel does alter antitumor effect, the 2 studies suggest that the higher dose of carboplatin used in the GOG trial is needed to overcome that interaction and optimize therapeutic results. While this issue is important since the increased carboplatin dose causes more neuropathy, no trials are underway to evaluate this. Such studies seem unlikely to evolve in light of the large number of promising new agents available for testing.

For now, it would seem prudent for the physician to initiate chemotherapy for advanced ovarian carcinoma at the higher carboplatin dose of area under the curve of 7.5 and to reduce the dose in subsequent courses as required by toxicity.

J. T. Thigpen, MD

Phase III Randomized Trial of 12 Versus 3 Months of Maintenance Paclitaxel in Patients With Advanced Ovarian Cancer After Complete Response to Platinum and Paclitaxel-based Chemotherapy: A Southwest Oncology Group and Gynecologic Oncology Group Trial

Markman M, Liu PY, Wilczynski S, et al (Cleveland Clinic Found, Ohio; Ohio State Univ, Columbus; Southwest Oncology Group Statistical Ctr, Seattle; et al)

J Clin Oncol 21:2460-2465, 2003 3–8

Background.—Standard initial treatment for ovarian cancer generally includes 5 to 6 courses of a platinum/taxane regimen. Limited randomized study data show no advantage of additional treatment or a consolidation strategy in ovarian cancer or other malignant tumors. However, findings of nonrandomized studies suggest that more protracted treatment with paclitaxel may benefit patients with ovarian cancer. An effort was made to determine whether continuing paclitaxel for an extended period prolongs progression-free survival (PFS) and improves survival in women with advanced ovarian cancer who had obtained a clinically defined complete response to a platinum/paclitaxel–based chemotherapy.

Methods and Findings.—By random assignment, 277 patients received 3 or 12 cycles of single-agent paclitaxel every 28 days. Fifty-four PFS events occurred in 222 patients during follow-up. The regimens did not differ significantly in toxicity except for peripheral neuropathy. The median PFS was 21 months in the 3-cycle group and 28 months in the 12-cycle group. The

Cox model–adjusted 3-cycle progression hazard ratio compared with the 12-cycle progression was 2.31. These findings resulted in trial discontinuation. As of the date of study termination, overall survival did not differ between groups.

Conclusions.—A 12-cycle course of single-agent paclitaxel significantly prolongs PFS in women with advanced ovarian cancer who attain a clinically defined complete response to initial platinum/paclitaxel–based chemotherapy.

► With few exceptions, maintenance therapy has not proved to be useful in malignant disease. In general, patients "win or lose" in the early phases of treatment. This was a relatively straightforward article in which patients who achieved a remission with 5 or 6 cycles of a platinum/paclitaxel regimen were randomly assigned to 3 additional cycles or 12 additional cycles of paclitaxel and cisplatin. The discussion in the article by Dr Markham and the accompanying editorial by Tate Thigpen clearly delineates the problems with this study. The study was terminated early by a Data Monitoring Safety Committee when the relapse-free survival was found to be highly significant statistically. Overall survival may yet show a difference but has not yet done so. The article does not produce a paradigmship for the treatment of ovarian cancer, but it should lead to points of discussion between physicians and those patients who achieve a complete remission after induction chemotherapy with cisplatin and paclitaxel. With longer follow-up, this may indeed become the standard of care.

P. J. Loehrer, Sr, MD

Extraovarian Peritoneal Serous Papillary Carcinoma: A Phase II Trial of Cisplatin and Cyclophosphamide With Comparison to a Cohort With Papillary Serous Ovarian Carcinoma—A Gynecologic Oncology Group Study

Bloss JD, Brady MF, Liao SY, et al (Univ of Missouri, Columbia; Roswell Park Cancer Inst, Buffalo, NY; Univ of California at Irvine; et al)

Gynecol Oncol 89:148-154, 2003 3–9

Introduction.—The condition was first described in 1959, yet the etiology, pathogenesis, cell of origin, and clinical characteristics of extraovarian peritoneal serous papillary carcinoma (EPSPC) remain obscure. The probability of response and progression-free and overall survival of a well-defined group of women with EPSPC treated with a combination of cisplatin and cyclophosphamide after cytoreduction surgery were examined in a Gynecologic Oncology Group phase II investigation and compared with those of a group of women with papillary serous ovarian carcinoma (PSOC) who received identical therapy.

Methods.—After primary surgery, patients underwent treatment with cisplatin 75 mg/m^2 and cyclophosphamide 750 mg/m^2 every 21 days for 6 cycles. Patient demographics, tumor characteristics, clinical and surgical response to treatment, progression-free survival, and overall survival were assessed. Patients with EPSPC were compared with patients with PSOC who received identical treatment on a separate protocol.

Results.—Women with a diagnosis of EPSPC tended to be older than the PSOC cohort (median age, 65.8 years vs 60.3 years; $P = .04$). The estimated probabilities of complete and partial clinical responses to the treatment regimen were 65% (95% confidence interval [CI], 41%-85%) for EPSPC versus 59% (95% CI, 47%-71%) for women with PSOC. Surgical complete response rates (20% vs 19%) were similar for the 2 groups. Death rates were similar for the 2 groups (hazard ratio, 1.25; 95% CI, 0.834-1.88).

Conclusion.—Women with EPSPC and PSOC have a similar probability of response to treatment with cisplatin and cyclophosphamide and a similar overall survival rate. It is reasonable to include EPSPC patients in future large-scale treatment trials assessing patients with advanced ovarian cancer.

▶ What most people mean when they refer to ovarian carcinoma is the most common type, celomic epithelial carcinoma of the ovary, which arises from the celomic epithelium and invests the ovary during development to form a "capsule." This same epithelium lines the entire peritoneal cavity, and prior studies have reported celomic epithelial carcinomas arising from portions of this epithelium other than that which invests the ovary. These "primary peritoneal neoplasms" have been excluded from studies of ovarian carcinoma in the past. This study of primary peritoneal neoplasms by Bloss et al in the Gynecologic Oncology Group demonstrates that these lesions exhibit similar response rates to chemotherapy as that observed with ovarian carcinoma. These results have led to the inclusion of these lesions in studies of ovarian carcinoma in more recent studies.

J. T. Thigpen, MD

Paclitaxel Plus Platinum-Based Chemotherapy Versus Conventional Platinum-Based Chemotherapy in Women With Relapsed Ovarian Cancer: The ICON4/AGO-OVAR-2.2 Trial

The ICON and AGO Collaborators (MRC Trials Unit, London)

Lancet 361:2099-2106, 2003 3–10

Background.—Treatments for ovarian cancer have improved greatly, yet most patients with ovarian cancer still have recurrence within 3 years of diagnosis. Platinum-based chemotherapy (PBC) is the usual first-line treatment and is often used to treat relapses occurring 6 months or more after first-line PBC. Whether adding paclitaxel to PBC would be more effective as second-line treatment than conventional PBC for women whose recurrence develops 6 months or more after initial treatment was examined.

Methods.—Between January 1996 and March 2002, 802 women were enrolled from 119 centers in 5 countries. All patients had epithelial ovarian cancer that had been treated with PBC but recurred 6 months later. All patients in the Arbeitsgemeinschaft Gynaekologische Onkologie (AGO) OVAR-2.2. trial had previously received paclitaxel plus either carboplatin or cisplatin. All patients in the International Collaborative Ovarian Neoplasm 4 (ICON4) trial had previously received PBC, with or without paclitaxel. Patients were randomly assigned to receive either conventional PBC or paclitaxel + PBC. Treatments were given every 3 weeks for at least 3 cycles; 72% received at least 6 cycles. Patients were followed up for a mean of 42 months to compare disease-free and overall survival between the 2 groups.

Results.—As of March 2003, 530 patients (66%) had died and 717 (89%) had shown disease progression or died. Two-year survival was better in the paclitaxel + PBC group (57% vs 50%), as was median survival (29 vs 24 months). Kaplan-Meier analyses showed a significant overall survival advantage with the paclitaxel + PBC regimen (mortality hazard ratio, 0.82). One-year progression-free survival was also better in the paclitaxel + PBC group (mean, 50% vs 40%; median duration, 9 vs 12 months), and the risk of disease progression was significantly lower in this group (hazard ratio, 0.76). Subgroup analyses confirmed the benefits associated with paclitaxel + PBC both for patients with previous exposure to taxanes and for those without previous taxane exposure. The most common adverse events were alopecia (25% vs 86%, conventional PBC vs paclitaxel + PBC), hematologic toxicity (46% vs 29%, respectively), and neurologic toxicity (1% vs 20%, respectively).

Conclusion.—For patients with platinum-sensitive recurrent ovarian cancer, second-line paclitaxel + PBC improves progression-free and overall survival compared with conventional PBC.

▶ This major article reports the results of an intergroup study of therapy in patients with platinum-sensitive recurrent ovarian carcinoma. Patients were randomized to either non–taxane-containing platinum-based therapy (the vast majority received carboplatin alone) or a regimen including a taxane plus a platinum compound (the vast majority received paclitaxel plus carboplatin). Results show a statistically significant improvement in both progression-free and overall survival for those patients receiving the taxane/platinum regimen. This marks the first randomized trial to demonstrate a survival advantage for second-line chemotherapy. The study has been criticized because approximately half of the patients did not receive a taxane as a part of their front-line therapy. Such critics believe that the improvement with the combination is entirely a taxane effect that would not apply to patients who received both a taxane and a platinum compound front-line. The investigators, however, did assess the effects of the treatments in both those who did and those who did not receive a taxane front-line and found no differences in the 2 subgroups with the advantage for the taxane/platinum regimen present in both.

Some have criticized the conclusions of the study on the basis that 75% of the patients had a treatment-free interval before recurrence of more than 12 months and that no significant difference between the 2 arms could be detected in the subgroup of patients who had a treatment-free interval before recurrence of 6 to 12 months. Such criticism is without basis since the subgroup with a 6- to 12-month treatment-free interval is too small to permit any conclusions to be drawn.

There are 2 practical implications of this study. First, the study establishes that, at least for now, the treatment of choice in platinum-sensitive recurrent ovarian carcinoma is a taxane/platinum combination. Second, the results suggest that improvement in survival is now a valid goal of second-line therapy in the subset with platinum-sensitive disease.

J. T. Thigpen, MD

Phase II Trial of Carboxyamidotriazole in Patients With Relapsed Epithelial Ovarian Cancer

Hussain MM, Kotz H, Minasian L, et al (Natl Cancer Inst, Bethesda, Md)
J Clin Oncol 21:4356-4363, 2003 3–11

Background.—First-line treatments for ovarian cancer usually cause persistent end-organ toxicity. Carboxyamidotriazole is a cytostatic agent developed to stabilize disease while the patient recovers from end-organ toxicity and to maintain an optimal therapeutic response or remission. Its efficacy and tolerability in this regard were examined.

Methods.—The subjects were 39 women (aged 29-80 years) with persistent or recurrent epithelial ovarian cancer. All patients had good end-organ function and measurable disease and had received fewer than 3 prior treatments. Patients were treated with daily oral carboxyamidotriazole according to a pharmacokinetic model to maintain plasma concentrations between 2 and 4 μg/mL. Treatment was interrupted if grades 3 or 4 toxicity developed and resumed at a 50% lower dose when toxicity decreased to grades 0 to 1. Response was assessed by physical examination and noninvasive imaging every 2 months. A positive response was defined as stabilization or improvement of disease for 6 months or more. A partial response was defined as a more than 50% decrease in lesion diameters in the absence of new lesions. A minor response was defined as a 25% to 50% decrease in lesion diameters without new lesions. Toxicity was assessed according to the National Cancer Institute Common Toxicity Criteria.

Results.—Response could be evaluated in 38 patients. Eleven patients (31%) had stabilization or improvement of disease for 6 months or more (range, 6-13 months); 10 of these 11 responders had platinum-sensitive disease. Additionally, there was 1 partial response (lasting 8 months) and 3 minor responses (lasting 8, 12, and 13 months). The median progression-free interval was 3.6 months. Carboxyamidotriazole was well tolerated; there were no grade 4 adverse events, and the only grade 3 adverse events were fatigue (5%), vomiting (2%), neutropenic fever (2%), and neutropenia (2%).

Conclusion.—Oral carboxyamidotriazole has a low toxicity profile compared with other second-line treatments for recurrent ovarian cancer. Approximately one third of patients achieved disease stabilization for 6 months or more. Thus, carboxyamidotriazole may have a role in prolonging the chemotherapy-free interval in patients with significant end-organ toxicity after previous treatment.

► This study by Hussain et al evaluated the activity of an antiangiogenic agent, carboxyamidotriazole. By the prospective standards of the study design, carboxyamidotriazole has significant activity in ovarian carcinoma. It must be noted, however, that the traditional response rate was 3% (1 partial response among 36 patients). The standard of stable disease for 6 or more months in 11 of 36 patients represents a new approach to evaluating biologic or targeted agents that are believed to be cytostatic. Time will tell whether the new definitions produce meaningful evaluations. In the meantime, carboxyamidotriazole will move forward for further evaluation in ovarian carcinoma.

J. T. Thigpen, MD

A Phase II Trial of ZD0473 in Platinum-Pretreated Ovarian Cancer

Gore ME, Atkinson RJ, Thomas H, et al (Royal Marsden Hosp NHS Trust, London; Belfast City Hosp, Northern Ireland; Royal Surrey Hosp, Guildford, England; et al)

Eur J Cancer 38:2416-2420, 2002 3–12

Background.—ZD0473 is a new platinum agent developed to treat platinum-resistant ovarian cancer. Its efficacy and tolerability in both platinum-resistant and platinum-sensitive recurrent ovarian cancer were examined.

Methods.—The subjects were 94 women (aged 27-75 years) with recurrent ovarian cancer who had received first-line platinum-based chemotherapy (PBC). Patients whose relapse occurred less than 26 weeks after the end of PBC were defined as platinum resistant (n = 59 [63%]), whereas those whose relapse occurred more than 26 weeks after the end of PBC were defined as platinum sensitive (n = 35 [37%]). Patients were treated with IV ZD0473, 120 to 150 mg/m^2, on day 1 of a 3-week cycle. To continue treatment, all patients had to have an absolute neutrophil count of 1.5 × 10^9 cells/L or greater, a platelet count of 100 × 10^9 cells/L or greater, serum creatinine and bilirubin levels less than 1.25 times the upper limit of normal, and no grades 2, 3, or 4 nonhematologic toxicity. Response was assessed according to revised National Cancer Institute Response Evaluation Criteria in Solid Tumors guidelines. Clinical benefit was defined as complete or partial response or stable disease lasting 6 weeks or greater. Toxicity was assessed according to the National Cancer Institute Common Toxicity Criteria.

Results.—Patients received 1 to 8 cycles of ZD0473 (median, 3 cycles) for a total of 337 cycles. Dose reduction was required in 35 patients (37%), and cycles were delayed because of toxicity in 41 patients (44%). Response could be evaluated in 38 platinum-resistant patients and 34 platinum-sensitive patients. Objective response rates were 8.3% for the platinum-resistant patients and 32.4% for the platinum-sensitive patients. Clinical benefit was seen by 43.3% of platinum-resistant patients and 76.5% of platinum-sensitive patients. Disease was stable in 32 patients (39.0%) and progressed in 35 (42.7%). The median progression-free interval was shorter in the platinum-resistant patients than in the platinum-sensitive ones (57 vs 180 days), as was survival (median, 242 vs 402 days). Grades 3 to 4 thrombocytopenia occurred in 58 patients (62%), grades 3 to 4 neutropenia occurred in 35 patients (37%), and grades 3 to 4 anemia occurred in 33 patients (35%). The most common nonhematologic grade 3 to 4 adverse reactions were lethargy in 16 patients and vomiting in 11 patients. No patient had clinically significant ototoxicity, nephrotoxicity, or neurotoxicity.

Conclusion.—The toxicity profile of ZD0473 as second-line treatment for ovarian cancer compares favorably with that of other forms of therapy and avoids the nephrotoxicity, ototoxicity, and neurotoxicity associated with cisplatin and carboplatin. The drug was more effective against platinum-sensitive disease than against platinum-resistant disease, and in this latter setting it does not appear to offer a significant therapeutic advantage over conventional platinum-based agents.

▶ This study by Gore et al evaluates ZD0473, a platinum compound designed to overcome platinum resistance in patients with platinum-sensitive and platinum-resistant ovarian carcinoma. Response rates reported included 8% in platinum-resistant patients and 32% in platinum-sensitive patients. The authors conclude that the drug has promising activity in platinum-sensitive ovarian carcinoma, similar to other agents. The only caveat to this conclusion is that cisplatin and carboplatin have even better activity reported in platinum-sensitive disease. If the treatment-free interval for all of the platinum-sensitive patients falls between 6 and 12 months, then the 32% response rate would be in line with that reported for cisplatin and carboplatin and better than that seen with other agents. The authors, however, do not provide this information. Despite the rather optimistic conclusions, it would seem that an agent designed to overcome resistance should have better activity in resistant patients than that observed and activity in sensitive patients at least as good as that expected from cisplatin or carboplatin.

J. T. Thigpen, MD

A Phase II Trial of Capecitabine (Xeloda) in Recurrent Ovarian Cancer

Vasey PA, McMahon L, Paul J, et al (Western Infirmary, Glasgow, Scotland; Royal Marsden Hosp, Sutton, England)

Br J Cancer 89:1843-1848, 2003 3–13

Background.—Oral capecitabine is an effective treatment for advanced colorectal cancer and metastatic breast cancer. Its efficacy and tolerability as a single agent in recurrent ovarian cancer were examined in a phase II study.

Methods.—The subjects were 29 women (aged 38-78 years) with recurrent epithelial ovarian cancer and CA 125 levels 100 kU/L or greater. All patients had previously been treated with platinum but had relapsed less than 12 months after their last course of chemotherapy. Patients were treated with oral capecitabine, 1250 mg/m^2, twice a day on days 1 to 14 of a 21-day cycle. Treatment was interrupted when grades 2, 3, or 4 toxicity developed, and reinstated at 50% to 75% of the initial dose once toxicity resolved to grades 0 or 1. Response was defined as a 50% decrease in serum CA 125 levels compared with 2 previous measurements or a serial decrease in CA 125 levels more than 75% over 3 samples.

Results.—The platinum-free interval was less than 6 months in 9 patients (30%) and more than 6 months in 20 patients (70%). Patients received 1 to 9 cycles of capecitabine (median, 4 cycles) for a total of 121 cycles. Dose reduction was required in 7 patients (24%), and 6 cycles were delayed because of treatment-related toxicity. Twenty-eight patients could be evaluated for response; 8 patients responded for a response rate of 29%. The median progression-free interval was 3.7 months, and the median overall survival was 8.0 months. Of note, after 6 months of treatment 28% were still progression free and 62% were still alive. Response rates did not differ significantly according to the platinum-free interval (44% for <6 months vs 21% for >6 months) or the treatment-free interval (24% for <6 months vs 33% for >6 months). The most common adverse events were hand-foot syndrome (grade 3 in 4 patients [14%]), nausea (grade 3 vomiting in 3 patients [10%]), and diarrhea. The only grade 4 toxicity was leukopenia in 1 patient (3%).

Conclusion.—The efficacy and tolerability of oral capecitabine compare well with those of other forms of monotherapy for the treatment of platinum-resistant epithelial ovarian cancer. The safety profile with this regimen was better than that with IV therapies, and its oral route of administration makes it much more convenient.

► Vasey et al report results with the treatment of platinum-pretreated ovarian carcinoma with capecitabine. Unfortunately, it is not clear whether the patients in this study were platinum sensitive or platinum resistant since patients with treatment-free intervals of less than 12 months were allowed in the study, and the most recent treatment (from which the treatment-free interval was assessed) did not have to contain platinum. Additionally, the investigators report serologic responses rather than responses from the assessment of measurable disease. Given these caveats, a 29% response rate is reported; 28% were noted to remain progression-free after 6 months. The authors conclude that capecitabine is significantly active in ovarian carcinoma. The relative merits of this activity, however, are unclear because of the nonstandard definitions used to characterize the patient population and to assess response.

J. T. Thigpen, MD

Altretamine (Hexamethylmelamine) in the Treatment of Platinum-Resistant Ovarian Cancer: A Phase II Study

Keldsen N, Havsteen H, Vergote I, et al (Herning Hosp, Denmark; Århus Univ Hosp, Denmark; Univ Hosps, Leuven, Belgium; et al)

Gynecol Oncol 88:118-122, 2003 3–14

Introduction.—Despite an initial good response to chemotherapy, ovarian cancer recurs in most patients and the long-term prognosis is dismal. The response to second-line chemotherapy tends to be poorer, particularly if the disease has progressed during treatment or recurs within a treatment-free interval of 6 to 12 months after initial therapy. A 14% response rate has been reported in 50 patients with platinum-resistant disease treated with altretamine (hexamethylmelamine). The activity of altretamine in women with epithelial ovarian carcinoma who responded (partial response or complete response) to first-line chemotherapy and relapsed within 6 months was evaluated in this multicenter phase II trial. This protocol was later amended to include women with relapse within 12 months.

Methods.—All patients had measurable disease (World Health Organization performance status 2 or below [Karnofsky index >60] and adequate bone marrow function and liver function) and had no more than 1 prior chemotherapy regimen. Altretamine 250 mg/m^2 per day was administered in 4 divided doses for 2 weeks; this was repeated every 4 weeks. Patient response was assessed after every 2 courses.

Results.—Thirty-one patients received a median of 3 courses of altretamine (range, 1-12 courses). Hematologic toxicity was minimal and gastrointestinal toxicity was common. Twenty-six patients were able to be evaluated for response. Three patients (9.7% intent-to-treat) had a partial response, 8 patients had stable disease, and 15 patients had progressive disease after 2 courses of treatment. Median time to progression was 10 weeks (range, 5-51 weeks) and median survival was 34 weeks (range, 7-112 weeks).

Conclusion.—Altretamine should not be used as standard treatment in patients with platinum-resistant recurrent ovarian cancer. This drug may be a useful alternative in patients who prefer oral therapy or when socioeconomic considerations are important.

▶ This study by Keldsen et al evaluated the activity of altretamine in platinum-resistant patients. The response rate of 9.7% is sufficiently low that one can conclude that altretamine has little useful activity in patients who are platinum resistant. This is particularly true since the investigators allowed 7 patients into the study with treatment-free intervals between 6 and 12 months rather than the more standard 6 months or less. Although altretamine clearly has activity in platinum-sensitive patients, its order of activity is considerably less effective than that seen with retreatment with a platinum-based regimen. This effectively means that altretamine has little role in the current management of patients with ovarian carcinoma.

J. T. Thigpen, MD

Phase II Evaluation of Three-Day Topotecan in Recurrent Platinum-Sensitive Ovarian Carcinoma: A Gynecologic Oncology Group Study

Miller DS, Blessing JA, Lentz SS, et al (Univ of Texas, Dallas; Roswell Park Cancer Inst, Buffalo, NY; Wake Forest Univ, Winston-Salem, NC; et al)

Cancer 98:1664-1669, 2003 3–15

Background.—IV topotecan, at a dose of 1.5 mg/m^2 daily for 5 days every 3 weeks, is effective for treating recurrent ovarian cancer. However, this regimen is associated with major toxicity, primarily myelosuppression. The effectiveness and tolerability of a 3-day topotecan regimen were investigated.

Methods.—The subjects were 30 women (aged 41-81 years) with ovarian cancer recurrence detected 6 months or more after first-line treatment with platinum-based chemotherapy. Patients were treated with IV topotecan, 2.0 mg/m^2 for 3 consecutive days on a 21-day cycle. The dose was adjusted to a maximum of 2.5 mg/m^2 if no grade 3 or 4 toxicity developed. The dose was reduced by 0.25-mg/m^2 increments in cases of neutropenia with fever, grade 4 thrombocytopenia, or grade 4 neutropenia lasting 7 days. Granulocyte colony stimulating factor, erythropoietin, and thrombopoietin were used as needed. Response was assessed by physical examination and imaging before each cycle. A complete response was defined as the disappearance of macroscopic disease for at least 4 weeks. A partial response was defined as a 50% or greater reduction in lesion diameters for at least 4 weeks. Toxicity was assessed according to the revised National Cancer Institute Common Toxicity Criteria.

Results.—Patients received 1 to 11 cycles of topotecan (median, 5 cycles). One patient discontinued treatment because of toxicity. Two patients had a complete response and 2 patients had a partial response, for an overall response rate of 14%. Disease was stable in 16 patients (55%) and progressed in 9 (31%). The median progression-free interval was 4.2 months. Nine patients (30%) had grade 3 neutropenia, whereas 18 (60%) had grade 4 neutropenia; 6 patients (20%) required granulocyte colony stimulating factor. Grades 3 to 4 anemia developed in 4 (13%) and 1 (3%) patients, respectively, whereas grades 3 to 4 thrombocytopenia developed in 3 (10%) and 1 (3%) patients, respectively. Ten patients (33%) had grade 3 leukopenia develop, but none had grade 4 leukopenia develop.

Conclusion.—Response rates with the standard 5-day topotecan regimen are 19% to 33% in platinum-sensitive patients. The current 3-day regimen was less effective, with an overall response rate of 14%. However, the hematologic safety profile was better with the abbreviated regimen, suggesting a 3-day topotecan regimen could be combined with platinum or paclitaxel as second-line therapy for recurrent ovarian cancer.

Three-consecutive-day Topotecan Is an Active Regimen for Recurrent Epithelial Ovarian Cancer

Brown JV III, Peters WA III, Rettenmaier MA, et al (Hoag Mem Hosp, Newport Beach, Calif; Univ of Washington, Seattle; Pacific Gynecology Specialists, Seattle)

Gynecol Oncol 88:136-140, 2003 3–16

Background.—A 3-day regimen of topotecan may be more convenient and less toxic for treating recurrent ovarian cancer than the standard 5-day regimen if the abbreviated regimen maintains its efficacy. This question was examined in a phase II trial.

Methods.—The subjects were 31 women (aged 32-84 years) with recurrent epithelial cancer of the ovary, peritoneum, or fallopian tube. Patients were treated with IV topotecan, 2.0 mg/m^2 for 3 consecutive days on a 21-day cycle. The dose was increased to a maximum of 2.5 mg/m^2 if no grade III or IV toxicity developed. The dose was decreased by 0.25-mg/m^2 increments in cases of grade 4 neutropenia complicated by fever or infection, grade 4 thrombocytopenia complicated by bleeding, grade 4 neutropenia or grade 4 thrombocytopenia lasting 7 or more days, or if the cycle was delayed by 7 or more days. Granulocyte colony stimulating factor and interleukin 11 were given as needed. Response was assessed by clinical and serologic criteria. A complete clinical response was defined as the disappearance of all known disease, including normalization of CA 125 levels. A partial clinical response was defined as a 50% or greater decrease in lesion diameters. A complete serologic response was defined as the normalization of CA 125 levels and the absence of symptoms associated with ovarian cancer. A partial serologic response was defined as a 50% decrease in serum CA 125 levels measured at least twice compared with baseline.

Results.—Patients received 2 to 8 cycles of topotecan (median, 6 cycles) for a total of 165 cycles. Twenty-eight patients could be evaluated for response. Among the 18 clinically evaluable patients, there were 2 complete responders and 2 partial responders, for an overall clinical response rate of 22.2%. Among the 10 serologically evaluable patients, there were 1 complete responder and 4 partial responders, for an overall serologic response rate of 50.0%. Thus, the overall response rate was 32.1%. Disease was stable in 14 patients (50.0%) and progressed in 5 (17.9%). Eighteen patients were platinum sensitive (ie, recurrence developed ≥6 months after their last platinum-containing treatment). Of these 18 patients, 12.5% had a complete response and 31.3% had a partial response, for an overall response among platinum-sensitive patients of 43.4%. The median progression-free interval for platinum-sensitive patients was 3 months longer than that for all patients (18.5 vs 15.5 weeks). Grade 3 neutropenia developed in 29.1% of cycles and grade 4 neutropenia in 23.6% of cycles, but only 3.6% of cycles required granulocyte colony stimulating factor. Grades 3 to 4 thrombocytopenia developed in 2% and 1% of courses, respectively.

Conclusion.—An abbreviated 3-day course of topotecan is an effective regimen with acceptable toxicity for treating recurrent ovarian cancer. Most patients do not require granulocyte colony stimulating factor support, and nonhematologic toxicity is mild and infrequent.

► These 2 studies evaluate a 3-day schedule of topotecan in patients with recurrent ovarian carcinoma. The Gynecologic Oncology Group (GOG) study by Miller et al (Abstract 3–15) used topotecan 2 mg/m^2 per day for 3 days every 3 weeks in platinum-sensitive ovarian carcinoma and noted a response rate of 14%, a rate half that of a prior GOG study with a 5-day schedule of 1.5 mg/m^2 per day every 3 weeks. Although the dose was 20% lower in this study, dose has not been identified as a major determinant of response with topotecan. This would suggest that a 3-day schedule decreases the activity of topotecan. The study by Brown et al (Abstract 3–16), using the same schedule, reports a considerably higher response rate of 32%. Among the 18 patients with platinum-sensitive disease, a 43% response rate was observed, whereas 2 of 12 patients with platinum-resistant disease responded (17%).

At first glance, these 2 studies would seem to contradict each other. Closer examination, however, reveals that the study by Brown et al included responses by CA-125 only in patients with no measurable masses. In fact, 18 patients were assessed by the same response criteria as those used in the GOG study, and the response rate in this group was 22% (4 of 18), which is more in line with the 14% reported by the GOG. In contrast, the group with serologic responses exhibited a 50% response rate (5 of 10). When assessing phase II data in recurrent or persistent ovarian carcinoma, it is important to read the fine print of the study to determine how response is assessed and to see how the investigators define drug resistance. Both studies are consistent with the view that shortening the schedule of topotecan reduces its efficacy in ovarian carcinoma.

J. T. Thigpen, MD

A Phase II Study of Docetaxel in Paclitaxel-Resistant Ovarian and Peritoneal Carcinoma: A Gynecologic Oncology Group Study

Rose PG, Blessing JA, Ball HG, et al (Case Western Reserve Univ, Cleveland, Ohio, Roswell Park Cancer Inst, Buffalo, NY; Univ of Massachusetts, Worcester; et al)

Gynecol Oncol 88:130-135, 2003 3–17

Introduction.—Docetaxel is an inhibitor of microtubule depolymerization and has shown activity in paclitaxel-resistant breast cancer and gynecologic cancer. It has also been observed in several human ovarian cancer long-term cell culture lines to be more cytotoxic than paclitaxel on a milliliter to milliliter basis. This increased toxicity may be from docetaxel's higher achievable intracellular concentration, higher affinity for microtubules, and slower cellular efflux. The Gynecologic Oncology Group performed a large, multi-institutional phase II trial to better determine the antitumor activity, nature, and degrees of toxicity in patients with paclitaxel- and platinum-resistant ovarian cancer deemed as progressive while receiving or within 6 months of therapy.

Methods.—Patients were eligible if they had measurable disease and had not received more than 1 chemotherapy regimen. Docetaxel, 100 mg/m^2, was administered IV over a 1-hour period every 21 days. A prophylactic regimen of oral dexamethasone, 8 mg twice a day, was initiated 24 hours before docetaxel administration and continued for 48 hours thereafter. Hepatic function was followed closely.

Results.—Sixty patients underwent a total of 256 courses. All 60 patients were evaluable for toxicity and 58 were evaluable for response. Of 22.4% of patients with response, 5.2% were complete responses and 17.2% were partial (95% confidence interval, 12.5%-35.3%). The median response duration was 2.5 months. The likelihood of a response did not seem to be associated with the length of the prior paclitaxel-free interval or the duration of prior paclitaxel infusions. Seventy-five percent of patients had grade 4 neutropenia, and there was 1 treatment-related death. A decrease in dose was necessary in 36% of patients.

Conclusion.—Docetaxel is active in paclitaxel-resistant ovarian cancer and peritoneal cancer. The significant hematologic toxicity necessitates further investigation to ascertain the optimal dose and schedule.

▶ This Gynecologic Oncology Group study evaluated the activity of docetaxel in patients with platinum/paclitaxel-resistant disease and observed a response rate of 22%. These data suggest that docetaxel and paclitaxel are not cross-resistant and that a change in the taxane can cause responses. Similar data are available for a switch to weekly paclitaxel in patients who proved resistant to paclitaxel given on an every 3 weeks schedule. In other words, a "modulated" taxane therapy is a valid option in patients with paclitaxel/platinum-resistant disease.

J. T. Thigpen, MD

Gemcitabine Reverses Cisplatin Resistance: Demonstration of Activity in Platinum- and Multidrug-Resistant Ovarian and Peritoneal Carcinoma

Rose PG, Mossbruger K, Fusco N, et al (Case Western Reserve Univ, Cleveland, Ohio)

Gynecol Oncol 88:17-21, 2003 3–18

Background.—Treatment success rates in patients with recurrent ovarian cancer who did not respond to first-line platinum-based chemotherapies are poor. In animal studies of ovarian cancer, survival is better with a combination of gemcitabine and cisplatin than with either drug alone. Whether this synergistic effect also occurs in women with platinum-resistant ovarian or peritoneal cancer was examined.

Methods.—The subjects were 36 women aged 44 to 82 years with ovarian (n = 33) or peritoneal (n = 3) cancer who had not responded to first-line platinum, paclitaxel, or other drugs. Patients received an IV infusion of gemcitabine (750 mg/m^2) followed by cisplatin (30 mg/m^2) on days 1 and 8 of each 3-week cycle. Therapy on day 8 was canceled when the absolute neutrophil count was less than 1000 cells/mm^3 or the platelet count was less than 75,000 cells/mm^3. Subsequent doses of gemcitabine were sequentially reduced to 600, 400, and 300 mg/m^2 until neutrophil and platelet counts normalized. A complete response was defined as resolution of signs, symptoms, biochemical parameters, and measurable disease without clinical evidence of progression for 4 or more weeks. A partial response was defined as a 50% or greater reduction in lesion diameters without any increase in lesion size or new lesions for 4 or more weeks.

Results.—Response to treatment could be evaluated in 35 patients. Nineteen patients (52.7%) required dose reductions caused by adverse events. Four patients (11.4%) had a complete response and 11 (31.4%) had a partial response, for an overall response rate of 42.9%. Of the 6 patients who had not responded to gemcitabine as a single agent, 4 had a response to combination therapy. Most of the responders (73%) had been platinum free for more than 12 months. The median response duration among the responders was 11 months. For all patients, the median progression-free interval was 6 months, and median survival was 12 months. The most common adverse events were thrombocytopenia (93.2%) and neutropenia (77.8%).

Conclusion.—The combination of gemcitabine and cisplatin appears to have a synergistic effect in platinum- and multidrug-resistant ovarian and peritoneal cancer. In fact, the combination showed activity in 4 of 6 patients who had not previously responded to gemcitabine alone. The regimen is tolerable, but hematologic toxicity and cisplatin-associated adverse events worsen as treatment continues.

Phase II Trials of Gemcitabine Plus Cisplatin Repeating Doublet Therapy in Previously Treated, Relapsed Ovarian Cancer Patients

Nagourney RA, Brewer CA, Radecki S, et al (Rational Therapeutics Inc, Long Beach, Calif; Univ of Illinois, Peoria; California Pacific Med Ctr, San Francisco; et al)

Gynecol Oncol 88:35-39, 2003 3–19

Background.—The combination of cisplatin and gemcitabine has a synergistic effect in patients with non–small cell lung cancer or advanced breast cancer. The potential role of combined cisplatin and gemcitabine therapy in patients with recurrent ovarian cancer was examined.

Methods.—The subjects were 27 women (aged 35-82 years) with recurrent ovarian cancer. Fourteen patients had platinum-resistant disease, whereas 13 patients had platinum-sensitive disease. Patients received an IV infusion of cisplatin (30 mg/m^2) followed by gemcitabine (600-750 mg/m^2) on days 1 and 8 of each 3-week cycle. Drug doses were reduced when hematologic toxicity (gemcitabine) or nausea, vomiting, neuropathy, or renal toxicity (cisplatin) developed. Complete and partial responses were evaluated according to Gynecologic Oncology Group criteria or (for patients whose only indication of disease was elevated serum CA-125 levels) Rustin's criteria. Additionally, 17 patients provided tumor samples for the ex vivo determination of tumor susceptibility to the combination.

Results.—Of the 27 patients, 7 (26.0%) had a complete response to combined gemcitabine plus cisplatin, whereas 12 patients (44.4%) had a partial response, for an overall response rate of 70.4%. Disease was stable in 7 patients (26%) and progressed in 1 (4%). Among the 13 patients with platinum-sensitive disease, 4 had a complete response and 7 had a partial response (overall response rate, 84%). Among the 14 patients with platinum-resistant disease, 3 had a complete response and 5 had a partial response (overall response rate, 57%). Among the responders, the median progression-free interval was 7.9 months. For all patients, the mean progression-free interval was 6.0 months and mean survival was 20.2 months. The most common grade III or IV adverse events were thrombocytopenia in 96.3% of patients, neutropenia in 81.5%, and leukopenia in 44.4%. In the ex vivo analyses, responders were significantly more likely than nonresponders to have a positive sensitivity assay (90% vs 29). Progression-free and overall survival rates were also significantly longer in patients with a positive assay, even after adjusting for platinum sensitivity status and the number of previous therapies received.

Conclusion.—The combination of gemcitabine and cisplatin appears to have a synergistic effect in patients with recurrent ovarian cancer. In fact, the combination was effective in 8 of 14 patients with platinum-resistant disease. Results of ex vivo sensitivity analyses correlated significantly with response, progression-free survival, and overall survival.

▶ These 2 phase II studies evaluate the combination of gemcitabine plus cisplatin in patients with recurrent or persistent ovarian carcinoma. In the Nagourney et al study (Abstract 3–19), almost half the patients had platinum-sensitive disease; whereas in the Rose et al study (Abstract 3–18) all patients were reported to be platinum resistant. Both studies report high response rates among the patients with platinum-resistant disease (43% in the Rose et al study and 57% in the Nagourney et al study). The explanation offered for these observations is that the 2 drugs are synergistic in such a way that resistance is effectively overcome. Although these observations require further study and confirmation (especially since the Nagourney et al study includes only 14 platinum-resistant patients), this combination certainly can be added to those approaches that can be tried in patients with platinum-resistant disease. Can carboplatin be substituted for cisplatin with the same results? The answer is not known.

J. T. Thigpen, MD

Phase II Study of Gemcitabine in Recurrent Platinum- and Paclitaxel-Resistant Ovarian Cancer

D'Agostino G, Amant F, Berteloot P, et al (Univ Hosp, Leuven, Belgium; Catholic Univ of the Sacred Heart, Rome)

Gynecol Oncol 88:266-269, 2003 3–20

Background.—The effectiveness and tolerability of gemcitabine for treating platinum- and paclitaxel-resistant ovarian cancer was examined in a phase II trial.

Methods.—The subjects were 50 women (aged 24-83 years) with ovarian cancer whose disease progressed despite up to 5 previous platinum- and/or paclitaxel-based chemotherapy treatments. Patients were treated with IV gemcitabine, 1000 mg/m^2, on days 1, 8, and 15 of a 28-day cycle. The dose was decreased by 20% to 50% if grade 4 neutropenia or grade 4 thrombocytopenia developed. Treatment was delayed 1 week in patients with a hemoglobin level less than 9 gm/dL, an absolute neutrophil count less than 1000 cells/5 L, or a platelet count less than 100,000 cells/5 L. Granulocyte colony stimulating factor and other hematologic support were given as needed. Clinical responses were evaluated according to the National Cancer Institute Response Evaluation Criteria in Solid Tumors guidelines. Toxicity was assessed according to the National Cancer Institute Common Toxicity Criteria.

Results.—The median platinum-free interval was 3 months (range, 1-11 months), and the median paclitaxel-free interval was 6 months (range, 1-36 months). Patients received 1 to 10 cycles of gemcitabine (median, 4 cycles) for a total of 210 cycles. Dose reduction was required in 36 patients (72%; 55% of cycles). Forty-one patients could be evaluated for response; 9 patients died of disease after only 1 cycle. Of these 41 patients, 7 (17%) had a partial response, 15 (36.6%) had stable disease for 16 or more weeks, and 19 (46.3%) had disease progression. The median progression-free interval was 18 weeks. Grades 3 to 4 hematologic toxicity occurred in 27 patients (54%); 16% and 2% had grades 3 to 4 anemia, respectively; 24% and 18% had grades 3 to 4 neutropenia; and 8% and 0% had grades 3 to 4 thrombocytopenia. Yet only 4 patients (8%) required granulocyte colony stimulating factor. Fifteen patients (30%) required blood transfusion, and 2 patients (4%) required erythropoietin. Four patients (8%) had grade 3 hepatic toxicity.

Conclusion.—Disease stabilized or partially responded in approximately 50% of these patients with resistant ovarian cancer. These patients were heavily pretreated; all but 4 had undergone at least 2 prior chemotherapy regimens. About half of the patients had grades 3 to 4 hematologic toxicity develop, and almost three fourths required a dose reduction. Yet despite this toxicity profile, gemcitabine is one of the safer agents for the salvage treatment of platinum- and paclitaxel-resistant ovarian cancer, and its efficacy may warrant its inclusion in platinum/paclitaxel regimens in chemotherapy-naive patients with ovarian cancer.

► The study by D'Agostino et al evaluated the activity of gemcitabine in patients with recurrent ovarian carcinoma. The investigators describe their patient population as platinum and paclitaxel resistant, but they report the median platinum-free interval as 3 with a range of 1 to 11 months and the median paclitaxel-free interval as 6 with a range of 1 to 36 months. By definition, therefore, many of the patients were platinum or paclitaxel sensitive. The response rate of 17% establishes that gemcitabine is active in previously treated patients, but it is impossible to determine what this means since we do not know whether the responses occurred in platinum-sensitive or platinum-resistant patients. In assessing such studies as this, it is imperative that the patient population be correctly described in terms of platinum sensitivity or platinum resistance; it is imperative that each of these 2 groups be treated as separate and different patient populations.

J. T. Thigpen, MD

Clinical Implications of a Rising Serum CA-125 Within the Normal Range in Patients With Epithelial Ovarian Cancer: A Preliminary Investigation

Wilder JL, Pavlik E, Straughn JM, et al (Univ of Kentucky, Lexington; Univ of Birmingham, Ala)

Gynecol Oncol 89:233-235, 2003 3–21

Background.—Many patients with epithelial ovarian cancer achieve remission. Disease status is monitored by periodic clinical examinations with serum marker assays for CA-125. The relapse rate of patients in remission who have progressively rising CA-125 levels within the normal range was examined.

Study Design.—The study group consisted of 11 women who were in remission from ovarian cancer and had progressively rising CA-125 levels, within the normal range, during follow-up. Recurrent cancer was documented by histologic disease on fine-needle biopsy or appearance of lesions on CT scans.

Findings.—All the 11 patients identified with rising serum CA-125 levels had ovarian cancer recur. The average time from the third increasing CA-125 value during follow-up to confirmation of recurrence was 189 days. The average time from complete remission was 21 months.

Conclusions.—This small preliminary study indicates that progressively rising serum CA-125 levels, even within the normal range, are associated with a high risk of tumor recurrence. If these results are confirmed, these patients should undergo thorough investigation to identify their tumor recurrence and initiate treatment as early as possible.

► The issue of the diagnosis of recurrent ovarian carcinoma and the timing of treatment has become a major controversy recently because of the widespread use of CA-125 as a marker in following patients. The 2 compelling questions have been (1) what constitutes a significant change in the CA-125, and (2) should treatment be initiated solely on the basis of a rising CA-125 level? The answer to the first question is the subject of the study of Wilder et al. Their data suggest that 3 successive rising values within the normal range of 0 to 35 U/mL are associated with a high likelihood of recurrence. Other reports have suggested that the criteria for recurrence based on CA-125 should require 3 successive rising values with at least the highest at a level more than 100 U/mL. Regardless of which set of criteria one chooses to use, the other question remains as to whether treatment should be started solely on the basis of a rising marker. At least for now, evidence of benefit for starting therapy at that point rather than waiting for either symptoms or CT scan evidence of recurrent masses is lacking.

J. T. Thigpen, MD

Usefulness of FDG PET for Assessment of Early Recurrent Epithelial Ovarian Cancer

Cho S-M, Ha HK, Byun JY, et al (Catholic Univ of Korea, Seoul; Univ of Ulsan, Seoul, South Korea)

AJR 179:391-395, 2002 3–22

Background.—Recurrence of epithelial ovarian carcinoma is a major problem. In the early postoperative period, a peritoneal disseminated lesion is the most common form of recurrence. Imaging is a requisite for the evaluation of these tumors, as clinical evaluation with tumor markers or physical examination has little diagnostic value in the early detection and localization of recurrent ovarian tumor. CT is the most commonly used diagnostic imaging technique before second-look surgery but is limited in its ability to reveal small lesions. And if a small lesion is detected, CT cannot confirm the lesion as a tumor recurrence if it is too small. This study evaluated the diagnostic accuracy of fluorodeoxyglucose (FDG) positron emission tomography (PET) in comparison with CT for the detection of recurrent ovarian carcinoma and its ability to reveal small tumor recurrence.

Methods.—A review was conducted of the records for 31 consecutive patients with pathologically proved epithelial carcinoma who underwent FDG PET 1 month before second-look surgery for the assessment of recurrent tumor. Of these patients, 21 also underwent CT 1 month before second-look surgery. The diagnostic accuracy of FDG PET alone was compared with that of combined FDG PET and CT in 21 patients using Bennett's test. The detection rates of individual tumors relative to their sizes were compared between FDG PET and CT by means of the McNemar test.

Results.—FDG PET had a sensitivity, specificity, and accuracy of 45.3%, 99.7%, and 91%, respectively. By comparison, CT alone had a sensitivity, specificity, and accuracy of 54.5%, 99.6%, and 91.7%, respectively; the combination of FDG PET and CT yielded a sensitivity, specificity, and accuracy of 58.2%, 99.6%, and 92.4%, respectively (Fig 2). Thus, there was no

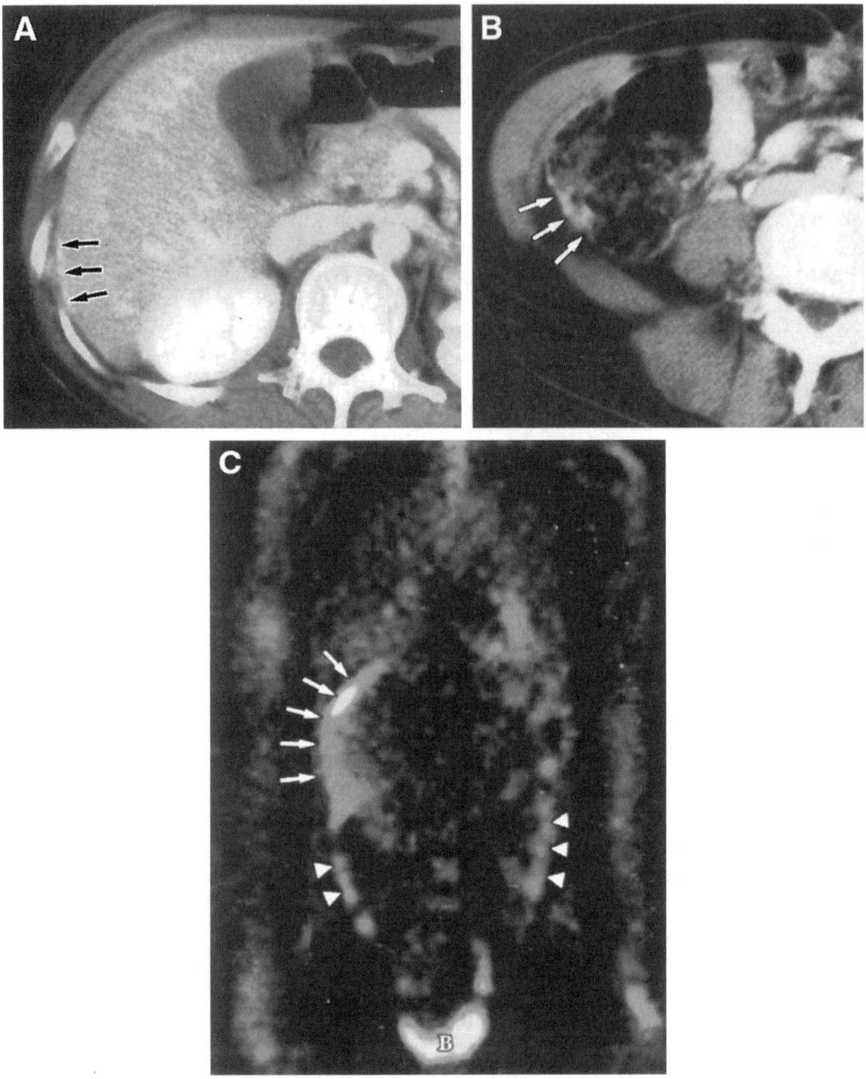

FIGURE 2.—A 39-year-old woman with recurrent ovarian cancer in the peritoneum. **A**, Contrast-enhanced CT scan obtained at level of liver shows smooth linear contrast enhancement (*arrows*) along hepatic surface. **B**, Contrast-enhanced CT scan obtained at level of mid abdomen shows subtle nodular linear contrast enhancement (*arrows*) at peritoneum along right paracolic gutter. **C**, Whole-body coronal image of fluorodeoxyglucose (FDG) positron emission tomogram shows strong FDG uptake at hepatic surface (*arrows*) and peritoneum (*arrowheads*) along both paracolic gutters. Urine in bladder (**B**) also shows FDG uptake. (Courtesy of Cho S-M, Ha HK, Byun JY, et al: Usefulness of FDG PET for assessment of early recurrent epithelial ovarian cancer. *AJR* 179:391-395, 2002. Reprinted with permission from the *American Journal of Roentgenology*.)

TABLE 1.—Diagnostic Accuracy of Fluorodeoxyglucose Positron Emission Tomography and CT for Revealing Recurrent Ovarian Tumor at 15 Specific Sites

Accuracy	Sensitivity (%)		Specificity (%)		Accuracy (%)		Positive Predictive Value (%)		Negative Predictive Value (%)	
	(*n* = 31)	(*n* = 21)	(*n* = 31)	(*n* = 21)	(*n* = 31)	(*n* = 21)	(*n* = 31)	(*n* = 21)	(*n* = 31)	(*n* = 21)
FDG PET (*n* = 31) and (*n* = 21*)										
Lesion-based	45.3 (34/75)	36.4 (20/55)	99.7 (389/390)	99.6 (259/260)	91.0 (423/465)	88.6 (279/315)	97.1 (34/35)	95.2 (20/21)	90.5 (389/430)	88.1 (259/294)
Patient-based	81.3 (13/16)	81.8 (9/11)	93.3 (14/15)	90.0 (9/10)	87.1 (27/31)	85.7 (18/21)	92.9 (13/14)	90.0 (9/10)	82.4 (14/17)	81.8 (9/11)
CT (*n* = 21*)										
Lesion-based		54.5 (30/55)		99.6 (259/260)		91.7 (289/315)		96.8 (30/31)		91.2 (258/283)
Patient-based		100 (11/11)		90.0 (9/10)		95.2 (20/21)		91.7 (11/12)		100.0 (9/9)
Combined FDG PET and CT (*n* = 21*)										
Lesion-based		58.2 (32/55)		99.6 (259/260)		92.4 (291/315)		97.0 (32/33)		91.8 (259/282)
Patient-based		100 (11/11)		90.0 (9/10)		95.2 (20/21)		91.7 (11/12)		100.00 (9/9)

Note: Numbers in parentheses are the data used to calculate the percentages.

*Overall diagnostic accuracies of fluorodeoxyglucose positron emission tomography (*FDG PET*) and CT were compared in 21 cases in which both FDG PET and CT were performed using Bennett's test (Bennett BM: On comparisons of sensitivity, specificity and predictive value of a number of diagnostic procedures. *Biometrics* 28:793-800, 1972.). There was no statistically significant difference in diagnostic accuracies between FDG PET and CT when both sensitivity and specificity were simultaneously compared ($\chi^2 < 5.991$).

(Courtesy of Cho S-M, Ha HK, Byun JY, et al: Usefulness of FDG PET for assessment of early recurrent epithelial ovarian cancer. *AJR* 179:391-395, 2002. Reprinted with permission from the *American Journal of Roentgenology*.)

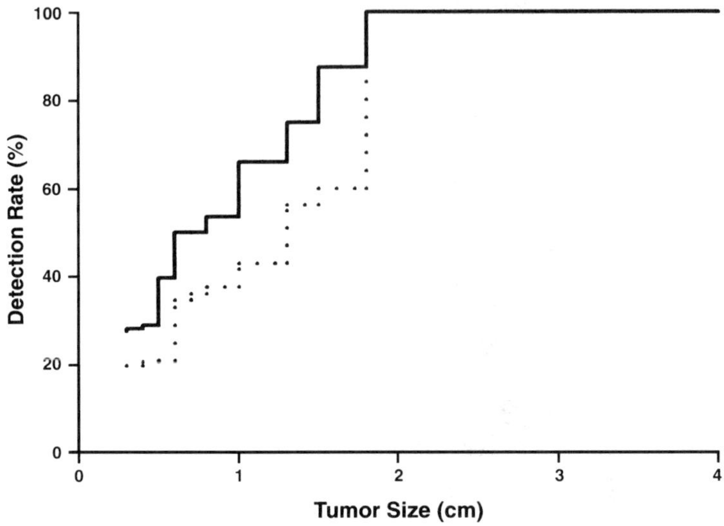

FIGURE 3.—Graph shows detection rate for specific tumor sizes on fluorodeoxyglucose (FDG) positron emission tomography (*dotted line*) and CT (*solid line*). To calculate detection rates for specific tumor size, all nodules in denominator that were larger than tumor size were included. Tumor detection rates on CT for tumors of diameters 0.3, 0.4, 0.5, 0.6, and 0.7 cm significantly exceeded those for FDG positron emission tomography ($P < .05$). (Courtesy of Cho S-M, Ha HK, Byun JY, et al: Usefulness of FDG PET for assessment of early recurrent epithelial ovarian cancer. AJR 179:391-395, 2002. Reprinted with permission from the *American Journal of Roentgenology*.)

statistically significant difference in the diagnostic accuracy of these 3 modalities (Table 1). However, the detection rates of tumor nodules on CT were significantly greater than those on FDG PET when the size of the nodule measured 0.3 cm to 0.7 cm (Fig 3).

Conclusion.—The use of FDG PET did not improve the overall diagnostic accuracy of detection of recurrent ovarian carcinoma compared with CT. FDG PET was, in fact, inferior to CT in the ability to reveal small-tumor recurrence.

► These investigators from Korea have studied the usefulness of FDG and PET scanning in the evaluation of patients with documented recurrent epithelial carcinoma of the ovary at the time of a second-look surgery. To everyone's disappointment, adding PET to CT did not appear to significantly increase the rate of detection of tumor nodules over CT alone. The problem is that the nodules seen are frequently less than 1 cm and that is actually below the typical resolution for a PET scan. This is another example of a great idea brought down to earth by factual reality (as opposed to virtual reality, which is obviously not reality at all).

E. Glatstein, MD

The Differential Diagnostic Potential of a Panel of Tumor Markers (CA 125, CA 15-3, and CA 72-4 Antigens) in Patients With a Pelvic Mass

Schutter EMJ, Davelaar EM, van Kamp GJ, et al (Vrije Universiteit, Amsterdam; Medisch Spectrum Twente, Enschede, The Netherlands)

Am J Obstet Gynecol 187:385-392, 2002 3–23

Background.—Patients who have a pelvic mass present a difficult diagnostic situation, with the origin and character of these findings problematic despite advances in imaging technology. Tumor markers may aid in diagnosis, but benign and malignant pelvic masses are not sufficiently distinguished by the CA 125 assay, the most widely used tumor marker for gynecologic (especially ovarian) neoplasms. The usefulness of a combined panel of serum tumor markers was evaluated, including the highly specific CA 15-3 and CA 72-4 with CA 125.

Methods.—Four hundred twelve patients with pelvic masses were assessed retrospectively.

Results.—Benign tumors were found in 171 patients, malignant tumors in 226 patients, and borderline tumors in 15 patients. There were 129 benign ovarian tumors and 133 ovarian carcinomas. Patients with benign disease were significantly younger than those with malignancies. CA 15-3 levels were normal in all cases of borderline tumors, but CA 125 levels were elevated in 9 cases and CA 72-4 levels were higher than normal in 4 cases.

For discriminating between benign pelvic masses and ovarian carcinoma, CA 125 alone was better than CA 72-4 or CA 15-3 alone (Fig 1); however, the various tests did not differ in the ability to discriminate between any benign and any malignant disease (Table 3). The highest sensitivity for a single test was with the CA 125 test, while the highest specificity and positive pre-

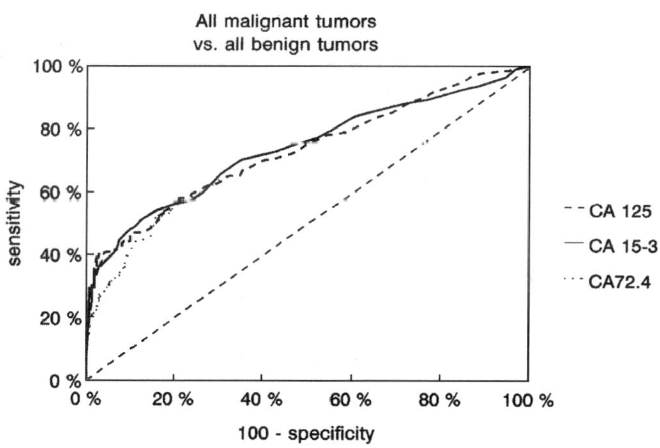

FIGURE 1.—Actual receiver operating characteristic curves for CA 125 (*hatched line*), CA 15-3 (*solid line*), and CA 72-4 (*dotted line*) assays that were used to discriminate between malignant (226 patients) and benign (171 patients) tumors. (Reprinted by permission of the publisher from Schutter EMJ, Davelaar EM, van Kamp GJ, et al: The differential diagnostic potential of a panel of tumor markers (CA 125, CA 15-3, and CA 72-4 antigens) in patients with a pelvic mass. *Am J Obstet Gynecol* 187:385-392, 2002. Copyright 2002 by Elsevier.)

TABLE 3.—Test Results for the Main Possible Combinations of Serum CA 125, CA 15-3, and CA 72-4 in the Discrimination of All Malignant Pelvic Masses (226 Patients) From All Benign Pelvic Masses (171 Patients)

CA 125*	CA 15-3†	CA 72-4‡	N§	Sensitivity	95% CI	Specificity	95% CI	PPV	95% CI	NPV	95% CI	Overall Test Accuracy	95% CI
+	+	+	64	28	22-33	99	97-100	97	89-100	51	45-56	58	53-63
+	+	No‖	85	36	29-42	97	95-100	94	87-98	53	48-59	62	57-67
+	**No**	**No**	**175**	**60**	**53-66**	**76**	**69-82**	**77**	**70-83**	**59**	**52-65**	**67**	**62-71**
+	No	+	100	40	34-47	95	91-98	91	85-97	55	49-60	64	59-69
–	–	–	168	27	21-32	36	29-44	36	28-43	27	22-33	30	26-35
–	–	No	211	38	31-44	25	19-32	40	34-47	24	18-30	32	28-37
–	No	No	220	40	34-47	24	18-31	41	35-48	23	17-30	33	29-38
–	No	–	176	29	23-35	35	28-42	37	33-47	27	21-33	32	27-36
No	+	**No**	**95**	**38**	**32-45**	**95**	**92-98**	**92**	**84-96**	**54**	**48-60**	**63**	**58-68**
No	+	+	66	28	22-34	99	97-100	97	89-100	51	46-56	59	54-64
No	–	–	223	38	31-44	19	13-25	38	32-44	19	13-25	30	25-34
No	–	No	302	62	55-68	5	2-8	46	40-52	8	4-16	37	32-42
No	**No**	+	**145**	**52**	**46-59**	**84**	**79-90**	**81**	**75-88**	**57**	**51-63**	**66**	**61-71**
No	No	–	252	48	41-54	16	10-21	43	37-49	19	12-25	34	29-39

Note: Single tests are in bold. *No* indicates that this method is not involved in this combination.

*+ = more than 35 U/mL; – = less than 35 U/mL.

†+ = more than 30 U/mL; – = less than 30 U/mL.

‡+ = more than 3.5 U/mL; – = less than 3.5 U/mL.

§True positives + false positives.

‖This method is not involved in this combination.

(Reprinted by permission of the publisher from Schutter EMJ, Davelaar EM, van Kamp GJ, et al: The differential diagnostic potential of a panel of tumor markers (CA 125, CA 15-3, and CA 72-4 antigens) in patients with a pelvic mass. *Am J Obstet Gynecol* 187:385-392, 2002. Copyright 2002 by Elsevier.)

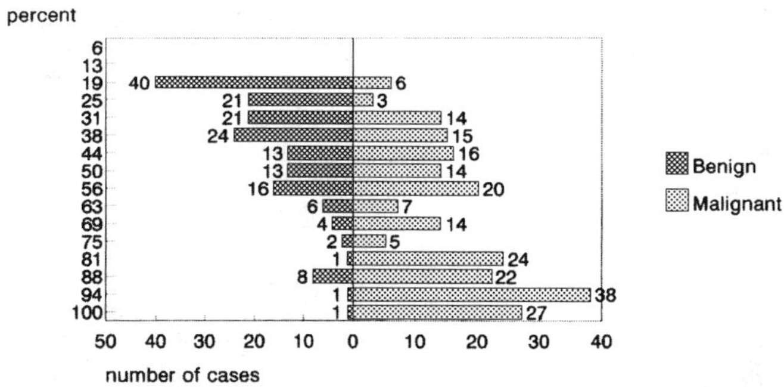

FIGURE 2.—Histogram of estimated probabilities of malignancy that were determined by logistic regression analysis. The *black bars* on the left side of center represent the number of cases actually with benign tumors at each level of probability; the *gray bars* on the right side of center represent the malignant tumors at each level of probability. (Reprinted by permission of the publisher from Schutter EMJ, Davelaar EM, van Kamp GJ, et al: The differential diagnostic potential of a panel of tumor markers (CA 125, CA 15-3, and CA 72-4 antigens) in patients with a pelvic mass. *Am J Obstet Gynecol* 187:385-392, 2002. Copyright 2002 by Elsevier.)

dictive value (PPV) were with the CA 15-3 test. A PPV of malignancy of 97% was obtained when elevated levels of all 3 markers were combined, but this condition only occurred in 28% of the malignant tumors and 41% of the ovarian carcinomas. Combining all 3 serum tumor markers with values less than cutoff level produced a false-positive PPV for malignancy of 12% to 36%, corresponding to a correct prediction of benign conditions of 64% to 88%.

Of all malignant and all benign tumors, 72.5% were correctly predicted; of ovarian carcinoma and benign tumors, 82.9% were correctly predicted (Fig 2). The most significant contribution to the logistic model in predicting malignancy was made by CA 15-3, whose odds ratio was 3.86; the odds ratios for CA 72-4, CA 125, and age group were 3.74, 1.74, and 1.28, respectively.

Conclusion.—Nearly all cases of malignant disease were identified when there were simultaneously elevated levels of CA 125, CA 15-3, and CA 72-4, but this condition occurred in few of the malignant tumors. The most significant contribution to the logistic regression analysis was made by the CA 15-3 antigen. The correct prediction was obtained by using the logistic model in 73% to 83% of cases.

► This multicenter retrospective Dutch study dealing with pelvic masses tried to study CA 125, CA 15-3, and CA 72-4 for the ability to diagnose ovarian cancer preoperatively. The findings are somewhat inconclusive, although the CA 15-3 antigen seemed to have the most specificity. On the other hand, the total marker panel was disappointing, for both specificity and sensitivity.

E. Glatstein, MD

Using the Expected Survival to Explain Differences Between the Results of Randomized Trials: A Case in Advanced Ovarian Cancer

Buyse M, for the International Collaborative Ovarian Neoplasm Collaborators and the Ovarian Cancer Meta-Analysis Project (Intl Drug Development Inst, Cambridge, Mass; et al)

J Clin Oncol 21:1682-1687, 2003 3–24

Background.—When the findings of different studies provide conflicting results, it can be difficult to draw conclusions. In 1989, a meta-analysis was performed of 6 randomized trials comparing a standard regimen of cyclophosphamide and cisplatin (CP) to CP plus doxorubicin (CAP) for patients with advanced ovarian cancer. The meta-analysis demonstrated that patients treated with CAP had a higher rate of response and a better survival rate than those treated with CP. The Second International Collaborative Ovarian Neoplasm Study (ICON2) was then performed to compare CAP with carboplatin alone. In contrast to the results of the meta-analysis, ICON2 found no difference between CAP and carboplatin alone. These discrepant results can be reconciled through the use of estimation of expected survival curves.

Study Design.—Analyses were based on individual patient data by an intent-to-treat approach. A proportional hazards regression model was fitted to the data of the meta-analysis, and covariates were eliminated with a step-down procedure. This model was used to construct the expected survival curve for each treatment arm of ICON2 by integrating the expected hazard rate over time. A nonparametric test was used to compare the expected with the observed survival curve.

Findings.—When the model derived from the meta-analysis was applied to the ICON2 data, there was no difference between the expected and observed curves for the CAP arm. For the carboplatin arm, the observed survival curve was significantly superior to the expected survival curve for CP.

Conclusions.—This analysis suggests that the difference between the results of the meta-analysis and the ICON2 trial are because of better results achieved with carboplatin alone compared with CP. An expected survival analysis may be useful to reconcile results of randomized trials with conflicting results.

First-Line Treatment for Advanced Ovarian Cancer: Paclitaxel, Platinum and the Evidence

Sandercock J, Parmar MKB, Torri V, et al (Univ of Birmingham, England; MRC Clinical Trials Unit, London; Istituto de Richerche Farmacologiche "Mario Negri," Milano, Italy)

Br J Cancer 87:815-824, 2002 3–25

Background.—The combination of carboplatin plus paclitaxel has become standard first-line therapy for women with advanced ovarian cancer in many countries but has been challenged by the results of a systematic review of 4 trials (GOG-111, OV10, GOG-132, and ICON3) that compared platinum plus paclitaxel to standard platinum-based treatment. GOG-111 and OV10 reported that paclitaxel/cisplatin was clearly better than cyclophosphamide/cisplatin, but GOG-132 suggested no benefit of paclitaxel/cisplatin compared with single-agent cisplatin. Reconciliation of the differing results of these trials involving 3588 patients was attempted.

Study Design.—There are 4 possible explanations for the differing results of these trials: differences in crossover between study arms, differences in patient type, differences in research arms, and differences in control arms between trials. Each hypothesis was considered regarding whether it was plausible, consistent with study data, and consistent with other evidence. A meta-regression approach was used to examine the consistency between each explanation and study data. Each trial was split along the key characteristic in question, and the heterogeneity between groups was compared with that within groups by the F-ratio.

Findings.—Only 1 explanation was consistent with the pattern of results observed in these 4 trials: the difference in the efficacy of the control arms. This suggests that the very positive results obtained with paclitaxel/cisplatin in GOG-111 and OV10 may have been caused by the use of suboptimal control arms. Specific concerns about the use of a cyclophosphamide/cisplatin control arm were raised before any discrepancy was detected.

Conclusions.—Four hypotheses have been suggested to explain the disparate results obtained from 4 randomized trials comparing paclitaxel plus platinum to a platinum-based control treatment for women with advanced ovarian cancer. Only the differences in control variables appear able to explain these discrepancies. On the basis of the results of these 4 trials, optimal dose single-agent carboplatin appears to be a safe and effective first-line treatment for women with advanced ovarian cancer.

► These 2 articles (Abstracts 3–24 and 3–25) examine presumed discrepancies among 4 randomized trials that have examined the addition of paclitaxel to front-line chemotherapy for ovarian carcinoma. Both articles attempt to make the same argument that single-agent carboplatin is as good as paclitaxel plus a platinum compound. The line of reasoning contends first that 2 of the trials (GOG 111 and OV 10), which randomized patients with advanced disease to either cyclophosphamide/cisplatin or paclitaxel/cisplatin, show an advantage for paclitaxel/cisplatin in terms of response, progression-free survival, and overall survival. The overall survival differences are large. Second, 2 of the trials (GOG 132 and ICON3) show no advantage for a paclitaxel/platinum combination compared with either single-agent cisplatin or carboplatin. Third, to determine which pair of trials is correct, one must look for an explanation that is consistent with the pattern of results. Finally, the only explanation, in the opinion of the authors, is that GOG 111 and OV 10 used an inferior control arm (cisplatin/cyclophosphamide), whereas GOG 132 (cisplatin) and ICON3 (carboplatin) used superior control arms. As a result, the authors conclude that single-agent carboplatin is the standard of care.

The problem with the 2 articles is that both ignore at least 3 randomized trials from the 1980s that showed either trends favoring cisplatin/cyclophosphamide over cisplatin or frank statistically significant advantages for cisplatin/cyclophosphamide over single-agent cisplatin. Why the authors would choose to ignore results of randomized trials and instead depend on indirect reasoning is difficult to understand. The better explanation for the observed discrepancies is more complex. First, GOG 111 and OV 10 were carefully designed and executed studies with good quality control and relatively homogeneous patient populations (large-volume advanced disease for GOG 111 and well-staged patients with stages IIB-IV disease for OV 10). It is not clear that the same can be said for ICON3. The study has never been audited; hence, quality control of data is lacking. All stages of disease were allowed in the trial; hence, the population of patients is heterogeneous and difficult to interpret. Delivery of the assigned regimen has never been confirmed in the patients. These factors make ICON3 very difficult to interpret. Second, GOG 132 suffers from a high rate of crossover in the single-agent arms prior to disease progression; hence, the study is probably not comparing single agents to concurrent combination therapy but rather sequential versus concurrent combination regimens. In short, by far the more credible trials are GOG 111 and OV 10; these 2 establish paclitaxel plus a platinum compound as the standard of care.

J. T. Thigpen, MD

Randomized Phase III Trial of Standard Timed Doxorubicin Plus Cisplatin Versus Circadian Timed Doxorubicin Plus Cisplatin in Stage III and IV or Recurrent Endometrial Carcinoma: A Gynecologic Oncology Group Study

Gallion HH, Brunetto VL, Cibull M, et al (Univ of Pittsburgh, Pa; Roswell Park Cancer Inst, Buffalo, NY; Univ of Kentucky, Lexington; et al)
J Clin Oncol 21:3808-3813, 2003 3–26

Background.—Most patients with endometrial cancer have potentially curable stage I disease at diagnosis, but a significant number have metastatic disease outside the pelvis or will have metastasis develop after primary therapy. Pelvic radiation therapy may be useful for the treatment of localized disease, but hormonal therapy or chemotherapy is generally used when distant metastasis is present. Whether circadian timed (CT) chemotherapy would provide improved response, progression-free survival, overall survival, and lower toxicity in comparison with standard timed (ST) chemotherapy was investigated.

Methods.—A total of 342 patients were included in this randomized phase III trial. Enrollment criteria included stage III or IV or recurrent endometrial cancer with poor potential for cure by radiation therapy or surgery, measurable disease, and no history of chemotherapy. Patients were randomly assigned to schedules of ST doxorubicin 60 mg/m^2 plus cisplatin 60 mg/m^2 (169 patients) or CT doxorubicin 60 mg/m^2 at 6 AM plus cisplatin 60 mg/m^2 at 6 PM (173 patients). The cycles were repeated every 3 weeks to a maximum of 8 cycles.

Results.—The objective response rate was 46% for the ST group and 49% for the CT group. The median progression-free survival and overall survival were 6.5 and 11.2 months, respectively, in the ST group and 5.9 and 13.2 months, respectively, in the CT group. The median total doses were 209 mg/m² doxorubicin and 349 mg/m² cisplatin in the ST group compared with 246 mg/m² doxorubicin and 354 mg/m² cisplatin in the CT group. Grade 3 or 4 leukopenia occurred in 73% of patients in the ST group and in 63% of patients in the CT group. Eight treatment-related deaths occurred.

Conclusions.—This phase III trial found no significant benefit from CT doxorubicin plus cisplatin in terms of response rate, progression-free survival, overall survival, or toxicity profile in patients with advanced or recurrent endometrial carcinoma.

► This Gynecologic Oncology Group randomized phase III trial evaluates the efficacy of CT chemotherapy administration in patients with advanced or recurrent endometrial carcinoma. Although the same drugs are used in both arms at the same doses, one arm administers the doxorubicin at 6 AM and the cisplatin at 6 PM to determine if this enhances the efficacy of the regimen. The concept of CT of chemotherapy administration has been widely studied in uncontrolled trials, but this represents the first time that the concept has been tested in a randomized phase III trial of a solid tumor. The study results show no advantage to CT. Since the approach does entail logistical problems, there would seem to be no reason to pursue the concept further.

J. T. Thigpen, MD

Activity of Paclitaxel as Second-Line Chemotherapy in Endometrial Carcinoma: A Gynecologic Oncology Group Study

Lincoln S, Blessing JA, Lee RB, et al (Rush Med College, Chicago; Roswell Park Cancer Inst, Buffalo, NY; Univ of Washington, Seattle; et al)

Gynecol Oncol 88:277-281, 2003 3–27

Background.—The number of chemotherapeutic agents effective in advanced or recurrent adenocarcinoma of the endometrium is limited. A previous phase II trial showed that paclitaxel was effective in patients with advanced or recurrent disease who had not undergone chemotherapy. Whether paclitaxel is effective for patients with advanced or recurrent disease who have already been exposed to chemotherapy was examined.

Methods.—The subjects were 50 women with persistent or recurrent adenocarcinoma of the endometrium. All patients had previously received chemotherapy (mainly doxorubicin/platinum–based therapy), and 20 patients had previously received radiotherapy. Paclitaxel was infused over a 3-hour period at an initial dose of 200 mg/m² (or 175 mg/m² for patients with prior pelvic radiation) every 21 days. Subsequent courses were not administered until the patient had fully recovered from any nonhematologic toxicity, the granulocyte count was more than 1500 cells/µL, and the platelet count was more than 100,000 cells/µL. Doses were modified based on nadir toxicity (both hematologic and nonhematologic) and adjusted to 200, 175, 135, or 110 mg/m^2.

Results.—Of the 50 patients, 2 were ineligible because of protocol, 3 withdrew from the study (1 had congestive heart failure develop, 1 had bleeding not related to hematologic toxicity, and 1 refused further treatment), and 1 died of toxicity. Of the 44 patients in whom response could be evaluated, 3 (6.8%) had a complete response and 9 (20.5%) had a partial response; thus, the overall response rate was 27.3%. Responders required a median of 2 courses of paclitaxel to respond (range, 1-4 courses), and their response lasted for a median of 4.2 months. Four of the 12 responders had received prior radiation. The median overall survival was 10.3 months.

Of the 48 patients in whom toxicity could be evaluated, 28 (58.3%) had at least 1 episode of grade 3 or 4 neutropenia, and 4 (8.3%) had grade 3 neurotoxicity develop. Three patients (6.3%) had grade 3 or 4 gastrointestinal symptoms, but only 1 patient had cardiac toxicity (grade 1). The 1 treatment-related death occurred in a 73-year-old patient who had undergone extensive surgery for endometrial cancer. Approximately 1 week after her initial paclitaxel treatment, she had weakness, thrombocytopenia, and febrile neutropenia develop. Despite resuscitation efforts, she died on day 11.

Conclusion.—Paclitaxel is effective for treating advanced or recurrent endometrial cancer in patients who have had prior chemotherapy. Studies are currently underway to determine the most effective starting dose of paclitaxel and to better define its role in endometrial cancer treatment.

► This Gynecologic Oncology Group (GOG) phase II study of paclitaxel in patients who had failed prior chemotherapy with doxorubicin-based regimens suggests significant activity even in this difficult patient population and confirms an earlier report from the GOG of activity for this drug in previously untreated patients with endometrial carcinoma. Both the prior GOG study (250 mg/m^2) and this trial (200 mg/m^2) used higher than usual doses of paclitaxel. This choice of higher doses is not based on any data that suggest the higher doses would be more effective. The GOG has subsequently reported at the annual meeting of the American Society of Clinical Oncology that a 3-drug combination of doxorubicin plus cisplatin plus paclitaxel is superior to the previous standard of doxorubicin plus cisplatin in terms of response, progression-free survival, and overall survival in randomized phase III trial comparing the 2 regimens.[1]

J. T. Thigpen, MD

Reference

1. Fleming GF, Brunetto V, Mundt AJ, et al: Randomized trial of doxorubicin (DOX) plus cisplatin (CIS) versus DOX plus CIS plus paclitaxel (TAX) in patients with advanced or recurrent endometrial carcinoma: A Gynecologic Oncology Group (GOG) study. *Proc ASCO* 21:202a (abstr 807), 2002.

A Phase II Trial of Arzoxifene, a Selective Estrogen Response Modulator, in Patients With Recurrent or Advanced Endometrial Cancer

McMeekin DS, Gordon A, Fowler J, et al (Univ of Oklahoma, Oklahoma City; Texas Oncology, Dallas; Ohio State Univ, Columbus; et al)

Gynecol Oncol 90:64-69, 2003 3–28

Background.—The prognosis for patients with endometrial cancer is very good because most patients are diagnosed with early stage disease. However, patients with advanced or recurrent disease account for almost 6000 deaths each year. The response rate was determined and the toxicity evaluated of LY353381 (arzoxifene) in patients with recurrent or advanced endometrial cancer.

Methods.—This phase II open-labeled study was conducted at 13 centers. Patients with measurable recurrent or advanced endometrial cancer that was amenable to curative therapies were eligible for inclusion in the study if the primary or recurrent tumor was estrogen receptor positive or progestagen receptor positive. If receptor status could not be determined, patients with well or moderately well-differentiated endometrial cancer were also eligible for inclusion. Patients were excluded if they had a history of salvage chemotherapy; however, patients with prior use of progestagens were included, and patients were stratified by prior exposure to progestagen. The patients received 20 mg/d by mouth and were treated for at least 8 weeks in the absence of disease progression or unacceptable toxicity. Efficacy was evaluated on the basis of the frequency of complete and partial responses, and a 95% confidence interval was calculated. The Kaplan-Meier method was used to analyze time to progression and duration of response.

Results.—Thirty-seven patients were enrolled from February 1999 to April 2001, of whom 34 received treatment. Efficacy was evaluated for the 29 patients who received at least 4 weeks of therapy and at least 1 tumor response assessment. Safety was assessed in all 34 patients who received treatment. Most of the patients (n = 30) were defined as progestagen sensitive, and 4 patients were defined as progestagen failures. There were 26 estrogen receptor–positive patients and 22 progestagen receptor–positive patients. Response to treatment was seen in 9 (31%) of 29 patients, with a median duration of response of 13.9 months. All the treatment responses occurred in progestagen-sensitive patients. In addition, 2 patients (1 from each progestagen cohort) had stable disease for 6 months or more. The median progression-free interval for all 29 patients was 3.7 months. Toxicity was minimal, and there were no grade 3 to 4 toxic effects; 9 patients had grade 1 to 2 toxic effects. The most common toxic effects were hot flashes, which were grade 1 in all 3 cases.

Conclusions.—This phase II trial found that arzoxifene demonstrated a high response rate, with the longest median duration of response of any phase II trial in this population. Further evaluation of arzoxifene is warranted in light of these findings.

▶ This phase II study of McMeekin et al evaluates a new selective estrogen receptor modulator, arzoxifene, in the treatment of advanced or recurrent endometrial carcinoma, which has known positive receptors for estrogen or progestagen in either the primary or recurrent tissue or is grade 1 or 2 if receptor status cannot be determined. The reported response rate of 31% suggests that this agent has significant activity. This is particularly noteworthy when one considers that recent data have shown little or no activity for tamoxifen in 2 phase II trials of the Gynecologic Oncology Group. Arzoxifene, an experimental agent from Eli Lilly, would appear to be a promising hormonal agent in the management of endometrial carcinoma.

J. T. Thigpen, MD

2001 Consensus Guidelines for the Management of Women With Cervical Intraepithelial Neoplasia

Wright TC Jr, for the 2001 ASCCP-Sponsored Consensus Workshop (Columbia Univ, New York; et al)

Am J Obstet Gynecol 189:295-304, 2003 3–29

Background.—Evidence-based guidelines for the management of cervical intraepithelial neoplasia (CIN) developed with the support of the American Society for Colposcopy and Cervical Pathology are presented.

Participants.—The guidelines were developed by an independent panel of 121 experts in professional organizations, federal agencies, national and international health organizations, and other groups. Guidelines were drafted by working groups based on formal literature reviews and an Internet-based bulletin board. The final version was approved by consensus in September 2001.

Management of CIN Grade 1.—Patients with biopsy-confirmed CIN-1 and a satisfactory colposcopic examination can be monitored without treatment or treated with ablation or excision. Under the first option, patients should undergo repeat cervical cytologic testing at 6 and 12 months or human papillomavirus (HPV) testing at 12 months. Colposcopy should be repeated if cytologic results reveal atypical squamous cells or greater risk or if high-risk types of HPV DNA are present. Annual cytologic screening can resume when cytologic findings are negative twice in a row or the 12-month HPV DNA test is negative. Alternatively, patients can be monitored with a combination of repeat cytologic testing and colposcopy at 12 months. Women with regression during follow-up should undergo repeat cytologic testing at 12 months. Acceptable treatment options include cryotherapy, laser ablation, and a loop electrosurgical excision procedure. Before ablation of CIN-1, endocervical sampling should be performed. If CIN-1 recurs after ablative therapy, excision should be performed. For patients whose colposcopic examination is unsatisfactory, a diagnostic excisional procedure is recommended. Follow-up alone may suffice for these patients, however, if they are pregnant, immunosuppressed, or adolescents.

Management of CIN Grades 2 and 3.—For patients with CIN-2 or CIN-3 and a satisfactory colposcopic examination, excision and ablation are both acceptable. Excision is preferred, however, for patients with recurrent CIN-2 or CIN-3. If the colposcopy examination is unsatisfactory, a diagnostic excisional procedure should be performed. Hysterectomy cannot be recommended as primary therapy for CIN-2 or CIN-3. After treatment, patients should be monitored with cytologic testing (with or without colposcopy) every 4 to 6 months until at least 3 cytologic results are negative, with annual cytologic testing thereafter. As with CIN-1, if cytologic testing reveals atypical squamous cells or greater risk, the patient should be referred for colposcopy. Alternatively, these patients may be monitored with HPV DNA testing at least 6 months after treatment. In this setting, annual cytologic exam is sufficient when HPV DNA test results are negative; however, colposcopy is recommended if high-risk types of HPV DNA are found. A single positive HPV test is not sufficient for performing a hysterectomy or repeat conization.

When CIN is identified at the margins of a diagnostic excisional procedure or in a postprocedure endocervical sample, endocervical sampling and colposcopy should be repeated 4 to 6 months later. A repeat diagnostic excisional procedure is acceptable in this setting, and hysterectomy can be performed if repeat diagnostic excision is not feasible or if CIN-2 or CIN-3 recurs or persists. Adolescents with CIN-2 whose colposcopic examinations are satisfactory and whose endocervical samples are negative should undergo colposcopy and cytologic testing every 4 to 6 months for 1 year. Adolescents with CIN-3 should undergo ablation or excision.

► This article summarizes the results of a consensus conference looking at the management of cervical intraepithelial neoplasia and provides guidelines for the management of these patients. It should be a useful guide for those involved in the management of preinvasive disease of the cervix.

J. T. Thigpen, MD

Randomized Trial of Cisplatin and Ifosfamide With or Without Bleomycin in Squamous Carcinoma of the Cervix: A Gynecologic Oncology Group Study

Bloss JD, Blessing JA, Behrens BC, et al (Univ of Missouri, Columbia; Washington Univ, St Louis; Roswell Park Cancer Inst, Buffalo, NY; et al)

J Clin Oncol 20:1832-1837, 2002 3–30

Background.—The optimal management for advanced, persistent, or recurrent squamous cell carcinoma of the cervix has not yet been defined. The results of phase II trials have suggested that the addition of bleomycin to the combination of cisplatin and ifosfamide may improve response rates and possible survival in this disease. The efficacy of this combination regimen was prospectively evaluated in women with histologically proven advanced recurrent or persistent squamous cell carcinoma of the cervix.

Methods.—From January 1994 to April 1997, 287 women were enrolled in this phase III trial and randomly assigned to receive either cisplatin (50 mg/m²), ifosfamide (5 g/m² over a 24-hour period), and mesna (6 g/m² during ifosfamide infusion and the following 12 hours) (CI regimen) or bleomycin 30 U over a 24-hour period on day 1 followed by cisplatin, ifosfamide, and mesna (CIB regimen).

Results.—There were no significant differences between the CI and CIB regimens in terms of response rates (32% vs 31.2%, respectively), progression-free survival, or overall survival. Progression-free survival and overall survival were associated with initial performance status. Patients with a performance status of 0 had a lower rate of failure and lower risk of death compared with patients with a performance status of 2. Leukopenia, neutropenia, anemia, thrombocytopenia, and nausea and vomiting were the most frequent grade 3 to 4 toxicities. No significant increase in the incidence of these toxicities was associated with either regimen.

Conclusions.—In this phase III trial among patients with histologically proven advanced recurrent or persistent squamous cell carcinoma, regimens of cisplatin and ifosfamide with or without bleomycin were found to have nearly identical rates of response, progression-free survival, overall survival, and toxicity. The addition of bleomycin to cisplatin and ifosfamide does not provide an improved outcome in patients with advanced cervical cancer.

► This randomized trial from the Gynecologic Oncology Group assigns women with stage IVB or recurrent carcinoma of the cervix to a doublet (ifosfamide/cisplatin) previously shown to be superior to cisplatin as a single agent in another randomized trial of this group or to a triplet (BIP), which has been widely used in the treatment of cervix carcinoma based on uncontrolled studies from the United Kingdom. The study noted no differences in efficacy and no significant differences in grade 3 to 4 toxicities. The conclusion of the study was that bleomycin did not contribute significant benefit when added to ifosfamide/cisplatin.

J. T. Thigpen, MD

Phase II Trial of Topotecan and Cisplatin in Persistent or Recurrent Squamous and Nonsquamous Carcinomas of the Cervix

Fiorica J, Holloway R, Ndubisi B, et al (H Lee Moffitt Cancer Ctr, Tampa, Fla; Florida Hosp, Orlando; Univ Med Ctr, Jacksonville, Fla; et al)

Gynecol Oncol 85:89-94, 2002 3–31

Background.—Cisplatin is a standard treatment for patients with advanced, recurrent cervical cancer. Topotecan is an established treatment for patients with gynecologic malignancies such as ovarian cancer, and it has shown nonoverlapping toxicity with cisplatin. The tolerability and antitumor activity of a cisplatin/topotecan doublet were evaluated in patients with persistent or recurrent cervical cancer.

Methods.—Thirty-two patients with bidimensionally measurable persistent or recurrent squamous cell and non–squamous cell cervical cancer and adequate bone marrow were included. Patients were administered 50 mg/m^2 of IV cisplatin over a 1-hour period on day 1 and 0.75 mg/m^2 of IV topotecan over a 30-minute period on days 1, 2, and 3 of 21-day cycles for 6 cycles or until disease progression. Gynecologic Oncology Group criteria were used to assess tumor response and regimen toxicity.

Results.—All but 2 of the 32 patients had received previous chemotherapy. The cisplatin/topotecan doublet was well tolerated, with 77% and 78% of courses without interruption or delay and at full doses, respectively. The most common toxicity was hematologic, with grades 3 to 4 neutropenia reported in 30% of cycles and thrombocytopenia reported in 10% of cycles. The overall response rate was 28%, with 3 complete and 6 partial responses. Nonirradiated fields showed an antitumor response rate of 30%, similar to the rate of 33% in previously irradiated fields, which was an indication of good drug penetration. The median duration of response was 5 months, with a range of 2 to 15 months. An additional 9 patients (28%) achieved stable disease. The median survival was 10 months, and 3 patients were in lasting remission.

Conclusions.—The combination of cisplatin and topotecan is safe, well tolerated, and active in patients with persistent or recurrent cervical cancer. A phase III multicenter trial is currently underway to confirm these findings.

► This phase II study of the Florida Society of Gynecologic Oncology evaluates a doublet of topotecan plus cisplatin in the treatment of carcinoma of the cervix. Both drugs had been previously identified as active by the Gynecologic Oncology Group (GOG). The doublet demonstrated a disappointing response rate of 28% in this trial (not much different from the overall 23% response rate observed by the GOG in studies of almost 800 patients treated with single-agent cisplatin), but the authors recommend further study in a phase III setting despite this. It is noteworthy that the study uses a 3-day schedule of topotecan despite evidence in other tumors that shortening of the schedule reduces the efficacy of the topotecan and despite the fact that a phase I study recommended use of the same daily dose of topotecan over a 5-day period in combination with cisplatin. This may account for the rather disappointing response rate. The GOG has recently completed a phase III trial comparing this doublet to single-agent cisplatin and showing a significant improvement in response rate, progression-free survival, and overall survival. One is left to wonder whether a 5-day topotecan schedule might have produced an even more striking result.

J. T. Thigpen, MD

4 Genitourinary

Screening Men for Prostate and Colorectal Cancer in the United States: Does Practice Reflect the Evidence?

Sirovich BE, Schwartz LM, Woloshin S (Dartmouth Med School, Hanover, NH)

JAMA 289:1414-1420, 2003 4–1

Background.—There has been a great deal of controversy in the medical literature and popular media regarding the debate about the efficacy of prostate-specific antigen (PSA) screening for prostate cancer. However, the extent to which men are actually screened for these cancers is not known. If cancer screening were evidence based, PSA screening would be less common than colorectal screening in men because colorectal cancer screening has broad acceptance and proved efficacy. The prevalence of PSA screening was compared with colorectal screening among men in the United States.

Methods.—This study used the 2001 Behavioral Risk Factor Surveillance System, an annual population-based telephone survey of US adults conducted by the Centers for Disease Control and Prevention. Data were gathered on a representative sample of 49,315 men 40 years or older from all 50 states and the District of Columbia. The main outcome measures were proportions of men ever screened and up to date on screening for prostate cancer (with PSA testing) and colorectal cancer (with fecal occult blood testing, flexible sigmoidoscopy, or colonoscopy).

Results.—The overall findings were that men 40 years and older are more likely to have ever been screened for prostate cancer (75% have had a PSA test) than for colorectal cancer (63% have had any colorectal cancer test). Men of all ages were more likely to have an up-to-date PSA screening than a colorectal cancer screening. The greatest consensus in favor of screening occurs among men aged 50 to 69 years; 54% of these men reported up-to-date testing for colorectal cancer. State-level analyses of this age group showed that men were significantly more likely to have an up-to-date screening compared with colorectal cancer screening in 27 states. Up-to-date colorectal cancer screening was more common in only 1 state.

Conclusions.—These findings indicate that prostate screening is more common than colorectal cancer screening among men in the United States. In light of these findings, it is recommended that physicians ensure that men who elect to be screened for cancer are made aware of the known mortality rate benefit of colorectal cancer screening and the uncertain benefits of screening for prostate cancer.

▶ This article doesn't address whether prostate cancer screening is less appropriate than colorectal cancer screening. It does suggest that ordering a blood test seems to be easier than passing out hemoccults or performing lower endoscopic procedures (flexible sigmoidoscopy or colonoscopy). The benefits of colorectal cancer screening as well as the limitations of prostate cancer screening need to be explained to our patients.

P. J. Loehrer, Sr, MD

Variation of Serum Prostate-Specific Antigen Levels: An Evaluation of Year-to-Year Fluctuations

Eastham JA, for the Polyp Prevention Trial Study Group (Mem Sloan-Kettering Cancer Ctr, New York, et al)

JAMA 289:2695-2700, 2003 4–2

Background.—Early detection programs for prostate cancer typically involve a digital rectal examination combined with a test for serum prostate-specific antigen (PSA) level. Since these tests have been introduced, epidemiologic data demonstrate an increase in the number of men diagnosed with prostate cancer and a shift to earlier stages of discovery. However, there has also been an increase in men undergoing radical prostatectomy for cancers that may be clinically insignificant. The reliability of PSA tests in a group of healthy men at risk for prostate cancer was retrospectively assessed.

Study Design.—Participants in the Polyp Prevention Trial had fasting blood samples drawn annually over a 4-year period. Samples from 972 men, aged 25 to 89 years, were tested for PSA level. The frequency of an abnormal PSA was estimated by PSA higher than 4 ng/mL, PSA higher than 2.5 ng/mL, age-specific PSA levels, free-to-total PSA ratio lower than 0.25 ng/mL among men with PSA levels between 4 and 10 ng/mL, and PSA velocity higher than 0.75 ng/mL per year.

Findings.—Prostate biopsy would have been recommended for 21% with at least 1 PSA level higher than 4 ng/mL, for 37% with a PSA level higher than 2.5 ng/mL, for 18% with a level above age-specific cutoffs, for 20% with a level between 4 and 10 ng/mL and a free-to-total ratio of less than 0.25 ng/mL, and in 15% of men with a velocity higher than 0.75 ng/mL. Among those men with an abnormal PSA test result, a subsequent test result was normal in 44% of those with a PSA level higher than 4 ng/mL, in 40% of those with a PSA level higher than 2.5 ng/mL, in 53% of those with a level between 4 and 10 ng/mL and a free-to-total ratio of less than 0.25 ng/mL, and 55% of those with a level above age-specific cutoffs.

Conclusions.—Because nearly half of the men who had an abnormal PSA test in this series had a subsequent normal test, fluctuating test results may result in many false-positive readings. This suggests that any single abnormal PSA level should be viewed with caution. A policy of waiting 4 to 6 weeks after an abnormal PSA test to repeat the test before proceeding with a diagnostic biopsy would decrease the number of unnecessary biopsies while permitting safe and timely diagnoses.

► Serum PSA testing is widely used as a screening tool for prostate cancer. When elevated, US and biopsies are performed. As this is associated with patient mortality and increasing health costs, proper interpretation of PSA is important. This is just one article that reminds physicians that one abnormal value should not be a "call to arms."

P. J. Loehrer, Sr, MD

Long-term Durability of PSA Failure-Free Survival After Radiotherapy for Localized Prostate Cancer

Yock TI, Zietman AL, Shipley WU, et al (Harvard Med School, Boston)
Int J Radiat Oncol Biol Phys 54:420-426, 2002 4–3

Background.—Prostate-specific antigen (PSA) testing serves both as a screening device and as a sensitive monitoring method for patients after treatment. The PSA level rises months to years before clinical failure is ap-

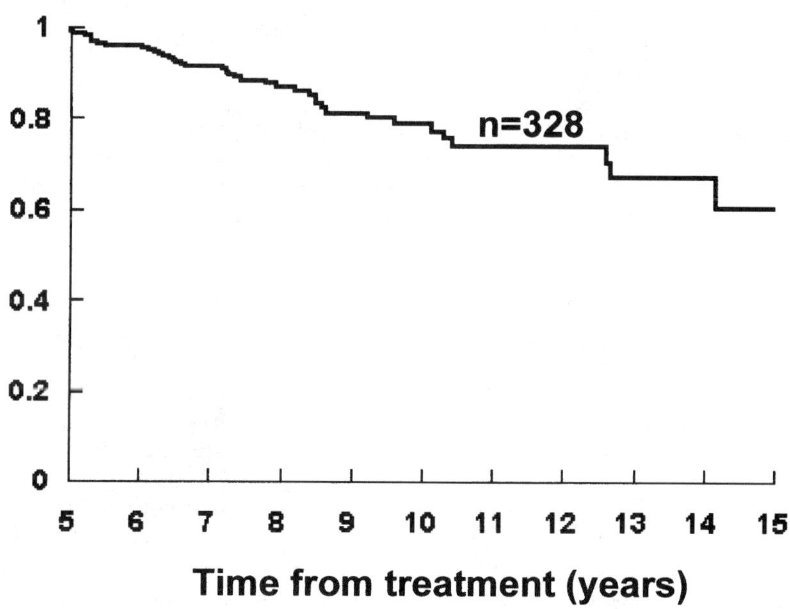

Year	5	6	7	8	9	10	11	12	13	14	15
# in Analysis	328	264	178	104	73	54	32	26	16	10	8

FIGURE 1.—Biochemical disease-specific survival in patients biochemically disease free at 5 years. (Reprinted from Yock TI, Zietman AL, Shipley WU, et al: Long-term durability of PSA failure-free survival after radiotherapy for localized prostate cancer. *Int J Radiat Oncol Biol Phys* 54:420-426, 2002. Copyright 2002, with permission from Elsevier Science.)

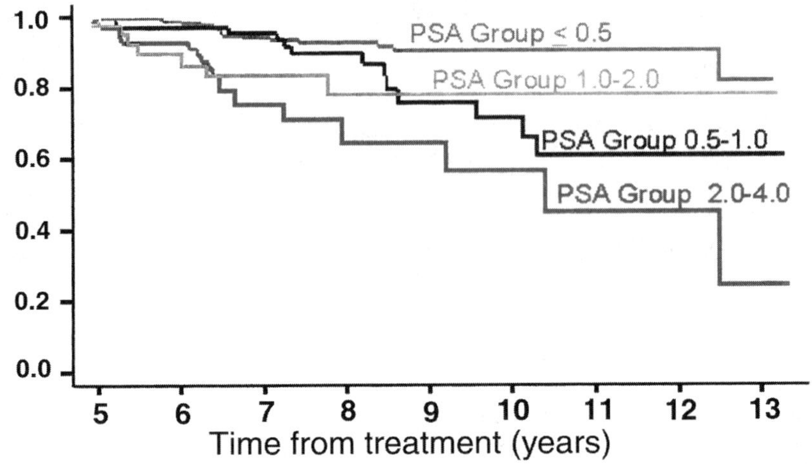

# in Analysis by year and PSA group	5	6	7	8	9	10	11	12	13
≤ 0.5 ng/ml	122	106	79	51	37	26	19	15	8
0.5-1.0 ng/ml	96	74	55	31	19	14	6	4	2
1.0-2.0 ng/ml	70	55	26	12	8	7	5	5	5
2.0-4.0 ng/ml	40	29	18	10	9	7	2	2	1

FIGURE 2.—Biochemical disease-free survival according to prostate-specific antigen (*PSA*) group. (Reprinted from Yock TI, Zietman AL, Shipley WU, et al: Long-term durability of PSA failure-free survival after radiotherapy for localized prostate cancer. *Int J Radiat Oncol Biol Phys* 54:420-426, 2002. Copyright 2002, with permission from Elsevier Science.)

parent. Having a low PSA for a long period may predict the subsequent disease-free survival. The disease-free survival for men who have undergone radiotherapy (RT) for prostate cancer was determined when the PSA levels remained low and showed no rising pattern 5 years after external beam radiotherapy (EBRT).

Methods.—Three hundred twenty-eight men who had EBRT to the prostate were studied. All were biochemically free of disease 5 years after EBRT; follow-up extended for a median of 7.4 years. Groups were formed based on PSA values at 5 years, including PSA 0.5 ng/mL or less, PSA 0.5 to 1.0 ng/mL, PSA 1.0 to 2.0 ng/mL, and PSA 2.0 to 4.0 ng/mL. The PSA progression-free rates were determined for all groups 10 years after treatment, and yearly hazard rates of progression for the 6 to 10 years after treatment were calculated.

Results.—Patients who were disease free at 5 years had an actuarial disease-free survival of 87% at 8 years, 79% at 10 years, and 67% at 13 years (Fig 1), but the lower the PSA value at 5 years, the greater the long-term disease-free survival rate. For the 122 patients with a PSA of 0.5 ng/mL or less, only 7 had failure, and their disease-free survival at 8 years was 97% and at 10 years, 92% (Fig 2). Patients who had T1-T2 tumors along with a Gleason score of 7 or higher had a greater likelihood of failure.

The initial PSA level predicted continued disease-free survival in patients free of disease after 5 years. The 5-year PSA level was significantly associated

TABLE 4.—Multivariate Analysis of Tumor Characteristics and Treatment Variables and Association With Biochemical Disease-Free Survival in Patients Biochemically Disease Free 5 Years After Treatment

Variable	Multivariate (*P* Value)	Multivariate (*P* Value) Without 5-y Group
T1-2 vs T3-4	0.02	0.22
GS ≤7 vs >7	0.32	0.31
PSA level at 5 y	<0.0001	
Initial PSA (≤10 vs >10 ng/mL)	0.25	0.03
Dose (≤68.4 vs >68.4 Gy)	0.43	0.40

(Reprinted from Yock TI, Zietman AL, Shipley WU, et al: Long-term durability of PSA failure-free survival after radiotherapy for localized prostate cancer. *Int J Radiat Oncol Biol Phys* 54:420-426, 2002. Copyright 2002, with permission from Elsevier Science.)

with late relapse, as was T stage (Table 4). The yearly hazard rates of PSA progression 6 to 10 years after RT showed no variation based on T stage or Gleason score, but an initial PSA of over 10 ng/mL was predictive of a higher rate of late progression of disease (Table 5). The hazard rates over 6 to 10 years after treatment for patients free of disease at 5 years after EBRT and for those having prostatectomy were comparable.

TABLE 5.—Hazard Rates of Biochemical Failure in Patients Biochemically Disease Free at 5 Years

Group	Yearly Hazard Rates						
	5-6	6-7	7-8	8-9	9-10	*P**	10-y PFS (%)
5-y PSA (ng/mL)							
<1.0	1.0	1.0	3.7	8.7	2.1		84
1.0 to ≤4.0	8.3	14.1	9.1	0	6.5	0.0001	68
T stage							
T1-2 (66%)	2.0	5.2	3.2	8.6	0		83
T3-4 (34%)	6.5	5.7	8.4	3.3	9.1		71
						0.06	
Initial PSA (ng/mL)							
≤10	2.9	3.0	3.6	10.3	0		82
>10	3.9	11.3	8.2	30	0		51
						0.008	
Gleason score							
≤7 (77%)	3.2	5.2	3.6	7.0	4.0		79
>7 (23%)	4.5	4.3	10.7	6.3	0		80
						0.51	
All patients	3.4	5.3	4.8	6.6	3.1		79
Prostatectomy series†	4.9	4.0	5.4	5.5	4.0		NA‡

*Log-rank test within the Statistical Analysis System Lifetest procedure.

†Data from Amling CL, Blute ML, Bergstralh EJ, et al: Long-term hazard of progression after radical prostatectomy for clinically localized prostate cancer: Continued risk of biochemical failure after 5 years. *J Urol* 164:101-105, 2000. This population included those patients with clinically stage T2b or lower disease and negative lymph nodes at surgery, who did not receive any adjuvant or neoadjuvant hormonal therapy or radiotherapy.

‡Direct comparison percentage not available.

Abbreviations: PFS, Progression-free survival; *PSA*, prostate-specific antigen; *NA*, not available.

(Reprinted from Yock TI, Zietman AL, Shipley WU, et al: Long-term durability of PSA failure-free survival after radiotherapy for localized prostate cancer. *Int J Radiat Oncol Biol Phys* 54:420-426, 2002. Copyright 2002, with permission from Elsevier Science.)

Conclusion.—An early therapeutic goal of treatment for prostate cancer is a low nadir PSA and its maintenance for at least 5 years. When patients who have RT are free of disease at 5 years and maintain low PSA levels, specifically, less than 2 ng/mL, most will be biochemically free of disease at 10 years. The hazard rates achieved with RT are comparable to those seen with prostatectomy for biochemical progression over the 6 to 10 years after treatment.

▶ This group of investigators from the Massachusetts General Hospital reports on a large series of patients treated with EBRT for prostate cancer. All the patients had more than 5 years of follow-up and, indeed, the maximum follow-up goes out to 15 years. The authors conclude that if the PSA level remains below 2 ng/mL 5 years after EBRT, the vast majority of patients will remain biochemically free of disease at 10 years, though initial T stage and PSA levels can predict for risk of late relapse. They also conclude that the hazard rates of biochemical progression are low in these irradiated patients and comparable to series treated by radical prostatectomy.

E. Glatstein, MD

Dose Response in Prostate Cancer With 8-12 Years' Follow-up

Hanks GE, Hanlon AL, Epstein B, et al (Fox Chase Cancer Ctr, Philadelphia)

Int J Radiat Oncol Biol Phys 54:427-435, 2002 4–4

Background.—The purpose of 3-dimensional conformal radiotherapy is to safely increase the dose of radiation that can be delivered to the target organ while restricting the dose to the surrounding normal tissues. This article reports on the long-term outcomes of prostate cancer patients who took part in the first radiation dose escalation study for which 8 to 12 years of follow-up is now available.

Methods.—In this prospective dose-escalation study, 232 patients with clinically localized prostate cancer received 3-dimensional conformal radiotherapy from March 1989 to October 1992. Data were available for 229 of these patients. The main outcome measures were the 8-, 10-, and 12-year actuarial rates of biochemical control (biochemically no evidence of disease [bNED]), freedom from distant metastasis (FDM), and morbidity.

Multivariate Cox proportional hazards modeling was used to determine the predictors of bNED control and FDM, including pretreatment prostate-specific antigen (PSA) level (continuous), tumor stage (T1/T2a vs T2b/T3), Gleason score 2-6 vs 7-10), and radiation dose (continuous). The patients received a median total dose of 74 Gy (range 67-81 Gy). The median follow-up for living patients was 110 months (range, 84-147 months). The bNED control was defined on the basis of the American Society for Therapeutic Radiology and Oncology consensus definition.

Results.—The overall actuarial bNED control in this series was 55% at 5 years, 48% at 10 years, and 48% at 12 years. Patients with pretreatment PSA levels of 10 to 20 ng/mL had statistically significant differences in bNED

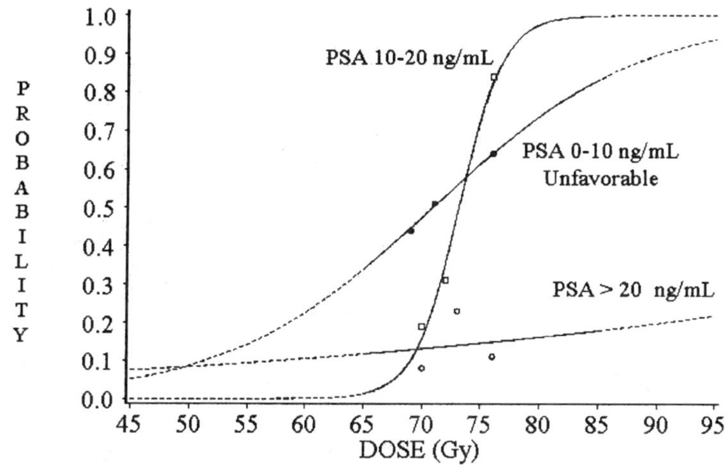

FIGURE 4.—Three-dimensional conformal radiotherapy dose-response function: Actuarial 8-year biologically no evidence of disease control. *Abbreviation: PSA*, Prostate-specific antigen. (Reprinted from Hanks GE, Hanlon AL, Epstein B, et al: Dose response in prostate cancer with 8-12 years' follow-up. *Int J Radiat Oncol Biol Phys* 54:427-435, 2002. Copyright 2002, with permission from Elsevier Science.)

control (19% vs 31% vs 84%) when stratified by dose (less than 71.5, 71.5-75.6, and more than 75.6 Gy, respectively) (Fig 4). Of the 229 patients for whom data were available, 124 (54%) patients had no clinical or biochemical evidence of disease (Fig 5). At last follow-up, 69 patients were alive and 55 were dead of recurrent disease.

Multivariate analysis showed that radiation dose was a statistically significant predictor of bNED control for all patients and for unfavorable patients with a PSA of less than 10 ng/mL. The radiation dose was a statistically sig-

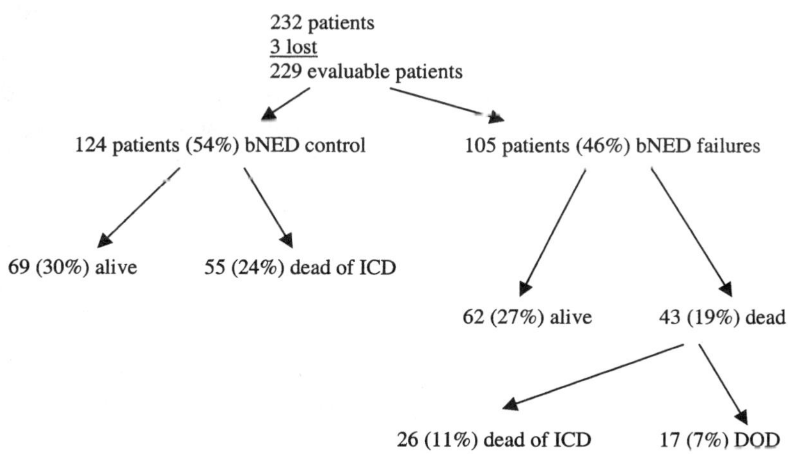

FIGURE 5.—Clinical outcome of 229 dose-escalation patients. *Abbreviations: ICD*, Intercurrent disease; *DOD*, dead of disease; *bNED*, biologically no evidence of disease. (Reprinted from Hanks GE, Hanlon AL, Epstein B, et al: Dose response in prostate cancer with 8-12 years' follow-up. *Int J Radiat Oncol Biol Phys* 54:427-435, 2002. Copyright 2002, with permission from Elsevier Science.)

nificant predictor across all groups for patients with a pretreatment PSA level of 10 to 20 ng/mL. The FDM rates for all patients in this series were 89%, 83%, and 83% at 5, 10, and 12 years, respectively. For patients with pretreatment PSA levels of less than 10 ng/mL, radiation dose, Gleason score, pretreatment PSA, and palpation T stage were significant predictors of distant metastasis.

Conclusion.—The long-term results of this radiation dose escalation study in patients with prostate cancer with more than 9 years of median follow-up confirmed that there is a dose response for both bNEd control and FDM. The absence of biochemical recurrence after 8 years is evidence of a lack of failure and suggests that the patient is cured.

▶ These investigators report the results of dose escalation and 3-dimensional conformal radiation therapy for patients with prostate cancer. They identified high-, intermediate, and low-risk patients. They conclude that there is a major dose response in prostate cancer. They show a fairly steep result in the intermediate group, but the evidence for dose response in the other 2 groups is unimpressive. They furnish estimates of morbidities of the gastrointestinal and genitourinary tracts, although this has become a complicated subject because they group all symptoms under a heading of severity (ie, grades 2 and 3), without detailing the precise complications.

This kind of lumping together under grade gives a fair amount of flexibility to the investigator to categorize morbidities. For example, there have been times in which investigators have called a need for transfusion a hematologic problem, rather than a gastrointestinal problem resulting from bleeding. The case for increasing doses is still somewhat unclear, as the morbidities reported here are not trivial in terms of their frequency. If one has a low stage T1 patient who is diagnosed by PSA only, the treatment has to be exceedingly safe. After all, that patient had no symptoms and by definition, nothing to palpate.

E. Glatstein, MD

Predictors of Biochemical Outcome With Salvage Conformal Radiotherapy After Radical Prostatectomy for Prostate Cancer

Katz MS, Zelefsky MJ, Venkatraman ES, et al (Mem Sloan-Kettering Cancer Ctr, New York)

J Clin Oncol 21:483-489, 2003 4–5

Introduction.—To determine which patients are most likely to respond to salvage radiation therapy, guidelines are necessary to predict whether a rising prostate-specific antigen (PSA) represents tumor confined to the prostate bed or whether it is an indicator of systemic disease. Clinicopathologic characteristics at initial presentation and at the time of recurrence that predict the efficacy of salvage radiotherapy (RT) were examined.

Methods.—One hundred fifteen patients with a rising PSA after radical prostatectomy were evaluated between January 1988 and June 2000. All patients received 3-dimensional conformal RT (3D-CRT) alone or in conjunc-

TABLE 3.—Multivariate Analysis of Prostate-Specific Antigen Failure after Salvage Radiation Therapy Based on Clinicopathologic Variables for 70 Patients Receiving Radiation Alone

	Risk Ratio	95% CI	*P*
Close/negative margins	1.42	1.03 to 1.97	.03
Absence of extracapsular extension	1.81	1.22 to 2.69	< .01
Presence of seminal vesicle invasion	1.68	1.20 to 2.35	< .01
Presalvage PSA >0.6 ng/mL	1.34	0.92 to 1.96	.13

Abbreviation: PSA, Prostate-specific antigen.

(Courtesy of Katz MS, Zelefsky MJ, Venkatraman ES, et al: Predictors of biochemical outcome with salvage conformal radiotherapy after radical prostatectomy for prostate cancer. *J Clin Oncol* 21(3):483-489, 2003. Reprinted with permission from the American Society of Clinical Oncology.)

tion with neoadjuvant androgen deprivation. Tumor- and treatment-related factors were assessed to ascertain predictors of subsequent PSA failure.

Results.—The mean follow-up after 3D-CRT was 42 months. The 4-year actuarial PSA relapse-free survival, distant metastasis–free survival, and overall survival rates were 46%, 83%, and 95%, respectively. Multivariate analysis was limited to 70 patients receiving radiation without androgen deprivation therapy and revealed that negative/close margins (P = .03), absence of extracapsular extension (P < .01), and the presence of seminal vesicle invasion (P < .01) were independently predictive of PSA relapse after RT (Table 3). Among the 70 patients who received RT alone, the 4-year PSA relapse-free survival was 77% (95% confidence interval [CI], 59%-100%) for those with no risk factors and 20% (95% CI, 10%-40%) among those with 1 or more risk factors (P < .01).

Of the 45 patients in the RT and neoadjuvant androgen deprivation therapy group, the rate was 91% (95% CI, 75%-100% for those with no risk factors and 43% (95% CI, 22%-82%) for patients with 1 or more risk factors (P = .02) (Fig 1). Neoadjuvant androgen deprivation did not improve the 4-year PSA relapse-free survival in patients who had positive margins, extracapsular extension, and no seminal vesicle invasion (P = .24). Neoadjuvant androgen deprivation improved PSA relapse-free survival when 1 or more of these variables was absent (P = .03).

Conclusion.—Salvage 3D-CRT can provide biochemical control in selected patients with a rising PSA after radical prostatectomy. Among patients with positive margins and no poor prognostic characteristics, 77% achieved PSA control after undergoing 3D-CRT. Salvage neoadjuvant androgen deprivation may enhance short-term biochemical control.

► These investigators from Memorial Sloan-Kettering in New York report their results with 115 patients who had a radical prostatectomy but then developed a rising PSA. It is difficult to generalize about these patients who represent chemical relapse. One needs a long time to know if they really achieve a good outcome or not. I am never quite certain myself exactly what to aim at since there is no real tumor target, and it is not always clear that the PSA is coming from the prostatic bed. In addition, once the prostate is in the bottle,

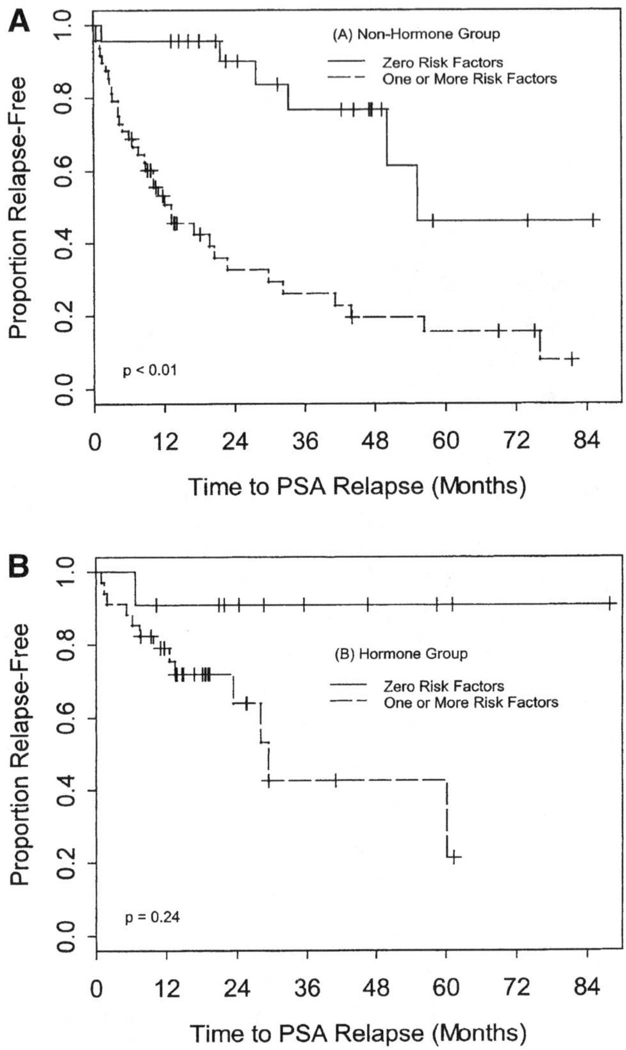

FIGURE 1.—Prostate-specific antigen (*PSA*) relapse-free survival according to a number of risk factors in 70 patients treated with radiation alone (**A**) and in 45 patients treated with radiation and neoadjuvant deprivation therapy (**B**). (Courtesy of Katz MS, Zelefsky MJ, Venkatraman ES, et al: Predictors of biochemical outcome with salvage conformal radiotherapy after radical prostatectomy for prostate cancer. *J Clin Oncol* 21(3):483-489, 2003. Reprinted with permission from the American Society of Clinical Oncology.)

tissues tend to fall together, filling in the former prostate space, and it is not really clear to me exactly where we should be putting the radiation.

Having said that, I have to say that the results these investigators report are really pretty good. They have identified margins, extracapsular extension, seminal vesicle invasion, and the presalvage PSA as important risk factors.

I think the fundamental question is whether radiation adds anything over what can be achieved with hormonal manipulation alone. It would be nice if one of the cooperative study groups could address this issue. The data presented here are interesting, but the real issue is what happens at 10 and 15 years. Prostate cancer is a notoriously sneaky disease, and the question remains whether any of these patients are truly cured. Only a longer follow-up will be able to clarify this issue.

E. Glatstein, MD

Changing Prostate-Specific Antigen Outcome After Surgery or Radiotherapy for Localized Prostate Cancer During the Prostate-Specific Antigen Era

D'Amico AV, Chen M-H, Oh-Ung J, et al (Brigham and Women's Hosp, Boston; Dana Farber Cancer Inst, Boston; Univ of Connecticut, Storrs)
Int J Radiat Oncol Biol Phys 54:436-441, 2002 4–6

Background.—There is evidence that prostate cancer is now diagnosed at smaller volumes, lower grades, and at a younger age. This shift has been attributed to the use of serum prostate-specific antigen (PSA) determination. This study evaluated the shift in PSA outcome after radical prostatectomy (RP) or external beam radiotherapy (EBRT) while controlling for follow-up during the PSA era.

Methods.—The study included 1440 patients with clinically localized prostate cancer managed with RP (1059 patients) or EBRT (381 patients) from 1989 to 2000. A single genitourinary pathologist reviewed all pathology specimens. For patients with a 2-year minimal follow-up, the 2-year actual PSA outcome stratified by risk group from low to high was calculated for 3 periods and compared for each treatment modality (Table 2). The American Society for Therapeutic Radiology and Oncology consensus definition of PSA failure was used, and comparisons were made with a χ^2 metric.

Results.—The proportion of patients with low-risk disease treated with RP and EBRT increased significantly over the course of the study, from 60%

TABLE 2.—Distribution of 1440 Study Patients Stratified by Treatment, Pretreatment Risk Group, and Period

	Radical Prostatectomy				External Beam Radiotherapy			
Risk Group	1/1/89-12/31/92 (n = 305)	1/1/93-12/31/96 (n = 486)	1/1/97-12/31/00 (n = 268)	P	1/1/89-12/31/92 (n = 27)	1/1/93-12/31/96 (n = 138)	1/1/97-12/31/00 (n = 216)	P
Low*	60	77	89	<0.0001	26	57	76	<0.0001
High†	40	23	11		74	43	24	

Note: Data presented as the percentage of patients. P values evaluated distribution of pretreatment risk groups across 3 periods using a χ^2 metric.

* Prostate-specific antigen (PSA) of ≤10 ng/mL and biopsy Gleason score of ≤6 and clinical stage T1c or T2a or ≤50% positive biopsy specimens and PSA >10 to 20 ng/mL or biopsy Gleason score 7 or clinical stage T2b.

† PSA >20 ng/mL or biopsy Gleason score 8 to 10 or clinical stage T2c or >50% positive biopsies and PSA >10 to 20 ng/mL or biopsy Gleason score 7 or clinical stage T2b.

TABLE 3.—Distribution of PSA Biopsy Gleason Score and Clinical T-Stage in High-Risk Patients Stratified by Interval and Treatment

	Radical Prostatectomy				External Beam Radiotherapy			
Clinical Factor	1/1/89-12/31/92 (n = 121)	1/1/93-12/31/96 (n = 113)	1/1/97-12/31/00 (n = 30)	P	1/1/89-12/31/92 (n = 20)	1/1/93-12/31/96 (n = 59)	1/1/97-12/31/00 (n = 51)	P
PSA (ng/mL)								
≤10	25	49	67	<0.0001	25	51	67	0.02
>10-20	37	28	27		40	28	24	
>20	38	23	7		35	22	10	
Gleason score								
≤6	64	29	13	<0.0001	55	27	24	0.05
7	22	42	57		25	40	41	
≥8	14	29	30		20	34	35	
Stage								
T1c or T2a	48	67	77	0.0007	10	41	43	0.009
T2b	31	19	13		10	27	20	
T2c	21	14	10		80	32	37	

Note: Data presented as the percentage of patients. P values evaluated distribution of pretreatment clinical factors across 3 periods using a χ^2 metric.

Abbreviation: PSA, Prostate-specific antigen.

(Reprinted from D'Amico AV, Chen M-H, Oh-Ung J, et al: Changing prostate-specific antigen outcome after surgery or radiotherapy for localized prostate cancer during the prostate-specific antigen era. *Int J Radiat Oncol Biol Phys* 54:436-441, 2002.)

to 89% and from 26% to 76%, respectively (Table 3). In addition, the 2-year actual PSA outcome also improved from 60% to 82% and from 67% to 91%, respectively. There was no significant difference in the 2-year actual PSA outcome in the low-risk patients, but this outcome improved during the 3 periods in the high-risk patients treated with RP (from 20% to 39% to 75%) and EBRT (from 50% to 59% to 83%). This improvement could be attributed to a shift toward a more favorable PSA level and clinical T-stage distribution for patients with a biopsy Gleason score 7 or greater disease (Table 4).

TABLE 4.—Distribution of PSA and Clinical Stage in High-Risk Patients With Biopsy Gleason Score of 7 or Greater Disease Stratified by Interval and Treatment

	Radical Prostatectomy				External Beam Radiotherapy			
Clinical Factor	1/1/89-12/31/92 (n = 44)	1/1/93-12/31/96 (n = 80)	1/1/97-12/31/00 (n = 26)	P	1/1/89-12/31/92 (n = 9)	1/1/93-12/31/96 (n = 43)	1/1/97-12/31/00 (n = 39)	P
PSA (ng/mL)								
≤10	27	59	69	0.0002	11	40	64	0.006
>10	73	41	31		89	60	36	
Stage								
T1c or T2a	48	71	85	0.0008	11	40	77	<0.0001
T2b or T2c	52	29	15		89	60	23	

Note: Data presented as the percentage of patients. P values evaluated distribution of pretreatment clinical factors across 3 periods using a χ^2 metric.

Abbreviation: PSA, Protein-specific antigen.

(Reprinted from D'Amico AV, Chen M-H, Oh-Ung J, et al: Changing prostate-specific antigen outcome after surgery or radiotherapy for localized prostate cancer during the prostate-specific antigen era. *Int J Radiat Oncol Biol Phys* 54:436-441, 2002.)

Conclusion.—Among patients with localized prostate cancer, a shift in presentation toward low-risk disease and earlier detection of high-grade disease has resulted in improved PSA outcome during the PSA era after radical prostatectomy or external beam radiotherapy.

► This report evaluates over 1400 patients with clinically localized prostate cancer managed with either RP or EBRT between 1989 and 2000. The important observation which they make is that during the study period, there was a significant increase in patients who had low-risk prostate cancer in both the RP group and the EBRT group. This era coincides with the standard use of PSA screener. It would appear that the use of PSA as a screening technique has shifted patients toward a lower risk category, as well as an earlier detection of those patients who had high-grade disease. The implications of this are important epidemiologically as well as in the interpretation of results reported from a wide variety of institutions. Long-term follow-up will tell us if this shift really means better outcome or not.

E. Glatstein, MD

Do Older Men Benefit From Curative Therapy of Localized Prostate Cancer?

Alibhai SMH, Naglie G, Nam R, et al (Univ Health Network, Toronto; Toronto Rehabilitation Inst; Univ of Toronto)

J Clin Oncol 21:3318-3327, 2003 4–7

Background.—The treatment of men with localized prostate cancer involves complex decision making. The role of age in this decision-making process is particularly problematic. Published studies have suggested that otherwise healthy older men with higher-grade prostate cancer may not be receiving potentially life-prolonging therapy because it is thought that these patients are unlikely to benefit from these therapies. However, prior decision-analytic models used in treatment decision making for these patients are based on outdated or suboptimal data on efficacy, patient preference, and comorbidity. Life expectancy and quality-adjusted life expectancy associated with available treatments for localized prostate cancer was estimated in men aged 65 years or older, with adjustments for Gleason score, patients preferences, and comorbidity.

Methods.—A decision-analytic Markov model was used to evaluate 3 treatments: a radical prostatectomy (RP), external beam radiotherapy (EBRT), and watchful waiting (Fig 1). Rates of treatment complications and pretreatment incontinence and impotence were obtained from published studies. Treatment efficacy was estimated by using cancer registry cohort data, pooled case series, and modern radiotherapy studies. Utilities were obtained from 141 prostate cancer patients and from published studies.

Results.—For men with well-differentiated tumors and few comorbidities, life expectancy up to age 75 years was prolonged with potentially curative therapy (RP or EBRT); however, quality-adjusted life expectancy was

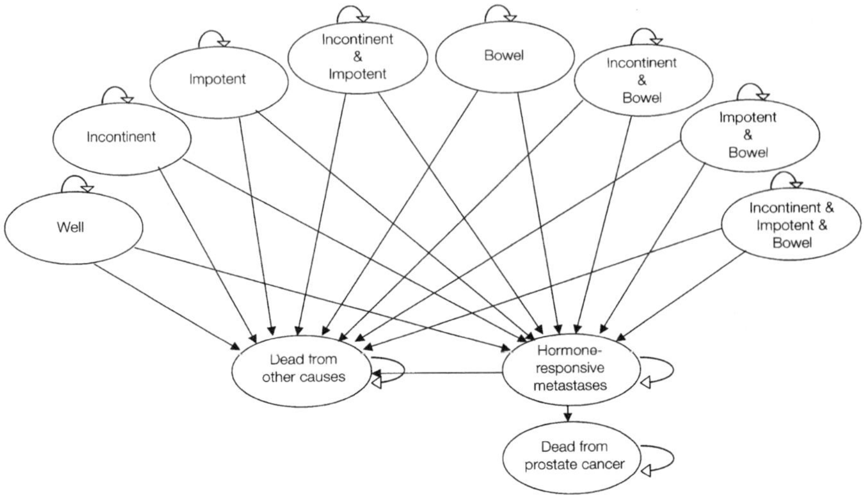

FIGURE 1.—Key health care states and transitions in Markov model, RP branch. After undergoing treatment, patients entered 1 of 8 posttreatment health care states. In each cycle, patients could remain stable, die as a result of other causes, or develop hormone-responsive metastases. Patients with metastases could either remain stable, die as a result of other causes, or die as a result of advanced prostate cancer. (Courtesy of Alibhai SMH, Naglie G, Nam R, et al: Do older men benefit from curative therapy of localized prostate cancer? *J Clin Oncol* 21:3318-3327, 2003. Reprinted with permission from the American Society of Clinical Oncology.)

not improved at any age with these treatments. In patients with moderately differentiated cancers, potentially curative therapy provided gains up to age 75 years. The benefits of potentially curative therapy were limited to men with no more than mild comorbidity (Fig 2). The use of cohort and pooled case series data showed that RP was preferred over EBRT in all groups but was comparable to modern radiotherapy.

Conclusions.—The use of potentially curative therapy in older men with localized prostate cancer and few comorbidities can provide significantly improved life expectancy and quality-adjusted life expectancy. It would appear from these findings that age should not be a barrier to the use of potentially curative therapy in these patients.

▶ In the absence of data, there seems to be a greater amount of dogma. The title of the article asks a good question and these authors try their best to answer it. In the absence of good randomized trials comparing treatment modalities, much of this is extrapolation. The essence is that age alone should not be the sole determining factor to treat men with prostate cancer. Fig 1 does a good job of describing the various health care states. This may be a helpful tool for discussion with elderly men with prostate cancer.

P. J. Loehrer, Sr, MD

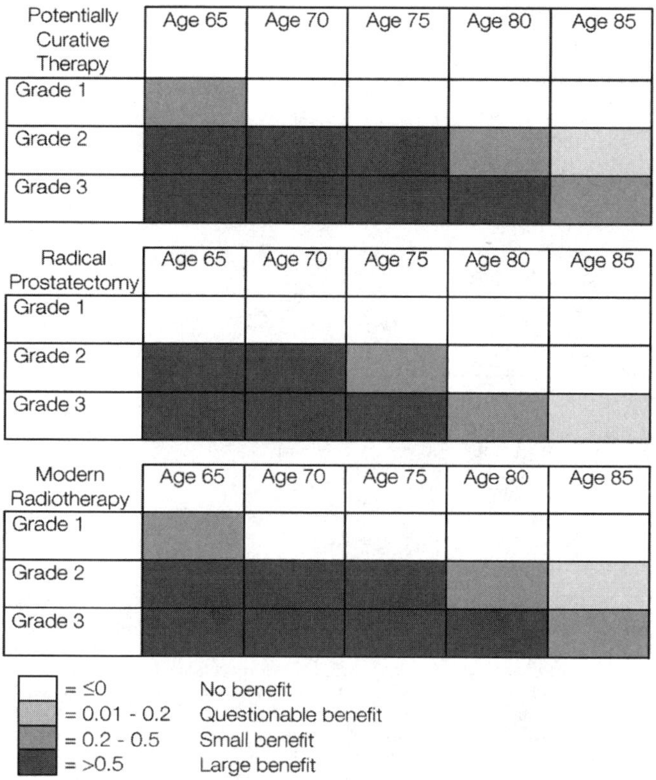

FIGURE 2.—Look-up table identifying patients who will gain in quality-adjusted life expectancy from potentially curative therapy, stratified by age and tumor grade. Illustrated are gains from potentially curative therapy (higher of RP or modern radiotherapy), RP, and modern radiotherapy compared with watchful waiting. Gains are stratified into 3 levels of benefit, which are stratified by tumor grade. Units are in quality-adjusted life-years. (Courtesy of Alibhai SMH, Naglie G, Nam R, et al: Do older men benefit from curative therapy of localized prostate cancer? *J Clin Oncol* 21:3318-3327, 2003. Reprinted with permission from the American Society of Clinical Oncology.)

Randomized, Double-blind, Controlled Trial of Mitoxantrone/Prednisone and Clodronate Versus Mitoxantrone/Prednisone and Placebo in Patients With Hormone-Refractory Prostate Cancer and Pain

Ernst DS, Tannock IF, Winquist EW, et al (Cross Cancer Inst, Edmonton, Alta, Canada; Princess Margaret Hosp, Toronto; London Regional Cancer Ctr; et al)

J Clin Oncol 21:3335-3342, 2003 4–8

Background.—For patients with hormone-resistant prostate cancer (HRPC), the combination of mitoxantrone and prednisone (MP) is a standard palliative treatment. Bisphosphonate drugs have shown promise in reducing time to progression and skeletal events in patients with HRPC, as well as hormone-sensitive prostate cancer. The effects of adding clodronate to MP for palliative treatment of HRPC were evaluated.

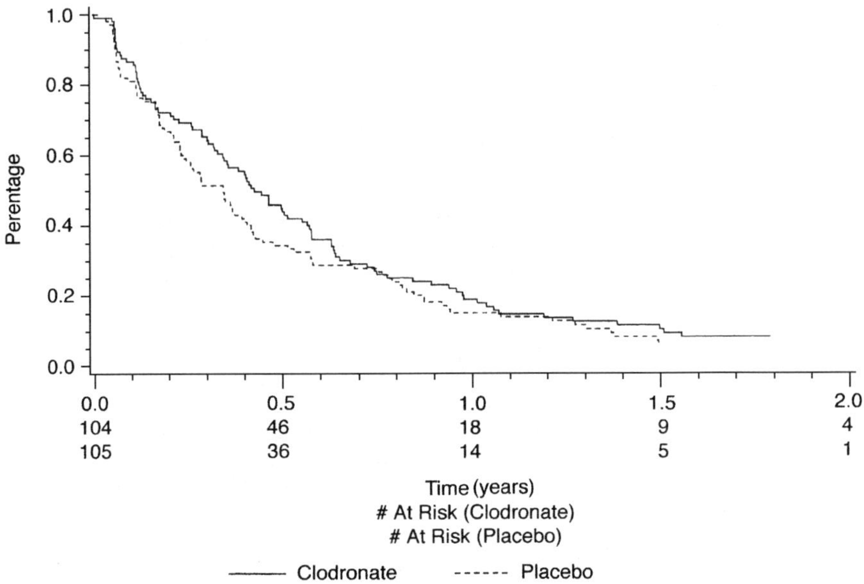

FIGURE 1.—Kaplan-Meier curve for symptomatic progression-free survival in the National Cancer Institute of Canada Clinical Trials Group Trial PR.6. Log-rank test for equality of groups, $P = .1362$; median for clodronate, 0.42 (95% confidence interval, 0.34-0.57); median for placebo, 0.33 (95% confidence interval, 0.24-0.41); hazard ratio of placebo/clodronate, 1.237 (95% confidence interval, 0.934-1.64). *Solid line*, clodronate; *broken line*, placebo. (Courtesy of Ernst DS, Tannock IF, Winquist EW, et al: Randomized, double-blind, controlled trial of mitoxantrone/prednisone and clodronate versus mitoxantrone/prednisone and placebo in patients with hormone-refractory prostate cancer and pain. *J Clin Oncol* 21:3335-3342, 2003. Reprinted with permission from the American Society of Clinical Oncology.)

Methods.—The randomized trial included 209 men with HRPC associated with bone metastases and bone pain. All patients received MP, consisting of mitoxantrone 12 mg/m^2 IV every 3 weeks and prednisone 5 mg orally twice daily. In addition, one group received clodronate 1500 mg IV or placebo every 3 weeks. Outcome measures included the present pain intensity index and a prostate-specific quality of life questionnaire, completed at each treatment visit, as well as a daily diary of analgesic use. A palliative response was defined as a reduction to 0 or of 2 points on the present pain intensity index or a 50% reduction in analgesic use.

Results.—Present pain intensity scores were 1 or 2 (mild pain) in 77% of patients and 3 or 4 (moderate pain) in 24%. A significant palliative response was reached for 46% of patients receiving clodronate compared with 39% receiving placebo. Other outcomes—including duration of response, survival, and quality of life scores—were similar between groups (Figs 1, 2, and 3). There was some evidence of benefit among patients with more severe pain.

Conclusions.—For patients with HRPC and bone metastases, adding clodronate to MP treatment does not increase the palliative response or improve quality of life. More study is needed to determine whether clodronate is of additional benefit to patients with moderate pain.

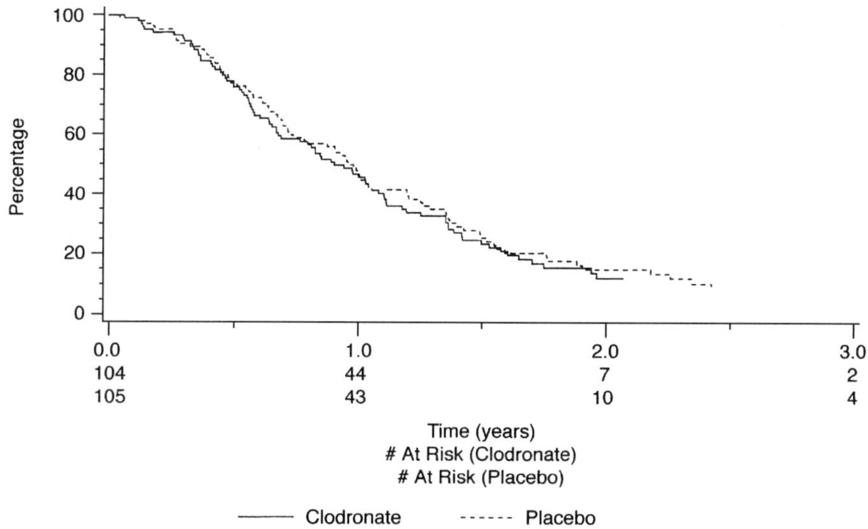

FIGURE 2.—Kaplan-Meier curve for overall survival in the National Cancer Institute of Canada Clinical Trials Group Trial PR.6. Log-rank test for equality of groups, $P = .7271$; observed events for clodronate, 87 (84%); observed events for placebo, 89 (85%); median for clodronate, 0.90 (95% confidence interval, 0.69-1.08); median for placebo, 0.96 (95% confidence interval, 0.74-1.20); hazard ratio of placebo/clodronate, 0.949 (95% confidence interval, 0.705-1.277). (Courtesy of Ernst DS, Tannock IF, Winquist EW, et al: Randomized, double-blind, controlled trial of mitoxantrone/prednisone and clodronate versus mitoxantrone/prednisone and placebo in patients with hormone-refractory prostate cancer and pain. *J Clin Oncol* 21:3335-3342, 2003. Reprinted with permission from the American Society of Clinical Oncology.)

▶ This group of investigators from Canada has performed many pivotal studies looking at impact of treatment on quality of life and costs. This is a nicely done study looking at an early generation bisphosphonate in hormone-refractory prostate cancer.

This trial fails to demonstrate a meaningful impact with clodronate in this heavily pretreated population. Whether earlier use of or more potent bisphosphonates would provide benefit is currently under investigation in the United States.

P. J. Loehrer, Sr, MD

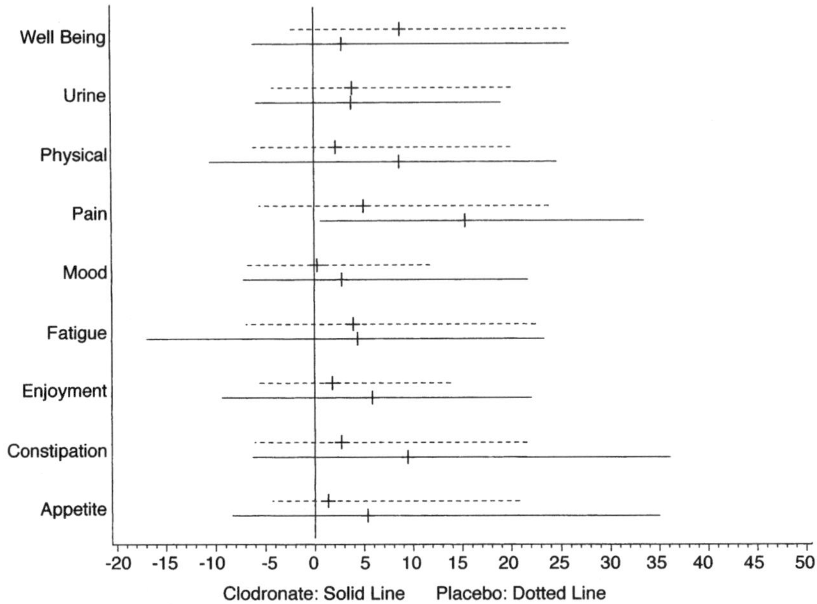

FIGURE 3.—Health-related quality of life: median change from baseline. Median and interquartile ranges are shown for patients randomly assigned to clodronate (*solid line*) or placebo (*broken line*). (Courtesy of Ernst DS, Tannock IF, Winquist EW, et al: Randomized, double-blind, controlled trial of mitoxantrone/prednisone and clodronate versus mitoxantrone/prednisone and placebo in patients with hormone-refractory prostate cancer and pain. *J Clin Oncol* 21:3335-3342, 2003. Reprinted with permission from the American Society of Clinical Oncology.)

A Randomized, Placebo-controlled Trial of Zoledronic Acid in Patients With Hormone-Refractory Metastatic Prostate Carcinoma

Saad F, for the Zoledronic Acid Prostate Cancer Study Group (Centre Hospitalier de l'Université de Montréal; et al)

J Natl Cancer Inst 94:1458-1468, 2002 4–9

Background.—Prostate carcinoma is 1 of the most common cancers in men, and a preferred metastatic site is bone. Patients with hormone-refractory metastatic prostate cancer are especially prone to progressive bone disease. Biphosphonates, pyrophosphate analogues that inhibit bone destruction, may be useful in the treatment of these patients. The effectiveness and safety of a new biphosphonate, zoledronic acid, in reducing skeletal events associated with metastatic bone disease in men with hormone-refractory prostate cancer was analyzed in a randomized, placebo-controlled, double-blind phase III trial.

Study Design.—The study group included 643 men with hormone-refractory prostate cancer and bone metastases who were randomly assigned to receive either 4 or 8 mg of zoledronic acid or placebo once every 3 weeks for 15 months. The 8-mg treatment arm was reduced to 4 mg because of renal toxicity. All patients also received calcium and vitamin D supplementation.

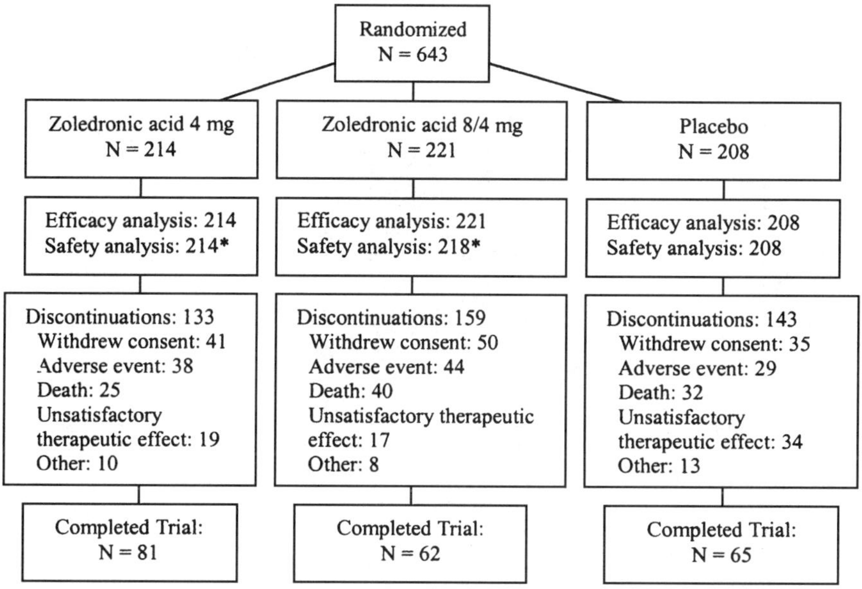

FIGURE 1.—CONSORT diagram. *Three patients, 1 randomly assigned to receive zoledronic acid at 4 mg and 2 randomly assigned to receive zoledronic acid at 8/4 mg, never received the study drug and were not included in the safety analysis. One patient randomly assigned to receive zoledronic acid at 8/4 mg incorrectly received 4 mg; this patient was included in the 8/4-mg group for efficacy and in the 4-mg group for safety analysis. (Courtesy of Saad F, for the Zoledronic Acid Prostate Cancer Study Group: A randomized, placebo-controlled trial of zoledronic acid in patients with hormone-refractory metastatic prostate carcinoma. *J Natl Cancer Inst* 94:1458-1468, 2002. By permission of Oxford University Press.)

The primary efficacy variable was the proportion of patients with at least 1 skeleton-related event, defined as pathologic bone fractures, spinal cord compression, bone surgery, bone radiotherapy, or a change in antineoplastic therapy to treat bone pain. Secondary efficacy variables included time to first skeleton-related event, skeletal morbidity rate, time to disease progression, objective bone lesion response, bone biochemical markers, and quality of life. All analyses were performed on an intention-to-treat basis. Safety was assessed by serial laboratory tests and adverse events.

Findings.—A greater proportion of patients who received placebo had skeleton-related events than those who received zoledronic acid (Fig 1). The median time to first skeleton-related event was 321 days for placebo patients and was not reached for patients receiving 4 mg of zoledronic acid (Fig 2). Urinary markers of bone resorption were significantly decreased in patients receiving zoledronic acid. Pain and analgesic scores were higher in placebo patients. No differences in disease progression, performance status, or quality-of-life scores were noted between placebo and treatment patients. Zoledronic acid was well tolerated at 4 mg, but the 8-mg dose was associated with renal toxicity.

Conclusions.—Patients with metastatic prostate cancer who received 4 mg of the biphosphonate, zoledronic acid, every 3 weeks tolerated it well and had fewer skeleton-related events than those who received placebo. The

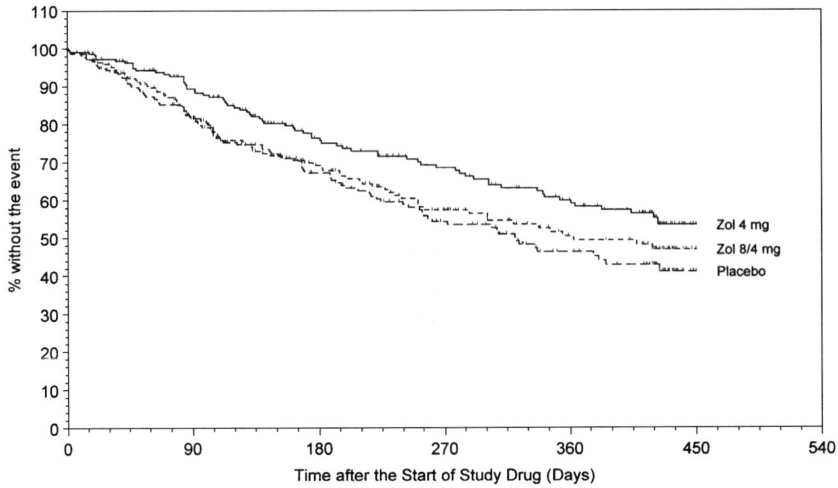

Zol 4 mg:	214	163	113	92	70	5	0
Zol 8/4 mg:	221	155	102	68	46	4	0
Placebo:	208	149	103	69	43	1	0

FIGURE 2.—Kaplan-Meier estimates of event rates for time to the first on-study skeleton-related event for all intent-to-treat patients with metastatic prostate cancer randomly assigned to receive zoledronic acid at 4 mg, zoledronic acid at 8/4 mg, or placebo. The number of patients at risk at each time point is shown in the table below the graph. Percentage of patients (95% confidence interval [CI]) without a skeleton-related event at 90 days; zoledronic acid at 4 mg, 90.0% (95% CI = 86.8% to 94.9%); zoledronic acid at 8/4 mg, 83.3% (95% CI = 78.2% to 88.4%); placebo, 83.5% (95% CI = 78.4% to 88.7%); at 270 days: zoledronic acid at 4 mg, 70.0% (95% CI = 63.0% to 76.9%); zoledronic acid at 8/4 mg, 58.0% (95% CI = 50.5% to 65.6%); placebo, 57.3% (95% CI = 49.7% to 64.8%); at 450 days: zoledronic acid at 4 mg, 55.1% (95% CI = 46.9% to 63.4%); zoledronic acid at 8/4 mg, 46.8% (95% CI = 38.2% to 55.4%); placebo, 42.8% (95% CI =34.4% to 51.2%). At the last study evaluation (450 days), *P* value (2-sided) from Cox regression = .011 for zoledronic acid at 4 mg versus placebo and *P* = 491 for zoledronic acid at 8/4 mg versus placebo. (Courtesy of Saad F, for the Zoledronic Acid Prostate Cancer Study Group: A randomized, placebo-controlled trial of zoledronic acid in patients with hormone-refractory metastatic prostate carcinoma. *J Natl Cancer Inst* 94:1458-1468, 2002. By permission of Oxford University Press.)

optimal role of zoledronic acid in the treatment of patients with metastatic prostate cancer is still being defined.

► Patients with prostate cancer experience develop skeletal complications from both malignant and nonmalignant causes. Androgen ablative therapy, which is being used more frequently and earlier in the course of prostate cancer, contributes significantly to osteoporosis. This article by Saad et al describes a landmark trial that proved to be the basis of approval of zoledronic acid by the FDA. The population studied was that of patients with hormonally refractory disease and known bone metastases. This incidence of skeleton-related events was significantly better for patients treated with zoledronic acid at 8 mg. Interestingly, the arm that initially used a higher dose of zoledronic acid and later cut back to 4 mg was not significantly different from the placebo arm. When we look back at the prestudy characteristics between the 3 treatment groups we find that the 4-mg group did have the fewest incidents of prestudy-related skeletal events and the shortest time from diagnosis to treatment (the latter suggesting a shorter exposure to androgen ablative therapy).

This is clearly an important trial; however, the impact of zoledronic acid in previously untreated patients with prostate cancer needs to be defined.

P. J. Loehrer, Sr, MD

Zoledronic Acid Exhibits Inhibitory Effects on Osteoblastic and Osteolytic Metastases of Prostate Cancer

Corey E, Brown LG, Quinn JE, et al (Univ of Washington, Seattle)

Clin Cancer Res 9:295-306, 2003 4–10

Introduction.—Bone is a frequent site for prostate cancer (PC) metastases. Bone metastases are responsible for most of the morbidity linked with PC. Bisphosphonates (BPs) are nonhydrolyzable pyrophosphate analogues that have inhibitory effects on osteoclast generation, maturation, and activity. They decrease osteoclastic bone resorption. The mechanisms underlying BP effects on cancer cells are not clearly elucidated. The effects of zoledronic acid (ZA), a new-generation BP, on PC cells in vitro and on both osteoblastic and osteolytic PC metastases were examined in a murine model.

Methods.—PC cells were treated with ZA in vitro and the effects on proliferation, cell cycle, and apoptosis were examined. In vivo, the PC-3 and LuCaP 23.1 subcutaneous cell lines and tibial tumors were treated with ZA. The effects on bone and tumor were evaluated by histomorphometry and immunohistochemistry.

Results.—Treatment with ZA reduced proliferation of PC cells and produced G_1 arrest and apoptosis of PC cells in vitro. In vivo, subcutaneous PC tumor growth was not affected by ZA. Growth of osteoblastic and osteolytic metastases of PC was inhibited markedly in vivo. Matrix metalloproteinase-2, matrix metalloproteinase-9, and Cathepsin K level were reduced in osteolytic bone metastases after ZA administration.

Conclusion.—ZA had direct antiproliferative and apoptotic effects on PC cells in vitro. The extent of inhibition of proliferation varied with the PC cell line. Antiosteolytic activity and the antitumor effects of this compound may benefit PC patients who have bone metastases.

► This article demonstrates a rationale to look at bisphosphonates in a broader sense than just building bone matrix. Randomized trials are needed to determine the true impact (therapeutic and financial) in the treatment of prostate cancer. This article must be placed in context with the one by Ernst et al (Abstract 4–8).

P. J. Loehrer, Sr, MD

Vertebral Metastases: Assessment With Apparent Diffusion Coefficient

Herneth AM, Philipp MO, Naude J, et al (Univ of Vienna; Univ of Technology, Graz, Austria; Stanford Univ, Palo Alto, Calif)

Radiology 225:889-894, 2002 4–11

Background.—Cancer patients often manifest vertebral metastases. MRI has evolved as the diagnostic method of choice for these patients because of its excellent tissue contrast on T1-weighted MR images. In the adult spine, this tissue contrast is evident after "yellow" bone marrow is replaced by hypercellular tissue or increased water content. The specificity of this characteristic is limited by similar signal intensity changes in both neoplasia and benign conditions such as inflammation, degeneration, or posttraumatic edema. This lack of specificity often results in diagnostic problems in elderly patients, in whom benign and pathologic fractures are common. The specificity of MRI may be increased with the use of diffusion-weighed MRI. The apparent diffusion coefficient (ADC) in the assessment of vertebral metastases and acute vertebral compression fractures was evaluated.

Methods.—The spines of 22 consecutive patients (19 women and 3 men) were prospectively investigated from June 1998 to December 1999. The patients ranged in age from 44.7 to 90.3 years, with a median age of 57.8 years. Both conventional and diffusion-weighted MRI were performed with a 1.0-T MRI unit. Vertebral metastases were diagnosed on the basis of findings at conventional radiography and/or CT, MRI, and scintigraphy.

Results.—There was a statistically significant difference between the mean ADCs of vertebral metastases (0.69×10^{-3} mm²/s ±0.24) and the mean ADCs of normal vertebrae (1.66×10^{-3} mm²/s±0.38) (Fig 1). The signal in-

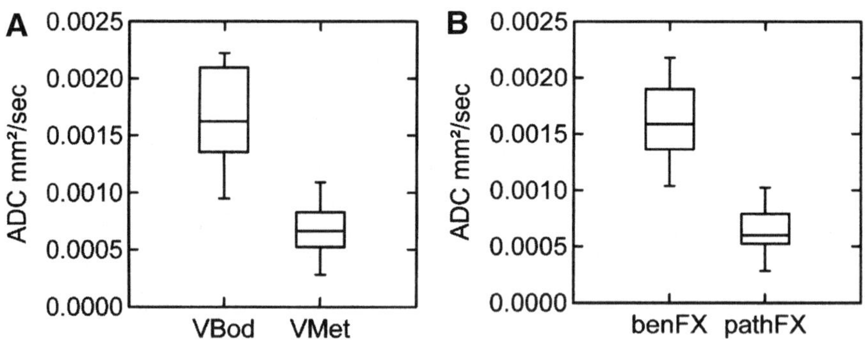

FIGURE 1.—Box plots of the apparent diffusion coefficients (*ADCs*) (**A**) in normal vertebrae (*Vbod*) and vertebral metastases (*Vmet*) and (**B**) in benign (*benFX*) and pathologic (*pathFX*) vertebral compression fractures. The *horizontal lines* are mean values, the *boxes* show minimum and maximum values, and the *whiskers* indicate plus or minus 2 standard deviations. Mean ADCs for the vertebral bodies and vertebral metastases are significantly different, and there is no overlap of absolute values. (Courtesy of Herneth AM, Philipp MO, Naude J, et al: Vertebral metastases: assessment with apparent diffusion coefficient. *Radiology* 225:889-894, 2002. Radiological Society of North America.)

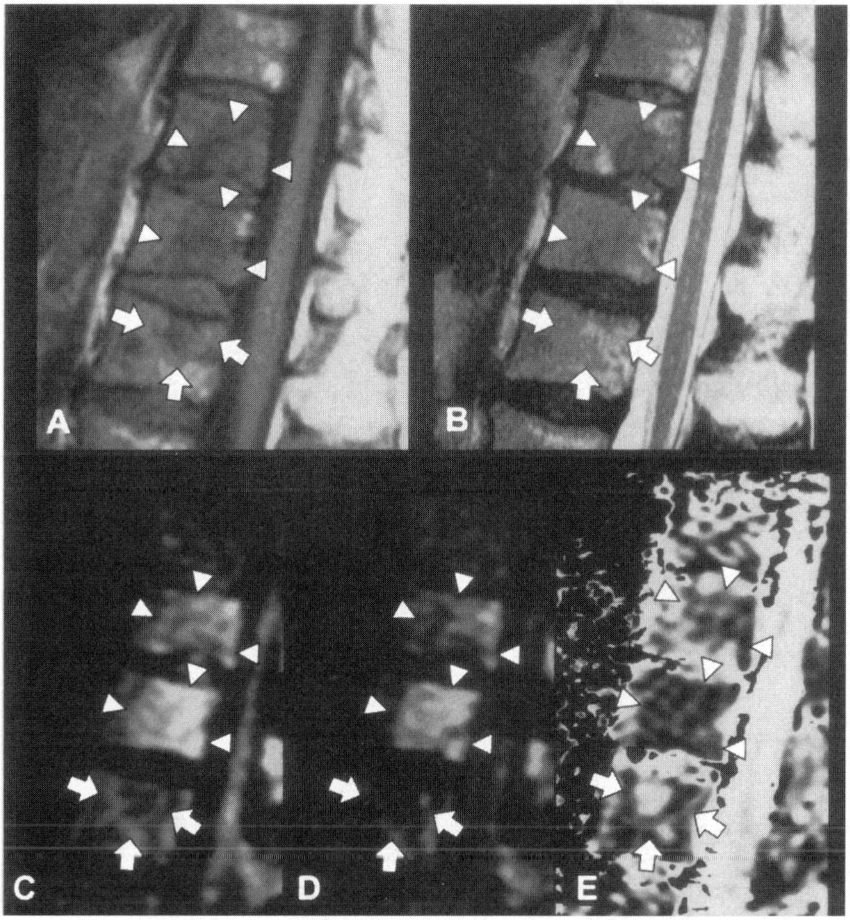

FIGURE 2.—Sagittal MR images of the lower thoracic and upper lumbar spine in a 63-year-old woman with breast cancer, known vertebral metastasis at L1 (*arrows*), and acute pathologic compression fractures at T11 and T12 (*arrowheads*). Vertebral compression fractures are (**A**) hypointense on T1-weighted MR image (500/14) and (**B**) hyperintense on T2-weighted MR image (2687/120). On diffusion-weighted echo-planar images (**C**, *b* value of 440 s/mm^2; **D**, *b* value of 880 s/mm^2), the vertebral metastasis and vertebral compression fractures appear hyperintense. **E**, Apparent diffusion coefficient map shows both vertebral metastasis and acute pathologic vertebral compression fractures with low apparent diffusion coefficients, which indicate hindered diffusion of water protons and the pathologic nature of these findings. Note the hyperintense area located centrally to the fracture of L1, which possibly indicates unhindered diffusion in an area of debris. (Courtesy of Herneth AM, Philipp MO, Naude J, et al: Vertebral metastases: assessment with apparent diffusion coefficient. *Radiology* 225:889-894, 2002. Radiological Society of North America.)

tensities of vertebral metastases and normal vertebrae were significantly different (Fig 2).

Conclusion.—Diffusion-weighted MRI is effective in permitting vertebral metastases and pathologic compression fractures to be distinguished from vertebral bodies and benign compression fractures on the basis of significantly different ADCs. The use of ADCs for patients with vertebral metastases may increase the specificity of MRI in these patients.

► These investigators from Austria and Stanford have carried out a small study on 22 patients, trying to distinguish vertebral metastatic disease with compression fracture from patients who have benign compression fractures. To do this, they have studied the ADC in assessing lesions. The idea of specificity of MRI can be increased with diffusion-weighted MRI by exploiting random translation motion of water protons. This random translational motion results in a loss of signal as a result of phased dispersion of spins, which in turn appears to be proportional to underlying ADC. The idea behind this concept is that the diffusion is minimized in tissues that have densely accumulated cells, such as tumor tissues.

In any event, this appears to be able to distinguish pathologic vertebral body collapse from benign collapse from osteoporosis or trauma. The small size of the study precludes the definitive conclusion, but this certainly looks like a promising way of making a very difficult clinical distinction.

E. Glatstein, MD

Postchemotherapy Retroperitoneal Surgery Remains Necessary in Patients With Nonseminomatous Testicular Cancer and Minimal Residual Tumor Masses

Oldenburg J, Alfsen GC, Lien HH, et al (The Norwegian Radium Hosp, Oslo, Norway)

J Clin Oncol 21:3310-3317, 2003 4–12

Background.—The retroperitoneal space is the primary site of metastases and residual tumor masses in patients with nonseminomatous germ cell tumors (NSGCTs). Complete resection usually requires retroperitoneal lymph node dissection (RPLND). Preoperative parameters predicting the histologic features of specimens obtained by RPLND were determined in patients with NSGCT with a residual mass of 20 mm in diameter or smaller after modern cisplatin-based induction chemotherapy.

Methods.—After cisplatin- or carboplatin-based induction chemotherapy, 87 patients with metastatic NSGCT underwent RPLND. The largest diameter of the residual mass on the transaxial plane was established to be 20 mm or less by abdominal CT immediately before RPLND.

Findings.—Sixty-seven percent of the patients were found to have complete fibrosis or necrosis; 26% had teratoma and 7% had vital malignant germ cell tumor. The latter group included 1 patient with rhabdomyosarcoma in the RPLND specimen. Also, in 5 of the 6 patients with vital malignant germ cell tumor, the residual lesion was 10 mm or less at pre-RPLND CT. No clinical or radiologic parameter before or after chemotherapy that significantly predicted the histologic characteristics of the residual mass could be identified.

Conclusions.—In this series, one third of retroperitoneal lesions 20 mm in diameter or smaller after chemotherapy were found to contain residual vital tumor tissue. Thus, postchemotherapy RPLND continues to be mandatory in patients with minimally sized residual lesions to reduce recurrences.

► The concept of surgical resection of "minimal" residual disease after chemotherapy for NSGCT is somewhat controversial. At Indiana University, the policy has been to resect patients with residual disease who have had nonseminomatous disease, less than a 90% reduction in the size of the pretreatment volume, and those patients with teratoma in the orchiectomy specimen.

This study suggests that even those patients with minimal disease may be considered for surgical resection. Of note is that 6 patients (7%) had persistent carcinoma in residual specimens. It should be noted, however, that 3 of 6 patients received carboplatin instead of cisplatin as primary induction therapy and that only 3 (4%) of 64 patients treated with bleomycin, etoposide, and cisplatin had residual cancer compared with 3 of 11 treated with carboplatin, etoposide, and bleomycin. Twenty-three (26%) had resected teratoma. Historically a 5% relapse rate has been seen in patients with a clinical complete remission from trials conducted at Indiana University, the Eastern Cooperative Oncology Group, and the Southeastern Cancer Study Group with cisplatin-based combination chemotherapy. It is possible that residual teratoma in some of these patients may represent an inert entity; however, the concerns for late relapse among these patients certainly exists. This is worthy of further evaluation.

P. J. Loehrer, Sr, MD

Update on Late Relapse of Germ Cell Tumor: A Clinical and Molecular Analysis

George DW, Foster RS, Hromas RA, et al (Indiana Univ Med Ctr, Indianapolis; Ohio State Univ, Columbus)

J Clin Oncol 21:113-122, 2003 4–13

Background.—Germ cell tumor (GCT), though rare, is the most common malignancy to develop in men aged 15 to 35 years. The cure rate for early stage testicular cancer is 95% to 100% with modern cisplatin-based chemotherapy and appropriate surgery. The cure rate for advanced disease is 70%. However, cancer relapses in up to 10% of men who become free of disease with initial chemotherapy. The clinical characteristics, outcomes, and molecular and cytogenetic features of patients with late relapses of GCT were reported.

Methods.—The review included 83 patients seen at 1 center from 1993 through 2000 for GCT relapse occurring more than 2 years after initial treatment. Some specimens were available for analysis for expression of the transcription regulator FoxD3 and apurinic/apyrimidinic endonuclease. The presence of chromosome 12 abnormalities was also investigated in these specimens.

Findings.—The median length of time between initial presentation and relapse was 85 months (Table 3). Of 49 patients with late relapse undergoing surgery, 43 achieved disease-free status. Twenty of this subgroup (46.5%) remained disease free. Of 32 patients given chemotherapy, only 6 (18.8%) achieved complete remission, 5 of whom remained disease free. Three of these 5 had not previously had chemotherapy. Eighteen of the 32 patients

TABLE 3.—Characteristics at Late Relapse

Characteristics	No. of Patients (%)
Time to late relapse	
2-5 years	23 (28)
> 5 years	60 (72)
Symptoms	50 (60)
Back/flank pain	20 (40)
Abdominal/pelvic pain	13 (26)
Patient-detected neck mass	5 (10)
Gastrointestinal bleeding	3 (6)
Dyspnea	3 (6)
Leg swelling	3 (6)
Other	8 (16)
Elevated tumor markers	
AFP	43 (52)
hCG	8 (10)
AFP + hCG	4 (5)
None	27 (32)
Unknown	1 (1)
Tumor sites	
Retroperitoneum	39 (47)
Lung/pleura	21 (25)
Retrocrural space	12 (14)
Abdomen/pelvis	12 (14)
Mediastinum	8 (10)
Marker only	7 (8)
Supraclavicular area	7 (8)
Liver	5 (6)
Other	9 (11)
Number of disease sites	
Marker only	7 (8)
One	47 (57)
Two	22 (27)
Three	3 (4)
Four	4 (5)
Histology	
Germ cell tumor	56 (66)
Pure teratoma	14 (17)
Transformed teratomatous elements	10 (12)
Sarcoma	5 (6)
Adenocarcinoma	5 (6)
Unknown	3 (4)
IGCC classification	
Good	56 (67)
Intermediate	13 (16)
Poor	13 (16)
Unknown	1 (1)

Abbreviations: AFP, Alphafetoprotein; *hCG*, human chorionic gonadotropin; *IGCC*, International Germ Cell Consensus.

(Courtesy of George DW, Foster RS, Hromas RA, et al: Update on late relapse of germ cell tumor: A clinical and molecular analysis. *J Clin Oncol* 21:113-122, 2003. Reprinted with permission from the American Society of Clinical Oncology.)

undergoing chemotherapy achieved disease-free status after postchemotherapy surgery, 12 of whom remained disease free. Overall, 85.2% of the 81 treated patients ultimately obtained disease-free status, with 46.9% remaining continuously free of disease at a median follow-up of 24.5 months. Another 9 patients are currently disease free after treatment for subsequent relapses. No definitive conclusions could be drawn from molecular and cytogenetic analyses.

Conclusions.—Lifetime follow-up is mandatory for men with GCT. Surgical resection alone continues to be the authors' preferred treatment for late relapse.

► The reality of late relapses in germ cell tumors has emerged during the last few years. Contraintuitively, patients who relapse greater than 2 years from initial diagnosis are less likely to be cured with chemotherapy alone than patients with earlier relapses. This study reviews a single institution's experience. The characteristics of patients with late relapses point out the findings that the vast majority have had prior nonseminomatous disease and on relapse are associated with elevated alphafetoprotein. Complete surgical resection of localized disease remains the primary treatment approach.

P. J. Loehrer, Sr, MD

Neoadjuvant Chemotherapy Plus Cystectomy Compared With Cystectomy Alone for Locally Advanced Bladder Cancer

Grossman HB, Natale RB, Tangen CM, et al (MD Anderson Cancer Ctr, Houston; Cedars-Sinai Comprehensive Cancer Ctr, Los Angeles; Southwest Oncology Group Statistical Ctr, Seattle; et al)

N Engl J Med 349:859-866, 2003 4–14

Background.—Patients with locally advanced cancer of the bladder are at a significant risk for metastases despite aggressive local therapy. A previous study by the Southwest Oncology Group showed that radiation therapy before radical cystectomy provided no improvement in outcome. Because of this finding, systemic chemotherapy has been explored in both neoadjuvant and adjuvant settings. The ability of neoadjuvant chemotherapy for improving outcome in patients with locally advanced bladder cancer who were treated with radical cystectomy was evaluated.

Methods.—A total of 307 patients with muscle-invasive bladder cancer (stage T2 to T4a) were randomly assigned to either surgery alone (154 patients) or combination of methotrexate, vinblastine, doxorubicin, and cisplatin followed by radical cystectomy (153 patients). The patients were stratified according to age (younger than 65 years vs 65 years or older) and stage (superficial muscle invasion vs more extensive disease). Analysis was by intention to treat.

Results.—Intention-to-treat analysis showed that the median survival among patients assigned to surgery alone was 46 months, whereas that of patients assigned to combination therapy was 77 months. Improved survival

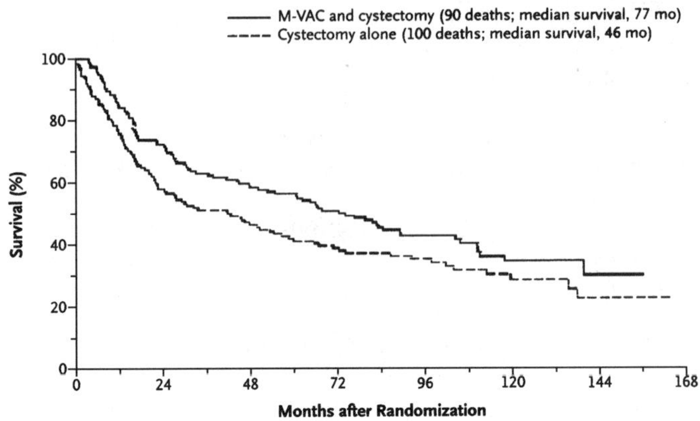

No. at Risk							
M-VAC and cystectomy	153	112	92	75	46	23	6
Cystectomy alone	154	88	67	50	37	18	7

FIGURE 1.—Survival among patients randomly assigned to receive methotrexate, vinblastine, doxorubicin, and cisplatin (M-VAC) followed by cystectomy or cystectomy alone, according to an intention-to-treat analysis. (Reprinted by permission of *The New England Journal of Medicine* from Grossman HB, Natale RB, Tangen CM, et al: Neoadjuvant chemotherapy plus cystectomy compared with cystectomy alone for locally advanced bladder cancer. *N Engl J Med* 349:859-866, 2003. Copyright 2003, Massachusetts Medical Society. All rights reserved.)

in both groups was associated with the absence of residual cancer in the cystectomy specimen (Fig 1). Significantly more patients in the combination-therapy group than in the cystectomy group had no residual disease (38% vs 15%).

Conclusions.—Among patients with locally advanced bladder cancer, the use of neoadjuvant methotrexate, vinblastine, doxorubicin, and cisplatin followed by radical cystectomy, in comparison with radical cystectomy alone, increased the likelihood of eliminating residual cancer in the cystectomy specimen. This combination therapy is associated with improved survival compared with cystectomy alone.

▶ Approximately 50% of patients with invasive bladder cancer will succumb to their disease despite surgical resection. As such, adjuvant therapy would appear logical. This study represents one of the first large trials demonstrating a therapeutic advantage with neoadjuvant methotrexate, vinblastine, doxorubicin, and cisplatin chemotherapy. Data from Europe using a cisplatin-based regimen before surgery or radiation therapy also show a survival advantage in a much larger population.[1] The authors are to be congratulated on their diligence in the completion of these trials. For patients with good performance status and organ function, this trial finally supports a role for systemic therapy.

P. J. Loehrer, Sr, MD

Reference

1. Hall RR: Updated results of a randomized controlled trial of neoadjuvant cisplatin (C), methotrexate (M) and vinblastine (V) chemotherapy for muscle-invasive bladder cancer [abstract]. *Prog Proc Am Soc Clin Oncol* 21:178a, 2002.

Expression of Thrombospondin-Derived 4N1K Peptide-Containing Proteins in Renal Cell Carcinoma Tissues Is Associated With a Decrease in Tumor Growth and Angiogenesis

Miyata Y, Koga S, Takehara K, et al (Nagasaki Univ, Japan)

Clin Cancer Res 9:1734-1740, 2003 4–15

Background.—The 4N1K peptide from thrombospondin (TSP) 1 has been found to have antiangiogenic activities. Whether the expression of 4N1K-containing proteins is associated with decreased growth of human renal cell carcinoma (RCC) was determined.

Methods and Findings.—One hundred nineteen surgically excised RCC tissues were analyzed for expression of 4N1K-containing proteins and TSP1, microvessel density, proliferation index, and apoptotic index by immunohistochemical methods. The antibody raised against the 4N1K peptide recognized protein fragments of matrix metalloproteinase 3-digested TSP1. In addition, it positively stained sections of renal cancer tissues. When the antibody was preincubated with immobilized 4N1K peptide, these reactions were not observed, indicating that the reactions may be 4N1K peptide specific. The expression of TSP1 was unassociated with various clinicopathologic features and tumor size. However, all 4N1K-positive tumors were confined locally and significantly smaller than 4N1K-negative tumors. Compared with 4N1K-negative tumors, 4N1K-positive tumors demonstrated significantly reduced microvessel density and a greater apoptotic index of tumor cells.

Conclusions.—The expression of 4N1K-containing proteins in tumor tissue appears to correlate with decreased angiogenesis and tumor growth. Thus, it may serve as a predictive marker for RCC progression.

► TSP1 is a naturally occurring antiangiogenic protein. It has been implicated as a critical factor in the body's antiangiogenic balance against factors such as vascular endothelial growth factor and fibroblast growth factor. The investigators assessed the expression of the 4N1K peptide from TSP1 in primary renal tumors from resected specimens. Using an antibody raised against these proteins, they were able to assess more than 100 surgical specimens. Among the parameters assessed were microvessel density and proliferation. There was no association between the expression of TSP1 protein and any of the biologic parameters studied. There did seem, however, to be an association with smaller primary tumors and 4N1K expression. In addition, 4N1K tumors did appear to be associated with a significantly lower microvessel density as well as a higher apoptotic index, suggesting that expression of this protein was associated with earlier, less aggressive tumors. The investigators have not yet extended their observation to paired samples with sites of metastases to determine whether primary tumors lacking TSP1 expression are associated with higher risk of distant metastatic disease, and this eventually needs to be done. The significance of this study relates to the fact that TSP1 mimetic therapies are being studied in RCC, and, as a result, a novel biologically active agent may have been identified for this disease.

M. S. Gordon, MD

Renal Cell Carcinoma With Retroperitoneal Lymph Nodes: Role of Lymph Node Dissection

Pantuck AJ, Zisman A, Dorey F, et al (Univ of California, Los Angeles)
J Urol 169:2076-2083, 2003 4–16

Background.—The benefits and morbidity of lymph node dissection in patients with localized and metastatic renal cell carcinoma have not been adequately defined. One experience was analyzed in a retrospective cohort study design.

Methods.—The charts of 1087 patients with renal cell carcinoma treated at 1 center were reviewed. Patients not receiving nephrectomy, patients with bilateral disease, and those with unknown nodal status were excluded from the analysis, leaving 900 patients meeting study criteria.

Findings.—Positive lymph nodes correlated with tumors that were larger, higher grade, locally advanced, and more commonly associated with sarcomatoid features. In addition, positive nodes were 3 to 4 times more common in patients with metastatic disease. Most of these patients could be identified preoperatively. Survival was identical in patients with regional lymph node involvement only and in those with distant metastases only. However, patients with both had a significantly worse survival than patients with one or the other. In patients with negative nodes, dissection could be performed without additional morbidity but conferred no survival advantage. Dissection was also safe in patients with positive nodes and correlated with improved survival and a trend toward improved immunotherapy response.

Conclusions.—Regional lymph node dissection is not necessary in patients with clinically negative lymph nodes. However, among patients with positive nodes, lymph node dissection in carefully selected patients undergoing cytoreductive nephrectomy and postoperative immunotherapy is associated with improved survival.

► The investigators performed a retrospective review of 900 cases of patients with unilateral renal cell cancers who underwent a nephrectomy to assess the role of lymph node dissection in this setting. They noted that clinically positive lymph nodes were typically seen in patients with metastatic disease and that patients with both metastatic disease and lymph node involvement had a somewhat poorer outcome that those with either setting alone. This may have to do with the fact that lymph node involvement was also associated with features that carry a poorer prognosis, such as more advanced primary tumor staging and the sarcomatoid histology. Importantly, patients in whom there was no clinical suspicion of lymph node involvement based on radiographic or surgical assessment rarely benefited from lymph node dissection. In contrast, there may be a value for debulking the patients with lymph node involvement prior to immunotherapy. In summary, the authors proposed that lymph node dissection be reserved only for patients in whom there is evidence of lymph node involvement and that patients with unilateral renal cell cancer without such evidence undergo the standard surgical procedure dictated by their primary tumor. This is important since the performance of nephron-sparing or laparoscopic surgery limits the ability to perform lymph node dissections.

M. S. Gordon, MD

Phase I Trial of Consensus Interferon in Patients With Metastatic Renal Cell Carcinoma: Toxicity and Immunological Effects

Hutson TE, Molto L, Mekhail T, et al (Cleveland Clinic Foundation, Ohio)
Clin Cancer Res 9:1354-1360, 2003 4–17

Background.—Metastatic renal cell carcinoma is refractory to standard chemotherapy. Consensus interferon (CIFN) is a novel synthetic type I IFN. The maximum tolerated dose, dose-limiting toxicities, and effects on chemokine/cytokine gene expression in peripheral blood mononuclear cells of CIFN was determined.

Methods.—Twenty-five patients, aged 38 to 76 years, were treated at different dose levels of subcutaneous CIFN in 4-week cycles between January 1999 and November 2000. Four received 9 μg/m^2 (group I); 14 received 15 μg/m^2 (group II); and 7 received 21 μg/m^2 (group III). Reverse transcription polymerase chain reaction was used to assess cytokine and chemokine gene expression in peripheral blood mononuclear cells.

Findings.—Dose-limiting toxicity occurred at the highest dose level. Toxicities included grade 3 or 4 respiratory distress or failure, occurring in 3 patients, and hypocalcemia, occurring in 1 patient, during the first treatment cycle. Grade 3 neutropenia, thrombocytopenia, fatigue, and nausea/vomiting were also documented. Cytokine and chemokine gene expression analyses of peripheral blood mononuclear cells from 8 patients showed induction of IFN-α, IP-10, and Mig. Administering CIFN IV induced a faster response but of a shorter duration. No responses were documented. However, 24 patients had stable disease for 4 to 32 weeks. These patients received a median of 3 treatment cycles, ranging from 1 to 8. The overall median survival was 13.5 months. In previously treated patients, the median survival was 12.7 months.

Conclusions.—These data show that the subcutaneous administration of CIFN at doses of up to 15 μg/m^2 3 times weekly is safe. None of the patients responded to treatment, yet the median survival was longer than that seen in previously treated patients with metastatic renal cell carcinoma.

▶ This phase I study assessed the safety and biologic effects of CIFN in patients with renal cell cancer. CIFN is an INF similar to INF-α and has antiviral activity superior to this latter agent. In this trial, the investigators assessed the safety of the drug, finding it to be associated with dose-limiting toxicities of respiratory failure and hypocalcemia. It did have typical INF toxicities. There were no objective responses, but many patients showed stable disease and the median survival of this previously treated group of patients was 13.5 months, which is longer than most second-line therapy studies in renal cell cancer. It is possible that this agent may have some superior effects to standard INF. However, the ease of administration of newer pegylated versions of INF may make this form of INF less desirable.

M. S. Gordon, MD

5 Hematologic Malignancies

Extramedullary Plasmacytoma: Clinical and Histopathologic Study

Strojan P, Šoba E, Lamovec J, et al (Inst of Oncology, Ljubljana, Slovenia: Maribor Teaching Hosp, Slovenia)

Int J Radiat Oncol Biol Phys 53:692-701, 2002 5–1

Background.—Among the B-cell neoplasms are plasma cell neoplasms, including solitary plasmacytoma of the bone, multiple myeloma, and extramedullary plasmacytoma (EMP). In EMP, infiltrates of plasma cells of diverse maturity and the resulting monoclonal immunoglobulin products are commonly noted. More than 80% of patients have EMP located in the upper aerodigestive tract, usually the nasal cavity, paranasal sinuses, nasopharynx, tonsils, and larynx. Most are male, and most are at advanced ages. Sixteen percent of patients progress to multiple myeloma. Treatment involves radiotherapy (XRT) or surgery. An analysis was conducted of the relationship between irradiation dose and local tumor control, the role of elective nodal irradiation, and the prognostic value of Bartl's histologic grading criteria.

Methods.—The 26 patients (5 women and 21 men; age range, 25-85 years; median age, 67 years) had 31 tumors. Follow-up extended a median of 5.1 years (range, 1.4-30.7 years).

Results.—According to Bartl's grading system, 12 tumors were grade 1, 12 were grade 2, and 2 were grade 3. Of 23 tumors having immunohistochemical analysis, 11 had clonality for immunoglobulin (Ig)G, 2 for IgM, and 1 for IgA; the 9 remaining tumors were negative for immunoglobulins. Lower 10-year disease-specific survival and a higher frequency of regional lymphadenopathy were noted in patients with high-grade tumors (Fig 1 and Table 2).

Eleven patients had XRT after diagnostic biopsy, with dosages of 40 to 50 Gy for macroscopic disease and 36 to 40 Gy for suspected microscopic disease; 18 patients had surgery, usually followed by postoperative XRT; and 2 patients had chemotherapy along with the primary XRT and nonradical surgery. For 87% of tumors, local control was achieved after the initial therapy. One patient required salvage surgery after XRT; this brought the overall rate of ultimate local control to 90%. Local recurrence developed in 3 patients

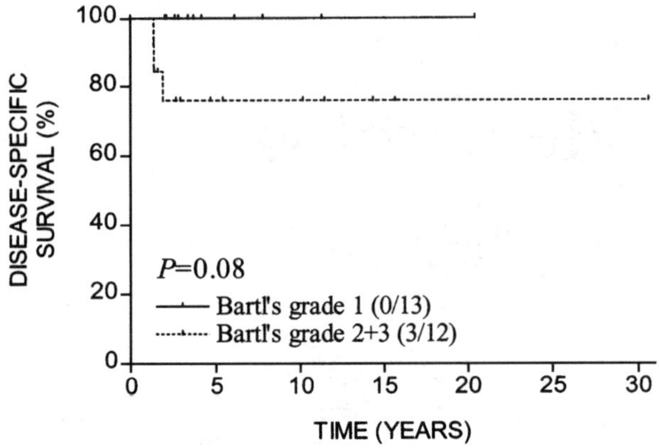

FIGURE 1.—Disease-specific survival according to Bartl's histologic grade. The *numbers in parentheses* indicate the number of events/total in each group. (Reprinted from Strojan P, Šoba E, Lamovec J, et al: Extramedullary plasmacytoma: Clinical and histopathologic study. *Int J Radiat Oncol Biol Phys* 53:692-701, 2002. Copyright 2002, with permission from Elsevier Science.)

with bulky disease and less XRT than had been planned. Of the 12 patients having surgery and postoperative XRT, none had local failure.

The overall rate of regional control was 97%, with 100% achieved for those having head and neck EMP and 80% for those with EMP in other locations. Elective nodal XRT was performed in 10 patients (Table 3). Two patients had multiple myeloma develop 22 and 25 months after EMP was diagnosed; both of these patients died, 1 after 1 month and the other after 72 months. After 2.1 to 30.7 years, 12 patients were alive without evidence of disease, 4 had died of tumor, and 9 had died of intercurrent diseases. Overall survival rates were 83% at 2 years, 78% at 5 years, and 61% at 10 years (Fig 2).

Conclusion.—When XRT is used with or without previous surgery, EMP can be highly curable, with few cases developing into multiple myeloma. Elective XRT was considered unnecessary for node-negative patients; for node-positive patients, the recommended treatment is nodectomy or neck

TABLE 2.—Prognostic Value of Bartl's Grading System

		No. of Events			
	No. of Cases	Local Failure and Multiple Myeloma	Lymph Nodes Involved at Diagnosis	Local Bone Destruction	Died of Disease
Grade					
Low	12	1	0	0	0
Intermediate	12	2	4	2	2
High	2	1	1	0	1
P value*	—	NS	0.04	NS	NS

*Fisher's exact test (2 × 2 table, low vs intermediate + high).
Abbreviation: NS, Not significant.
(Reprinted from Strojan P, Šoba E, Lamovec J, et al: Extramedullary plasmacytoma: Clinical and histopathologic study. *Int J Radiat Oncol Biol Phys* 53:692-701, 2002. Copyright 2002, with permission from Elsevier Science.)

TABLE 3.—Risk for Regional Relapse and Role of Elective Regional Nodal Irradiation: Review of the Literature

Author (Ref.)	No. of Cases	Lymph Nodes Involved at Diagnosis (%)	Elective XRT	Regional Relapse (%)	Outcome	Recommendation for Elective XRT
Knowling *et al.* (2)	25	7 (28)	No	3/25 (12)	NED,1 DODM and RD, 1 DORD, 1	Yes, selective*
Mayr *et al.* (3)	13	1 (8)	Yes, 2 No, 11	0/2 2/11 (18)	NED, 1 DODM, 1	Yes
Shih *et al.* (4)	10	3 (30)	n.r.	1/10 (10)†	n.r.	Yes
Liebross *et al.* (5)	22	n.r.	Yes, 7 No, 15	0/7 1/15 (7)	– DOMM, 1	Yes, selective‡
Susnerwala *et al.* (19)	25	2 (8)	No	1/25 (4)	RC and AWMM	No
Bush *et al.* (25)	10	2 (20)	Yes, 6 No, 4	0/10	–	Yes, selective§
Jyothirmayi *et al.* (27)	7	n.r.	No	0/7	–	No
Tsang *et al.* (31)	14	n.r.	n.s.	0/14	–	Yes, selective*
Bolek *et al.* (32)	10	2 (20)	Yes	0/10	–	Yes
Present series	31	7 (23)	Yes, 17 No, 14	1/17 (6) 0/14	DOLD & RD –	No

*For lymphatic involvement, including Waldeyer's ring presentations.
†Relapse in a lower cervical lymph node outside the previous radiation field.
‡For patients with extramedullary plasmacytoma of the oral cavity, oropharynx, nasopharynx, and larynx.
§For cases with bulky local disease only.

Abbreviations: XRT, Radiotherapy; *NED*, no evidence of disease; *DODM*, died of distant metastases; *RD*, regional disease; *DORD*, died of regional disease; *DOMM*, died of multiple myeloma; *RC*, regional control; *AWMM*, alive with multiple myeloma; *DOLD*, died of local disease; *n.r.*, not reported; *n.s.*, not specified.

(Reprinted from Strojan P, Šoba E, Lamovec J, et al: Extramedullary plasmacytoma: Clinical and histopathologic study. *Int J Radiat Oncol Biol Phys* 53:692-701, 2002. Copyright 2002, with permission from Elsevier Science.)

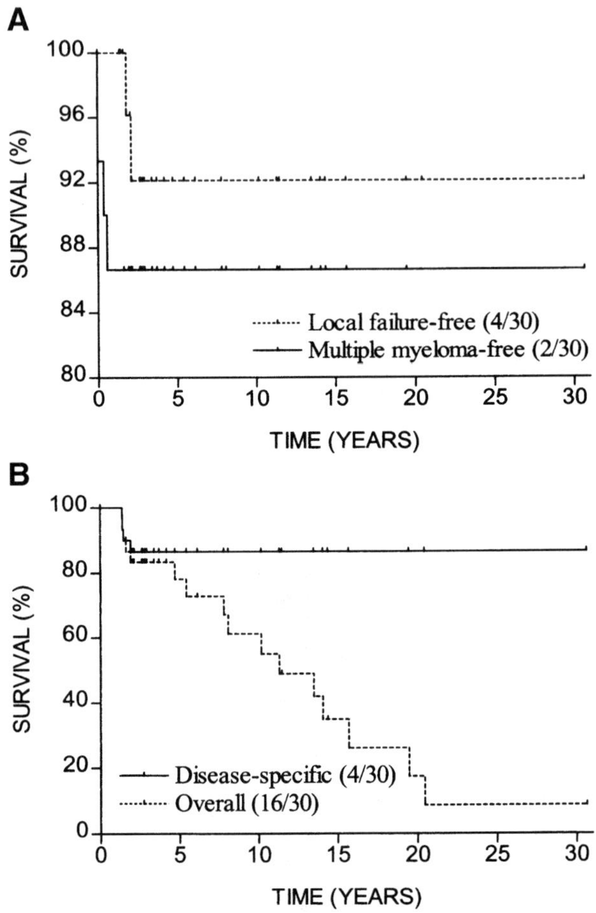

FIGURE 2.—Survival of patients with extramedullary plasmacytoma. **A**, Local failure-free survival and multiple myeloma-free survival. **B**, Disease-specific survival and overall survival. The *numbers in parentheses* indicate the number of events/total in each group. (Reprinted from Strojan P, Šoba E, Lamovec J, et al: Extramedullary plasmacytoma: Clinical and histopathologic study. *Int J Radiat Oncol Biol Phys* 53:692-701, 2002. Copyright 2002, with permission from Elsevier Science.)

dissection and then XRT with a dose of 36 to 40 Gy or XRT alone with a dose of 40 to 50 Gy. The surgical bed or affected nodal region(s) is included on the neck only. The usefulness of Bartl's grading system was undetermined.

► This is a modest size but interesting series from Slovenia with 26 patients and 31 EMPs over a 30-year period. Twenty-six patients make it a relatively large published series concerning radiation treatment. It should be noted, however, that it is only 26 patients, not 31 listed under Table 3.

One of the reasons I include this article is that it gives enough information to make the reader aware of how subtle statistics can be. Fig 1 talks about the disease-specific survival, giving the impression of a relatively favorable outcome. Fig 2A shows survival by whether or not there is failure or full multiple myeloma over time. The curve that needs to be called to the reader's attention is in Fig 2B, which gives the overall survival and shows that by 20 years, there are only approximately 10% of the patients who are still doing well. This is another example of radiation oncologists talking about local control and cancer-specific survival when they do not really want to talk about the true survival. Survival remains the most important issue in outcome, and that cannot be overemphasized.

E. Glatstein, MD

Combination Therapy With Thalidomide Plus Dexamethasone for Newly Diagnosed Myeloma

Rajkumar SV, Hayman S, Gertz MA, et al (Mayo Clinic, Rochester, Minn)
J Clin Oncol 20:4319-4323, 2002 5–2

Background.—Multiple myeloma (MM) is a plasma cell malignancy characterized by increased marrow angiogenesis. It is usually treated with a combination of vincristine, doxorubicin, and dexamethasone (VAD) for 4 to 6 months followed by autologous stem cell transplantation. Thalidomide has antiangiogenic activity and may be useful in the treatment of patients with MM. The safety and efficacy of combination dexamethasone and thalidomide therapy was examined as a less toxic alternative to VAD before transplantation induction therapy for patients with MM.

Study Design.—This study group consisted of 50 patients with newly diagnosed MM. The median serum M protein level before therapy was 3.8 g/dL. The bone marrow plasma cell percentage before therapy ranged from 10% to 97%. Thalidomide was administered orally at a dose of 200 mg/day. Birth control was required of all participants. Dexamethasone was administered orally at a dose of 40 mg on days 1 to 4, 9 to 12, 17 to 20 (odd cycles), and 1 to 4 (even cycles), repeated monthly. The primary end point was a confirmed response to therapy.

Findings.—Of the 50 treatment-naive MM patients, confirmed response was detected in 32, for a response rate of 64%. Of these patients, 31 proceeded to stem cell collection after 4 therapy cycles. Grades 3 and 4 toxicity occurred in 32% of patients. The most common were deep vein thrombosis, constipation, rash, and dyspnea. Three deaths occurred during therapy from pancreatitis, pulmonary embolism, and infection.

Conclusions.—The combination of thalidomide and dexamethasone is tolerated and effective as first-line treatment for multiple myeloma, providing an oral alternative to standard VAD therapy. The mechanism of action of thalidomide in MM is not yet understood and prognostic factors have not been defined. Long-term outcomes also await further study.

► This treatment of MM has rapidly moved beyond the old standards of alkylator-based chemotherapy. With this demonstration of antitumor activity for agents such as thalidomide in relapsed and refractory patients, application of these agents in earlier stage disease as well as in the front-line settings is being explored. In this study, Rajkumar et al assessed a regimen of pulse dexamethasone with thalidomide in newly diagnosed MM. This regimen showed promise with high response rates in patients with refractory disease. In this report, a response was seen in 32 of 50 patients, for a response rate of 64%. Complete response to this therapy was seen in approximately one fourth of patients. Predominant toxicities included those frequently seen with thalidomide, including thromboembolic events, rash, and constipation. Because the majority of patients proceeded to high-dose chemotherapy with stem cell transplant, no conclusions regarding the durability of dexamethasone/thalidomide responses can be made. Randomized trials of the regimen are ongoing.

M. S. Gordon, MD

Thalidomide Alone or With Dexamethasone for Previously Untreated Multiple Myeloma

Weber D, Rankin K, Gavino M, et al (Univ of Texas, Houston)
J Clin Oncol 21:16-19, 2003 5–3

Background.—Many treatments for multiple myeloma (MM) are useful. However, the disease eventually relapses and becomes treatment resistant. The effects of thalidomide in patients with asymptomatic MM and the effects of thalidomide-dexamethasone in patients with previously untreated symptomatic myeloma were assessed.

Methods.—Twenty-eight patients with previously untreated asymptomatic myeloma received 100 to 200 mg of thalidomide orally at bedtime. The dose was increased weekly by 50 to 100 mg, as tolerated, until a maximum of 600 mg was reached. In addition, 40 previously untreated patients with symptomatic myeloma were treated by this protocol, to a maximum dose of 400 mg, with the addition of dexamethasone, 20 mg/m^2, for 4 days beginning on days 1, 9, and 17. The second and third cycles of repeated dexamethasone were started on day 30. Treatment duration was at least 3 months in both patient groups.

Findings.—Patients given thalidomide alone had a response rate of 36%, and those given thalidomide plus dexamethasone was 72%. The latter group included complete remission in 16% of patients. The median time to remission was 4.2 months in the group receiving thalidomide only and 0.7 months in the group receiving thalidomide plus dexamethasone. Grade 3 toxicities included infections in 9 patients and thrombotic or embolic events in 7. Two patients died from MM, 1 from infection, 1 from an unknown cause, and 1 from a possible thromboembolic event.

Conclusions.—Thalidomide alone appears to be effective in treating newly diagnosed myeloma. When combined with dexamethasone, it induces a high frequency of response and a rapid onset of remission. The incidence of serious irreversible toxicity was low.

► Thalidomide is recognized as having activity in MM, with an approximately 30% response rate in relapsed patients. The addition of dexamethasone to previously treated patients raises the response rate to about 50%, and initial data suggested that the response rate is even higher in previously untreated patients. This study represents the second of 2 trials studying thalidomide in previously untreated patients either alone or in combination with dexamethasone. In 40 patients treated with the combination of thalidomide and dexamethasone, the response rate was 72%. Toxicity of the regimen included thrombotic events that were adequately prophylactically managed with oral anticoagulants. The remissions were rapid in nature with a median time to remission of less than 1 month. Patients treated with this combination maintained their ability to mobilize peripheral blood stem cells adequately. These results are superior to single-agent thalidomide, which demonstrated a response rate of 36% in a group of previously untreated patients. A current randomized trial in ECOG will define the role of this combination in first-line therapy, but the speed of response and the high response rate suggest that it will have significant value.

M. S. Gordon, MD

High-Dose Chemotherapy With Hematopoietic Stem-Cell Rescue for Multiple Myeloma

Child JA, for the Medical Research Council Adult Leukaemia Working Party (Univ of Leeds, England; et al)

N Engl J Med 348:1875-1883, 2003 5–4

Background.—High-dose therapy with supporting autologous stem-cell transplantation for treating cancer continues to be controversial. First-line regimens with high-dose therapy in patients with multiple myeloma are associated with better remission rates than conventional-dose therapies. However, there is limited evidence that this translates to improved survival.

Methods.—Four hundred seven patients were enrolled in the Medical Research Council Myeloma VII Trial, a multicenter study. All had untreated disease and were younger than 65 years. Patients received either standard conventional-dose combination chemotherapy or high-dose treatment and an autologous stem-cell transplant. At the end of the study, 401 patients were evaluable.

Findings.—Complete response rates were higher in the patients receiving intensive therapy than in those receiving standard therapy: 44% and 8%, respectively. Partial response rates were 42% and 40%, respectively. The rates of minimal response were 3% in the intensive treatment group and 18% in the standard treatment group. In an intention-to-treat analysis, the intensive therapy group had a greater overall and progression-free survival than did the standard treatment group. The median survival was 54.1 months in the intensive treatment group and 42.3 months in the standard-therapy group. The survival benefit showed a trend to being greater in patients with a poor prognosis, defined by high β_2-microglobulin concentrations.

Conclusions.—High-dose autologous stem-cell rescue therapy appears to be an effective first-line approach for treating multiple myeloma in patients younger than 65 years. Further research is warranted.

▶ These investigators report on the results of a randomized trial of standard IV chemotherapy compared with a combination of standard therapy followed by high-dose chemotherapy. Over 400 patients were randomly assigned to this trial, which suffers from the fact that the standard therapy was not identical to the pretransplant therapy used in the high-dose arm. Patients in the high-dose arm who achieved a maximal response to standard induction therapy were then treated with stem cell mobilization and transplant. The authors present that there is a statistically significant survival advantage for patients undergoing high-dose chemotherapy compared with standard therapy and that this is associated with a higher rate of complete responders in the experimental arm. They do not define the responses at the 2 different stages of therapy in the experimental arm, and hence it is difficult to determine whether or not the standard arm with an 8% complete response rate acted significantly differently than the induction portion of the experimental arm. This is one potential confounder in the study. Given the fact, however, that multiple randomized trials of different chemotherapy regimens have failed to identify a clearly superior standard chemotherapy, it is likely that the greatest degree of benefit was derived from the high-dose chemotherapy. This study therefore identifies in a randomized fashion the standard for patients with multiple myeloma who are eligible for high-dose chemotherapy.

M. S. Gordon, MD

Response Rate, Durability of Response, and Survival After Thalidomide Therapy for Relapsed Multiple Myeloma

Kumar S, Gertz MA, Dispenzieri A, et al (Mayo Clinic, Rochester, Minn)

Mayo Clin Proc 78:34-39, 2003 5–5

Background.—In multiple myeloma (MM), a clonal proliferation of abnormal plasma cells in the bone marrow results in a variety of clinical manifestations. Osteolytic bone lesions, anemia, life-threatening hypercalcemia, and renal failure can occur. The efficacy of thalidomide in patients with MM relapse was investigated.

Methods.—Thirty-two patients with relapsed MM were enrolled in the study. Patient ages ranged from 36 to 78 years. In all patients, previous chemotherapy had failed. In 5, stem cell transplantation had failed. The patients received oral thalidomide, 200 mg/d, for 2 weeks. This dose was increased as tolerated to no more than 800 mg/d.

Findings.—Ten responses were confirmed for a rate of 31%. Also, 1 unconfirmed partial response and 7 minimal responses were reported. The median response duration was 11.9 months. Twenty patients died, and disease progressed in 26. Surviving patients were followed up for a median of 28.5 months. The median progression-free survival was 8.6 months. Treatment responders had a median progression-free survival of 15.7 months. For the whole group, median survival was 22 months. Grade 3 or greater treatment-related nonhematologic toxicities included neuropathy in 16%, sedation in 13%, febrile neutropenia in 6%, and constipation in 6%.

Conclusions.—Thalidomide appears to be useful in treating relapsed MM. In the current series, thalidomide yielded a durable response in approximately one third of the patients, the median response duration being nearly 1 year.

▶ The authors report on their experience in relapsed and refractory myeloma with the drug thalidomide. This agent has a known activity profile in this patient population. Thirty-two patients were accrued to a single institution study assessing the value of thalidomide in a previously treated group of patients. This group of patients was perhaps not as refractory as others, with only 10 patients having undergone a prior cycle of high-dose chemotherapy. Overall, the response rate was approximately 30%, which is similar to other reported series. The median follow-up for responding patients was 28.5 months, with a median progression-free survival of 8.6 months for all patients and twice as long (15.7 months) in responding patients. Side effects were typical for thalidomide and included constipation, neuropathy, and sedation. The use of thalidomide in myeloma has defined activity and can be considered a standard for patients with relapsed and refractory disease.

M. S. Gordon, MD

A Phase 2 Study of Bortezomib in Relapsed, Refractory Myeloma

Richardson PG, Barlogie B, Berenson J, et al (Dana-Farber Cancer Inst, Boston; Univ of Arkansas, Little Rock; Cedars-Sinai Med Ctr, Los Angeles; et al)

N Engl J Med 348:2609-2617, 2003 5–6

Background.—The boronic acid dipeptide bortezomib is a novel proteasome inhibitor. Preclinical and phase I studies have shown that bortezomib has antimyeloma activity. The effects of bortezomib were investigated in patients with relapsed, refractory myeloma.

Methods.—Two hundred two patients were enrolled in the multicenter, open-label, nonrandomized trial. All had relapsed myeloma refractory to most recent treatment. Treatment consisted of bortezomib, 1.3 mg/m^2 of body surface area, twice weekly for 2 weeks, followed by 1 week with no therapy, for up to 8 cycles. Oral dexamethasone was added to the treatment regimen of patients with a suboptimal response to bortezomib alone. At the end of the study, 193 patients were evaluable.

Findings.—Ninety-two percent of the evaluable patients had received 3 or more of the major classes of agents for myeloma. The bortezomib response rate was 35%. Among the responders were 7 patients in whom myeloma protein became undetectable and 12 in whom this protein was detected only by immunofixation. Overall, the median survival was 16 months. The median duration of response was 12 months. Fourteen percent of patients had grade 4 adverse events. Grade 3 events included thrombocytopenia in 28%, fatigue in 12%, peripheral neuropathy in 12%, and neutropenia in 11%.

Conclusions.—In this series of patients with relapsed, refractory myeloma, the novel proteasome inhibitor bortezomib was able to induce a clinically significant response with manageable toxic effects. Currently, an international, randomized, phase III trial is underway comparing bortezomib with high-dose dexamethasone in this patient population.

▶ Multiple myeloma is a complex hematologic disorder with limited available therapies. Front-line therapy typically consists of chemotherapy followed by high-dose chemotherapy with stem cell rescue. Even with this aggressive therapy, there is no cure for multiple myeloma. Recent studies have demonstrated that the class of drugs known as proteasome inhibitors has activity in multiple myeloma and may have use in the setting of relapsed and refractory disease. This phase II trial represents a large single-arm experience with the proteasome inhibitor bortezomib. The agent, administered twice weekly for 2 weeks followed by a week off, was able to induce objective responses in 35% of the 193 evaluable patients. Among these responders were 7 patients who attained complete responses with disappearance of their myeloma protein. The median overall survival in this heavily pretreated group was approximately 16 months. The agent was well tolerated, with mild myelosuppression as its principle toxicity. This study is critical for a number of reasons; first, it defines the activity of this agent in a significantly unmet need. Second, it represents the first evidence of activity for a new class of drugs, the proteasome inhibitors, and provides a rationale for further investigation of these agents in other malignancies. A phase III trial comparing bortezomib with standard pulse dexamethasone has been completed and the results are pending.

M. S. Gordon, MD

Should Adolescents With Acute Lymphoblastic Leukemia Be Treated as Old Children or Young Adults? Comparison of the French FRALLE-93 and LALA-94 Trials

Boissel N, Auclerc M-F, Lhéritier V, et al (Hôpital Saint-Louis, Paris; Hôpital Trousseau, Paris; Hôpital Edouard Herriot, Lyon, France; et al)

J Clin Oncol 21:774-780, 2003 5–7

Background.—There has been considerable progress in the treatment of childhood acute lymphoblastic leukemia (ALL) over the past few decades, and this has resulted in dramatic improvements in prognosis for these patients. However, this progress in pediatric therapy has also widened the gap between outcomes in children and adults. Recent pediatric trials have reported complete remission rates of 95% to 99% and estimated 5-year event-free survival (EFS) rates approaching 80%, but in adult trials only 80% to 85% of patients with ALL usually obtain complete remission, and only 30% to 40% are still alive 5 years later. The pediatric and adult therapeutic practices in the treatment of ALL in adolescents were compared.

Methods.—From June 1993 to September 1994, 77 and 100 adolescents were enrolled in the pediatric FRALLE-93 and adult LALA-94 protocols, respectively. The patients ranged in age from 15 to 20 years. The effects on the trial of achieving complete remission and EFS were evaluated.

Results.—The patients in the FRALLE-93 protocol were younger than those in the LALA-94 protocol (15.9 vs 17.9 years). However, other characteristics were similar, including median white blood cell count, B/T lineage, CD10-negative ALL, and poor-risk cytogenics. The rate of complete remission depended on white blood cell count and trial (Fig 1). Univariate analysis indicated that unfavorable prognostic factors for EFS were the trial, an in-

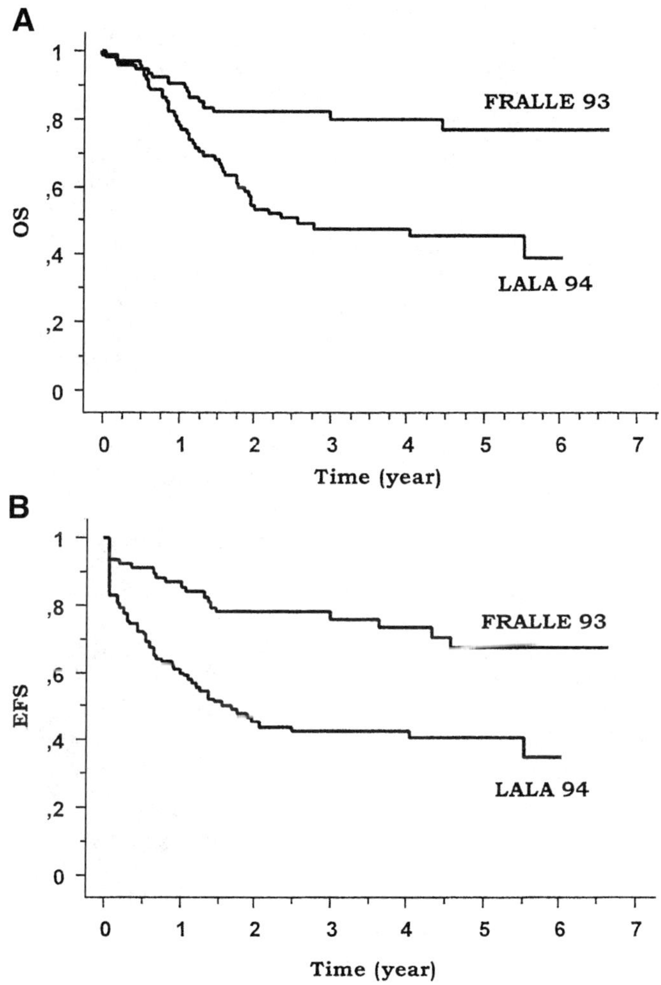

FIGURE 1.—Overall survival (A) and EFS (B) according to the protocol. (Courtesy of Boissel N, Auclerc M-F, Lhéritier V, et al: Should adolescents with acute lymphoblastic leukemia be treated as old children or young adults? Comparison of the French FRALLE-93 and LALA-94 trials. *J Clin Oncol* 21:774-780, 2003. Reprinted with permission from the American Society of Clinical Oncology.)

creasing white blood cell count, poor-risk cytogenics, and T lineage. The trial and white blood cell count persisted as significant prognostic factors for EFS on multivariate analysis. Lineage subgroup analysis showed an advantage for the FRALLE-93 trial for achievement of complete remission (98% vs 81%) and EFS in B lineage ALL and for EFS in T lineage ALL. Age was not a significant prognostic factor in this population.

Conclusions.—It would appear from these findings that adolescents should be included in intensive pediatric protocols. It is recommended that new trials for the treatment of young adults with ALL be designed on the basis of pediatric protocols.

► For many years, the issue of whether to treat adolescents and young adults with cancer according to more intensive pediatric approaches versus often less intensive protocols designed for adult patients has been controversial. In this study by Boissel et al, a group of adolescents and young adults with ALL were treated on either a pediatric protocol (FRALLE-93) or an adult protocol (LALA-94). When patient and leukemia characteristics were balanced, a major prognostic factor was the protocol that was used. That is, patients treated with the FRALLE-93 protocol had a significantly improved outcome in the rate of complete remission, overall survival, and EFS compared with patients treated on the LALA-94 protocol. Thus, for this group of patients with B- or T-lineage ALL, outcomes were significantly better when the FRALLE-93 pediatric protocol was used. It is unclear what the basis for the outcome differences is, but the intensity and more rapid timing of chemotherapy courses were felt to play important roles. Thus, adolescents with ALL are likely to have a better outcome when treated by intensive pediatric protocols. It remains unclear how far up the age spectrum this conclusion can be extended or whether such a recommendation will also help adults with ALL characterized by other features, such as the t(9;22) translocation.

R. J. Arceci, MD, PhD

The Lethal Effects of Pharmacological Cyclin-Dependent Kinase Inhibitors in Human Leukemia Cells Proceed Through a Phosphatidylinositol 3-Kinase/Akt-Dependent Process

Yu C, Rahmani M, Dai Y, et al (Virginia Commonwealth Univ, Richmond)
Cancer Res 63:1822-1833, 2003 5–8

Background.—Little is known about the signaling events underlying the induction of apoptosis by flavopiridol (FP) and other pharmacologic cyclin-dependent kinase (CDK) inhibitors. In addition, virtually nothing is known about the role of the phosphatidylinositol 3-kinase (PI3K) pathway in regulating apoptosis in cells subjected to CDK inhibition. The effects of disruption of the PI3K pathway on the response of human leukemia cells to pharmacologic CDK inhibitors were determined.

Methods and Findings.—U937 monocytic leukemia cells were exposed to minimally toxic levels of FP, roscovitine, or CGP74514A for 3 hours, in conjunction with the P13K inhibitor LY294002 (LY). A marked decline in Akt phosphorylation resulted. Co-exposing cells to LY and CDK inhibitors lead to a marked increase in mitochondrial damage within 3 hours, along with caspase activation and apoptosis. Similar interactions occurred in a variety of other leukemia cell types. Ectopic expression of Bcl-2 markedly blocked FP-LY-induced apoptosis, though to a much lesser extent than by dominant-negative caspase-8. Agents inhibiting protein kinase (PK) A, PKC, mitogen-activated protein (MAP)/extracellular signal-regulated kinase (ERK) kinase p38 MAP kinase, m-target of rapamycin, and ataxia-telangiectasia mutation did not enhance FP-induced apoptosis. However, the P13K inhibitor wortmannin had effects comparable to those of LY. Diminished Bad phosphorylation, Bcl-2 cleavage induction, and downregulation of X-linked IAP and Mcl-1 cells accompanied the striking potentiation of CDK inhibitor-induced apoptosis by LY. In addition, cells exposed to CDK inhibitors and LY demonstrated decreased phosphorylation of glycogen synthase kinase-3, forkhead transcription factor, $p70^{S6K}$, and ERK. However, $p34^{cdc2}$ and p38 MAPK activation was increased. Cells treated with LY/CDK also showed a reduction in pEb dephosphorylation on CDK2- and CDK4-specific sites as well as retinoblastoma protein cleavage and cyclin D_1 downregulation. Inducible expression of constitutively active Akt partially but significantly attenuated apoptosis in Jurkat leukemia cells treated by FP alone or combined with LY. Combined LY and FP treatment produced a marked elevation in apoptosis in primary leukemic blasts from a patient with acute myeloblastic leukemia.

Conclusions.—These data suggest that the PI3K/Akt pathway has an important role in regulating the apoptotic response of human leukemia cells to pharmacologic CDK inhibitors. The combined interruption of CDK- and P13K-related pathways may be a novel approach for treating hematologic malignancies.

► The cell cycle pathway is one of the most critical targets for anti-cancer therapy. It has long been recognized that a number of enzymatic pathways are critical to cells traveling in the cell cycle and that their inhibition can lead to apoptosis and cell death. What has not been clear is the specific mechanism of action of these agents. An example of one specific target is CDK. Inhibitors of CDK induce apoptosis of tumor cells, though the specific pathway associated with this effect is unclear. These investigators performed studies with a leukemia cell line demonstrating that CDK inhibition induces apoptosis by a PI3K/Akt pathway. The impact of this observation is significant since this pathway is affected by numerous agents that affect the HER growth factor signaling system. Hence, the rationale for the combination of CDK and PI3K/Akt inhibitors has been identified, and it is anticipated that such preclinical and clinical studies may provide enhanced antitumor activity.

M. S. Gordon, MD

Clinical Relevance of Internal Tandem Duplication of the *FLT3* Gene in Childhood Acute Myeloid Leukemia

Liang D-C, Shih L-Y, Hung I-J, et al (Mackay Mem Hosp, Taipei, Taiwan; Chang Gung Univ, Taipei, Taiwan; Chang Gung Children's Hosp, Linkou, Taiwan; et al)
Cancer 94:3292-3298, 2002 5–9

Background.—Outcomes in patients with childhood acute myeloid leukemia (AML) have improved significantly with the development of modern chemotherapy. Cytogenic studies have demonstrated the heterogeneity of AML and the prognostic impact of clonal chromosomal abnormalities. It has also been shown that the response to chemotherapy is significantly affected by the presence of specific genetic abnormalities; however, specific fusion transcripts resulting from chromosomal translocations that are of prognostic significance are present in only 40% of childhood AML. Thus, it would be beneficial if new molecular abnormalities other than specific fusion transcripts could predict the outcome of childhood AML. A recent study has identified an internal tandem duplication of the *FLT3* gene (*FLT3*/ITD) in approximately 20% of patients with adult AML that is associated with a poor outcome. The clinical significance of *FLT3*/ITD in childhood AML was investigated.

Methods.—Genomic DNA polymerase chain reaction (PCR) was used to identify *FLT3*/ITD in 80 children with de novo AML. Genescan analysis was then conducted to determine the allelic distribution of those PCR products with aberrant bands. Direct sequencing of PCR products was then performed in each sample with *FLT3*/ITD.

Results.—*FLT3*/ITD was identified in 9 of 80 patients with AML, for an incidence of 11.3%. The size of duplicated fragments ranged from 21 base pairs (bp) to 75 bp, and the mutant to wild-type ratio of *FLT3* ranged from 0.28 to 16.60 in the 9 patients with *FLT3*/ITD. The incidence of *FLT3*/ITD in childhood AML in patients older than 10 years was 24% compared with 5% of those patients 10 years or younger. There were 6 non-M3 AML patients with *FLT3*/ITD, all of whom were older than 10 years. In the 12 patients with acute promyelocytic leukemia, *FLT3*/ITD was found in 2 of 2 patients with S-form *PML/RARα* compared with 1 in 10 patients with non-S-form *PML/RARα*. No cytogenetic abnormalities or fusion transcripts derived from common specific translocations were found in non-M3 AML patients with *FLT3*/ITD. No correlation was found between the treatment outcome and the presence of *FLT3*/ITD in non-M3 AML patients; rather, all 3 patients with a mutant *FLT3* to wild-type ratio of greater than 2.0 died within 8 months of diagnosis, and 2 of these patients did not achieve complete remission.

Conclusions.—Mutant *FLT3* to wild-type ratio, not the presence of *FLT3*/ITD itself, may serve as a potential marker for improvement of risk assessment in childhood AML.

► Prognostic factors that can both predict outcome and direct therapy are important to identify in AML. The analysis of mutations in the *FLT3* receptor, a class III tyrosine kinase receptor, has been extensively studied in adult patients with AML and less well studied in children. In addition, recent data would suggest that internal tandem duplications of this receptor are associated with a poor prognosis, higher initial white blood cell count, and, in some studies, a lower remission rate. More recent studies have suggested that more important than the mere presence of an *FLT3*/ITD is the ratio of mutant to normal alleles. In this study by Liang et al, the impact of *FLT3* mutations in pediatric patients with AML was examined. This study raises several important points. First, the numbers of the study are small, thus compromising conclusions, despite some significant or nonsignificant *P* values. Second, the treatment that the patients received was not very similar to the best outcome therapies provided in North America or in Europe; this raises the issue of how different prognostic factors can correlate with different outcomes based on the therapy patients receive. Third, despite some limitations of the study, the data do suggest that in nonpromyelocytic leukemia, the ratio of ITD mutant to normal alleles for the *FLT3* gene may be a critical measurement and should be studied more closely and prospectively.

R. J. Arceci, MD, PhD

Identification of Gene Expression Profiles That Segregate Patients With Childhood Leukemia

Moos PJ, Raetz EA, Carlson MA, et al (Univ of Utah, Salt Lake City; Univ of New Mexico, Albuquerque; Univ of Colorado, Denver)

Clin Cancer Res 8:3118-3130, 2002 5–10

Introduction.—Emerging technologies, including DNA microarrays, facilitate gene expression analysis on an unprecedented scale. Important clinical applications of this technology include refinement of diagnoses, predictions of prognosis, assessment of disease progression, and detection of relevant pathways for the design of new therapeutics. To identify genes whose expression correlate with biologic characteristics of childhood leukemia, the expression profiles of 4608 genes by cDNA microarrays were prospectively examined in 51 freshly processed bone marrow samples from children with acute leukemia.

Methods.—Two supervised techniques of analysis were used to detect the 20 best discriminating genes between these cohorts: acute myelogenous leukemia (AML) versus acute lymphoblastic leukemia (ALL), B-lineage versus T-lineage ALL, newly diagnosed B-lineage standard-risk versus high-risk ALL, and B-lineage leukemia harboring the *TEL-AML1* fusion versus patients with no molecularly characterized translocation.

Results.—These techniques identified overlapping sets of genes that segregated patients within described subgroups. Cross-validation revealed that most patients could be correctly classified based on these genes alone. Hierarchical clustering grouped patients with similar and clinical disease characteristics. The potential for select genes to discriminate patients was verified by real-time polymerase chain reaction in samples that were examined by microarray profiling and in uniformly processed leukemia marrow samples.

Conclusion.—As expected, microarray technology can successfully segregate patients defined by traditional measures, including immunophenotype and cytogenetic alterations. Among specific subgroups, this preliminary analysis also indicates that microarrays can detect unanticipated similarities and diversity in persons and therefore may be helpful in future risk-group stratification.

► The use of microarray RNA expression analysis to discriminate among different types of leukemia or solid tumors is continuing to provide new information, especially in subtypes that have not been as easy to classify. The study by Moos et al used expression profiles that include about 4600 cDNAs to study 51 cases of acute leukemia. The results show that such an expression analysis can discriminate different classes of leukemia, such as AML versus ALL, B lineage versus T lineage and, of more interest, standard-risk versus high-risk ALL and B-lineage ALL with and without the *TEL-AML1* translocation. One could argue that simply determining whether *TEL-AML1* was present would be easier than doing microarray expression analysis. While such a conclusion would be true, the expression analysis provides the potential for deepening our understanding of the other characteristics of specific leukemias and potentially help to identify new pathways that could be therapeutically targeted. This latter point offers much more potential than for using this new technology simply to risk-group stratify.

R. J. Arceci, MD, PhD

Presence of Clone-Specific Markers at Birth in Children With Acute Lymphoblastic Leukaemia

Hjalgrim LL, Madsen HO, Melbye M, at al (Statens Serum Institut, Copenhagen; Natl Univ Hosp, Copenhagen; Univ of Aarhus, Denmark; et al)

Br J Cancer 87:994-999, 2002 5–11

Introduction.—B-precursor acute lymphoblastic leukemia (ALL) is the most common subtype of pediatric leukemia and is responsible for the peak in ALL incidence observed between the ages of 2 and 5 years in industrialized countries. Recent trials have suggested that the development of ALL may frequently be initiated in utero. Approximately 25% of all cases of B-precursor ALL are characterized by a translocation between chromosomes 12 and 21. This translocation fuses 2 putative transcriptional regulators, *TEL* and *AML1*, which are both important in the early hematopoiesis, producing a *TEL-AML1* transcript. A molecular biologic investigation was performed in 9 children with B-precursor ALL who carried the chromosomal translocation t(12;21).

Methods.—For each child, the nonconstitutive chromosomal sequences that made up the t(12;21) fusion gene were identified. Leukemia clone-specific DNA primers were constructed and applied in nested polymerase chain reaction analyses of DNA extracted from the patients' Guthrie cards obtained at birth.

Results.—Leukemia clone-specific fusion genes were identified in Guthrie card DNA in 3 children, aged 2 years, 11 months; 3 years, 4 months; and 5 years, 8 months at leukemia diagnosis.

Conclusion.—These findings are consistent with prior observations, thus providing further evidence that the development of t(12;21) B-precursor ALL may be initiated in utero. Review of the current literature suggests that age at leukemia may be inversely associated with the burden of cells with leukemia clonal markers (ie, leukemia predisposed cells at birth) and that particular types of childhood ALL develop as a multiple step process involving both prenatal and postnatal genetic events.

► The prenatal origin of some types of acute leukemia and solid tumors has been established with both molecular studies and radiographic methods. Such studies are important, particularly those involving molecular analyses, as they may point to clues of etiology and biologic behavior. The report by Hjalgrim et al demonstrates that 3 of 9 patients with ALL characterized by the chromosomal translocation t(12;21), which results in a *TEL-AML1* fusion transcript, had evidence on their newborn Duffy card blood samples of this precise translocation. These results thus provide evidence for prenatal development of this subtype of ALL. Future studies will hopefully be able to address the questions of when during embryogenesis such abnormal clones arise, what the subsequent changes are that lead to leukemia, and whether the leukemias that arise in utero differ in biologic behavior from those that arise postnatally.

R. J. Arceci, MD, PhD

Significant Correlation Between the Degree of *WT1* Expression and the International Prognostic Scoring System Score in Patients With Myelodysplastic Syndromes

Cilloni D, for the Piedmont Study Group on Myelodysplastic Syndromes (Univ of Turin, Italy; et al)

J Clin Oncol 21:1988-1995, 2003 5–12

Background.—The myelodysplastic syndromes (MDS) are clonal hematopoietic stem cell diseases characterized by ineffective dysplastic hematopoiesis, peripheral-blood cytopenia, and a high risk of progression to acute myeloid leukemia (AML). The International Prognostic Scoring System (IPSS) evaluates marrow blast cell percentage, karyotype, and degree of cytopenia to assess risk, facilitate clinical decision making, and assist in the design of clinical trials. The Wilms' tumor gene, *WT1*, is normally barely expressed in normal peripheral blood (PB) and bone marrow (BM) but is highly expressed in most acute forms of leukemia. Whether the pattern of *WT1* expression could represent a useful prognostic and progression marker for MDS was examined.

Study Design.—Bone marrow samples were obtained from 79 patients with refractory anemia (RA), 31 patients with RA with excess blasts (RAEB), 18 patients with secondary AML (s-AML) evolved from MDS, and 3 patients with 5q deletion as their only cytogenetic abnormality. PB samples were also collected from 42 of these patients. All these samples were tested for *WT1* expression, which was correlated with the IPSS score. Samples were also obtained during follow-up of 3 patients with RA and 7 patients with RAEB who were treated with supportive therapy only and progressed to acute leukemia. Two patients with RAEB who had intense eradicating chemotherapy were also monitored. Cytogenetic analysis was performed for all patients. A control group consisting of 31 normal BM samples, 46 normal PB samples, and PB samples from 2 patients with megaloblastic anemia, and 5 patients with erythroid hyperplasia caused by hemolytic anemia were also tested for *WT1* expression. The *WT1* expression pattern was determined by real-time quantitative polymerase chain reaction assay.

Findings.—*WT1* expression above the levels of normal controls was observed in 65% of BM and 78% of PB samples of patients with RA and 100% of both BM and RA samples from patients with RAEB and s-AML. The degree of *WT1* expression was well correlated with MDS type. It was higher in RAEB and s-AML than in RA and increased with disease progression. There was a significant correlation between *WT1* expression levels, blast cell percentage, and the presence of cytogenetic abnormalities. There was also a significant correlation between *WT1* expression levels and the IPSS score.

Conclusions.—The expression of *WT1* was examined in BM and PB from patients with MDS. These patients have excess expression of *WT1*, which increases with disease progression and is correlated with both blast percentage and cytogenetic alterations. There is a very high correlation between *WT1* expression and IPSS. This suggests that *WT1* is a useful molecular marker for MDS risk assessment and disease progression. The biologic significance of *WT1* overexpression in MDS remains to be elucidated.

► *WT1* is a tumor suppressor gene that is overexpressed in patients with AML. This study explores the relationship between *WT1* expression and the leukemic evolution of MDS. Samples from 131 patients with MDS were obtained and real-time quantitative polymerase chain reaction assay was performed for the *WT1* transcript. *WT1* expression was directly correlated with the number of BM blast cells present. As a result, *WT1* expression also directly correlated with the IPSS. Increased numbers of blasts, more complex cytogenetics, and worsened cytopenias all correlated with *WT1* expression. Specifically, what role *WT1* plays in the evolution from MDS to AML is unclear and, more importantly, the possibility that *WT1* could become a target for anticancer therapy needs to be explored. Further investigation of its actual role in MDS evolution is necessary.

M. S. Gordon, MD

Combined Treatment With Arsenic Trioxide and All-Trans-Retinoic Acid in Patients With Relapsed Acute Promyelocytic Leukemia

Raffoux E, Rousselot P, Poupon J, et al (Hôpital Saint-Louis, Paris; Hôpital Fernand Widal, Paris; Hôpital Necker, Paris; et al)

J Clin Oncol 21:2326-2334, 2003 5–13

Background.—Arsenic trioxide (ATO) can induce a high hematologic response rate in patients with relapsed acute promyelocytic leukemia (APL). Preclinical studies suggest that all-trans-retinoic acid (ATRA) may strongly enhance ATO response. ATO alone was compared with ATO plus ATRA in patients with relapsed APL.

Methods.—Twenty patients with relapsed APL were enrolled in the randomized study between 1998 and 2001. All had been previously treated with ATRA-containing chemotherapy.

Findings.—Eighty percent of the patients obtained a complete response after 1 induction cycle consisting of ATO with or without ATRA. Clinical and pharmacokinetic analyses showed that induction of APL cell differentiation was the main mechanism of action of ATO in vivo. The 2 treatment groups were comparable in hematologic and molecular response, time needed to reach complete response, and outcomes. Three of 16 patients obtaining a complete response who reached molecular remission after 1 induction cycle all received chemotherapy for treatment-induced hyperleukocytosis. Another 3 patients receiving further ATO with or without ATRA cycles later converted to molecular negativity.

Conclusions.—In these patients with APL relapse, ATRA did not appear to significantly improve responses to ATO. Further research is needed to assess other potential combinations, including ATO plus chemotherapy.

► APL is a rare hematologic malignancy that is characterized by the use of ATRA as a differentiating agent. This agent is highly effective in inducing complete remissions in patients with APL. A second differentiating agent that has activity in this disease is ATO. In this study, a small number of patients previously treated with ATRA were exposed either to ATO alone or in combination with ATRA. Overall, 20 patients were randomly assigned to the 2 arms. The complete remission rate was 80% regardless of whether patients received single-agent or combination therapy. No differences in molecular remissions were seen. The conclusion of the authors is that the addition of ATRA does not appear to add significantly to the treatment of patients with relapsed disease. A large intergroup US trial is currently being conducted that will address the role of arsenic in front-line therapy of APL.

M. S. Gordon, MD

Therapy-Related Acute Promyelocytic Leukemia

Beaumont M, Sanz M, Carli PM, et al (Service des Maladies du Sang, Lille, France; Hôpital du Bocage, Dijon, France; CHU, Strasbourg, France; et al)

J Clin Oncol 21:2123-2137, 2003 5–14

Background.—Until the early 1980s, most cases of therapy-related myelodysplastic syndromes (tMDS) and acute myeloid leukemia (tAML) developed 3 to 10 years after prolonged use of alkylating agents and presented as tMDS with complete or partial deletion of chromosome 7 or 5, often with other cytogenetic abnormalities. More recently, however, tAML has been described after the use of topoisomerase II inhibitors. These illnesses often showed normal karyotype or cytogenetic rearrangements specific to de novo AML, with 11q23 prearrangements predominating, yet t(8;21), inv(16), and 6(15;17) were less often seen. Acute promyelocytic leukemia (APL) is a specific subtype of AML that is characterized by the morphology of blasts (hypergranular cells with many Auer rods), t(15;17) translocation leading, at the molecular level, to promyelocytic leukemia–retinoic acid receptor alpha (PML-RARα) rearrangement, major coagulopathy, and specific differentiation of blast cells by all-*trans*-retinoic acid (ATRA). Patients with tAPL that developed after chemotherapy, radiotherapy, or both for a prior disorder, diagnosed in the last 20 years in 3 European countries were analyzed.

Methods.—This retrospective analysis reviewed the primary disorder and its treatment, the interval from primary disorder to development of tAPL, characteristics of tAPL, and its outcome in 106 patients.

Results.—Of the 106 cases of tAPL included in this study, 80 were diagnosed in the past decade, which is indicative of an increasing incidence of tAPL. The primary disorders were predominantly breast carcinoma (60 patients), non-Hodgkin's lymphoma (15 patients), and other solid tumors (25 patients). Chemotherapy alone was administered to 30 patients, 27 patients had received radiotherapy alone, and 49 patients had received both chemotherapy and radiotherapy. Chemotherapy included at least 1 alkylating agent in 68 patients and at least 1 topoisomerase II inhibitor in 61 patients, including anthracyclines (30 patients), mitoxantrone (28 patients), and epipodophyllotoxins (19 patients). The median interval from primary disorder to tAPL diagnosis was 25 months, with a range of 4 to 276 months. The characteristics of tAPL were found to be generally similar to those of de novo APL. The actuarial survival with treatment using anthracycline-cytarabine–based chemotherapy or ATRA combined with chemotherapy was 59% at 8 years.

Conclusions.—This retrospective study of tAPL found that tAPL is not exceptional and usually develops less than 3 years after a primary neoplasm, particularly breast carcinoma, is treated in particular with topoisomerase II–targeted drugs. The characteristics and outcome of tAPL appear to be similar to those of de novo APL.

► Therapy-related solid tumors and hematologic malignancies have increased in frequency over the last several decades. In proportion to more widespread usage of chemotherapy and radiation therapy, well known are the risks with chronic use of alkylating agents that result in myelodysplastic syndrome and acute myelogenous leukemia. These are usually associated with the lesions of chromosome 5, 7, and others. The usage of topoisomerase II inhibitors (etoposide, tenoposide) has also been shown to increase the risk of acute myelogenous leukemia but do so within 1 to 2 years of therapy. APL is a less common subtype of acute myelogenous leukemia, which is associated with the unique syndrome, specific translocations [t(15;17)] and differentiation induced by ATRA. This paper is a large analysis of patients who develop tAPL. Unlike the other therapy-related hematologic malignancies, these patients appear to do similarly well with ATRA compared with the de novo patients with APL.

P. J. Loehrer, Sr, MD

Prediction of Initial Cytogenetic Response for Subsequent Major and Complete Cytogenetic Response to Imatinib Mesylate Therapy in Patients With Philadelphia Chromosome-Positive Chronic Myelogenous Leukemia

Kantarjian H, Talpaz M, O'Brien S, et al (Univ of Texas, Houston)
Cancer 97:2225-2228, 2003 5–15

Background.—Molecular abnormalities associated with the Philadelphia chromosome (Ph) have been implicated as the main pathophysiologic events in the development of chronic myelogenous leukemia (CML). Obtaining a major or complete cytogenetic response correlates with excellent long-term survival. Early allogeneic stem cell transplantation may be associated with a better outcome. Thus, early parameters predicting subsequent cytogenetic responses would improve treatment decision making. Early cytogenetic responses may predict later major or complete cytogenetic responses to imatinib mesylate treatment in patients with Ph-positive CML.

Methods and Findings.—Two hundred sixty-one patients with Ph-positive, chronic-phase CML were enrolled in the study. Interferon therapy had failed in all patients, and imatinib mesylate treatment was initiated. Persistence of 100% Ph-positive cells after 6 or more months of imatinib mesylate treatment correlated with a major cytogenetic response rate ranging from 9% to 13%. The complete cytogenetic response rate ranged from 0% to 4%. A minor cytogenetic response after 3 to 12 months of treatment still correlated with high rates of major or complete cytogenetic response rates, ranging from 68% to 83% and from 35% to 54%, respectively.

Conclusions.—Current data suggest that only patients with no cytogenetic response after 6 or more months of imatinib treatment should be considered for alternative therapies. All others should continue with imatinib therapy until there is clear evidence of cytogenetic response loss or hematologic resistance.

► One of the most significant predictors of long-term benefit from imatinib therapy in patients with CML is the attainment of a major or complete cytogenetic response. Patients achieving these end points have more durable responses than those having no or minimal cytogenetic response. Given the fact that many patients with CML have the option of allogeneic bone marrow transplantation, the timing of these therapies becomes critical. The investigators in this study prospectively assessed the frequency with which early cytogenetic response predicted for later benefit. They concluded that patients who failed to achieve any cytogenetic response after 12 months of therapy, regardless of the hematologic response (which will be nearly 100%), almost never attain a major or better cytogenetic response. In contrast, those with at least a minor cytogenetic response anywhere from 3 to 12 months after initiating therapy still run a high chance of attaining a more substantial and clinically meaningful cytogenetic response. This paradigm suggests that patients with persistent 100% Ph positivity on cytogenetic studies at least 6 months after initiating imatinib therapy could be offered alloBMT regardless of their hematologic response since the major benefit for signal transduction inhibitor therapy will likely not be seen in their case.

M. S. Gordon, MD

The Effect of Imatinib Mesylate on Patients With Philadelphia Chromosome-Positive Chronic Myeloid Leukemia With Secondary Chromosomal Aberrations

Mohamed AN, Pemberton P, Zonder J, et al (Wayne State Univ, Detroit)
Clin Cancer Res 9:1333-1337, 2003 5–16

Background.—In patients with chronic myeloid leukemia (CML) with Philadelphia chromosome–positive (Ph+) karyotype, the acquisition of secondary chromosomal aberrations signals a clonal evolution correlated with disease progression to accelerated/blastic phase. The effects of imatinib mesylate in such patients were reported.

Methods.—Fifty-eight patients with secondary abnormalities as well as t(9;22)(q34;q11.2) or its variants were identified in a group of 137 patients with CML treated by imatinib mesylate. By clinical criteria, 12 patients were in the chronic phase of disease, 24 in the accelerated, and 21 in the blastic.

Findings.—The major routes of CML clonal evolution were evident in more than half the patients. The rest had minor routes of secondary abnormalities, with −17/17p−, 11p−/rearr(11p), and −7/rearr(7) being most common. In 1 patient, an inv(16)(p13q22) developed as a secondary anomaly during blastic transformation. Bone marrow consistently showed myelomonocytic morphologic features with eosinophilia. Cytogenetic responses to imatinib mesylate were noted in 26% of the patients. Twelve patients obtained complete cytogenetic remission. Two had a major response and 1 had a minor response. Most responses occurred within 3 to 6 months. At more than 17 to 30 months after treatment, 7 patients are still in remission. Two patients had a relapse 12 to 19 months after treatment initiation. One patient required bone marrow transplantation.

Conclusions.—Some patients with Ph+ CML with clonal evolution have a complete cytogenetic response to imatinib mesylate. However, responses tend to be brief. Such patients may benefit from subsequent stem cell transplantation. Thus, patients with CML with clonal evolution may need treatment in addition to imatinib mesylate to best eradicate Ph+ leukemic cells.

► The identification of clonal evolution in patients with CML is often a harbinger of transformation to accelerated or blast phase. Typically, patients who acquire additional chromosomal abnormalities or additional copies of Ph+ rapidly progress and are usually identified for more aggressive therapy such as stem cell transplant. The authors assessed the impact of imatinib on cytogenetics of patients with additional chromosomal aberrations. Fifty-eight cases of CML patients with additional chromosomal aberrations were identified in a series of 137 who were treated with imatinib. Among these, 13 were in chronic phase while the remainder were either in accelerated (n = 24) or blast (n = 21) phase. The additional cytogenetic abnormalities were varied and included additional Ph+ copies, additional of 8, and a patient with an M4e-type of blast crisis with an inversion of chromosome 16. Cytogenetic responses occurred in 15 (26%) of the 58 cases, with 12 of the cases attaining a complete cytogenetic response. The majority of the complete cytogenetic responders occurred in patients with additional abnormalities in chronic phase as opposed to accelerated or blast crisis. Overall, the duration of these major or complete cytogenetic responses was reasonably long lasting and seen within 3 to 6 months of therapy. Hence, patients with additional chromosomal abnormalities should be monitored closely and, given the relatively brief duration of the responses seen, these patients should be considered for early stem cell transplant if available.

M. S. Gordon, MD

Imatinib Compared With Interferon and Low-Dose Cytarabine for Newly Diagnosed Chronic-Phase Chronic Myeloid Leukemia

O'Brien SG, Guilhot F, Larson RA, et al (Univ of Newcastle, England; Centre Hospitalier Universitaire de Poitiers, France; Univ of Chicago; et al)

N Engl J Med 348:994-1004, 2003 5–17

Background.—Imatinib is a selective inhibitor of the BCR-ABL tyrosine kinase. Research has shown that it yields high response rates in patients with chronic-phase chronic myeloid leukemia (CML) who did not respond to interferon-α. The efficacy of imatinib and interferon-α combined with low-dose cytarabine in patients with newly diagnosed chronic-phase CML were investigated.

Methods and Findings.—By random assignment, 1106 patients received imatinib or interferon-α plus low-dose cytarabine, with crossover to the alternative treatment permitted. The median patient follow-up was 19 months. The estimated rate of a major cytogenetic response at 18 months was 87.1% in imatinib recipients and 34.7% in combination therapy recipients. Estimated rates of complete cytogenetic response in the 2 groups were 76.2% and 14.5%, respectively. The estimated rate of freedom from progression to accelerated-phase or blast-crisis CML at 18 months was 96.7% and 91.5% in the imatinib and combined treatment groups, respectively. Patients given imatinib tolerated treatment better than those receiving the combination.

Conclusions.—On several measures, imatinib has advantages over interferon-α plus low-dose cytarabine as first-line therapy in patients with newly diagnosed chronic-phase CML. Imatinib was superior in hematologic and cytogenetic response, tolerability, and the likelihood of progression to accelerated-phase or blast-crisis CML.

► The signal transduction inhibitor imatinib has revolutionized the care and management of patients with CML. Having already demonstrated the ability to induce responses in patients with CML who are intolerant of interferon, the next critical question was whether or not imatinib should replace interferon and low-dose cytarabine as the front-line standard therapy. To this end, this randomized trial was initiated. Patients with newly diagnosed CML in chronic phase were randomly assigned to standard interferon-α with low-dose cytarabine versus imatinib. More than 1100 patients were randomized and crossover was allowed. With a median follow-up of more than 1.5 years, the imatinib arm demonstrated a statistically significant improvement in major and complete cytogenetic responses as well as a significant decrease in migration from chronic phase to either accelerated phase or blast-crisis phase. This study establishes imatinib as the new standard for the first-line therapy of CML.

M. S. Gordon, MD

Imatinib Mesylate for Philadelphia Chromosome-Positive, Chronic-Phase Myeloid Leukemia After Failure of Interferon-α: Follow-up Results

Kantarjian HM, Talpaz M, O'Brien S, et al (Univ of Texas, Houston)

Clin Cancer Res 8:2177-2187, 2002 5–18

Background.—Molecular abnormalities associated with the Philadelphia chromosome (Ph) have been implicated in the pathophysiology of Ph+ leukemias, such as chronic myeloid leukemia. The suppression of Ph+ cells has become a goal of therapy. Imatinib mesylate (Gleevec, Glivec) was designed to selectively inhibit the *Bcl-Abl* tyrosine kinase. Long-term follow-up of 261 adult patients with CML who did not respond to interferon-α therapy and who were treated with imatinib was described.

Study Design.—Imatinib was given orally at 400 mg/d. Patients were followed up every 3 months. They were analyzed for hematologic and cytogenetic response, long-term prognosis, prognostic factors, and tolerability.

Univariate and multivariate analyses were performed to identify prognostic factors.

Findings.—Overall, there was a 94% complete hematologic response and a 71% cytogenetic response to imatinib in this study group. At a median follow-up of 17 months, 94% were still taking imatinib. The 18-month estimated freedom from progression rate was 93%, and survival rate was 96%. Multivariate analysis indicated that long chronic phase, marrow basophilia, a high percentage Ph+ cells, and prior hematologic resistance to interferon were associated with an adverse response to therapy. Univariate analysis identified that leukocytosis, a high percentage of peripheral and marrow blasts, marrow basophilia, and cytogenetic clonal evolution were associated with decreased survival. A cytogenetic response by 6 months of therapy was associated with increased survival. The survival rate was better for those who had been treated with imatinib mesylate than for historical controls.

Conclusions.—Imatinib mesylate is a safe and effective treatment for patients with chronic-phase myeloid leukemia who were previously unsuccessfully treated with interferon therapy. Imatinib must be considered the new standard of care for these patients. Combination therapy with imatinib should be investigated to further improve response rate and long-term prognosis for patients with chronic myeloid leukemia.

► This study provides long-term follow-up on imatinib treatment for patients with chronic-phase chronic myeloid leukemia refractory with intolerance to interferon-α. The complete hematologic response rate in this study is 94%, confirming the earlier data. Cytogenetic response, the gold standard for effective therapy, occurred in 71% of patients, with complete cytogenetic response seen in 45% of cases. Achievement of earlier cytogenetic response (by 3-6 months of treatment) is associated with a prolonged survival rate. The authors identified a number of clinical characteristics associated with higher rates of cytogenetic response and outcome. These include patients with prior hematologic response to interferon, longer duration of disease from time of diagnosis to initial time of imatinib treatment, low bone marrow basophil, and a high percentage of Ph+ bone marrow cells at start of therapy. These patients have a 93% chance of major cytogenetic response.

M. S. Gordon, MD

Extended Follow-up of Patients With Hairy Cell Leukemia After Treatment With Cladribine

Goodman GR, Burian C, Koziol JA, et al (Scripps Research Inst, La Jolla, Calif)
J Clin Oncol 21:891-896, 2003 5–19

Background.—Hairy cell leukemia (HCL) is an uncommon, indolent, chronic B-cell lymphoproliferative disorder. This disease, which accounts for approximately 2% of all adult leukemias in the United States, involves the marrow and spleen. Treatment includes splenectomy, interferon-α2a and -α2b, pentostatin, and cladribine. Extended follow-up of patients with HCL treated by cladribine was reported.

Methods.—Two hundred nine patients with 7 or more years of follow-up were included in the study. All had HCL treated by cladribine given in courses of 7-day continuous IV infusion at 0.1 mg/kg/d.

Findings.—Ninety-five percent of the patients obtained a complete remission and 5% a partial response after a single cladribine course. For all responders, the median duration of first response was 98 months. Thirty-seven percent of patients had a relapse after their first cladribine course, with a median time to this relapse of 42 months. At 108 months, the overall survival rate was 97%. A total of 58 second malignancies developed in 48 patients. Second malignancies had an observed-to-expected ratio of 2.03.

Conclusions.—A single course of cladribine can induce high response rates in patients with HCL. Most of these responses are complete remissions. Patients who have relapses can be retreated successfully with cladribine.

► HCL is a malignant condition with a number of highly effective treatments. Among these is the drug cladribine for which a single IV course of therapy is effective in producing long-lasting remissions. The largest volume of experience with this agent in this disease comes from Scripps Cancer Center. More than 200 patients with HCL were followed up for at least 7 years after cladribine therapy. Of these 207 patients, 95% achieved a complete remission, with another 5% achieving a partial remission after a single course of therapy. The median duration of first response was 96 months, and 66 patients relapsed after their first course of therapy. The overall survival rate was 97% at 108 months. No significant increase in second malignancies was seen, and relapsing patients could typically be re-treated and achieve another durable response. Patients with complete responses tended to do better than those with partial responses. These long-term follow-up data confirm the long-lasting benefit of cladribine in this patient population and raise questions with regard to the mechanism of the chemosensitivity of HCL to this agent, which should be studied in the modern era of genomics and proteomics to ascertain whether this could be translated to other diseases.

M. S. Gordon, MD

High Levels of Adenovirus DNA in Serum Correlate With Fatal Outcome of Adenovirus Infection in Children After Allogeneic Stem-Cell Transplantation

Schilham MW, Claas EC, van Zaane W, et al (Leids Universitair Medisch Centrum, Leiden, The Netherlands; Centro de Educatión Médica e Investigaciones Clínicas, Buenos Aires, Argentina)

Clin Infect Dis 35:526-532, 2002 5–20

Introduction.—Since 1995, the incidence of adenovirus infections among pediatric stem cell transplantation (SCT) recipients has risen markedly, making it crucial to find new ways to monitor adenovirus infection. A retrospective analysis was performed in 36 children with adenovirus infection after allogeneic SCT.

Methods.—The 36 patients were from a cohort of 328 children who underwent SCT between 1985 and 1998. All patients had 1 or more adenovirus-positive stool culture. Levels of adenovirus DNA in serum samples obtained from 36 transplant recipients with stool cultures positive for adenovirus were determined by polymerase chain reaction semiquantitatively by analyzing serial dilutions of the DNA template.

Results.—Six (86%) of 7 children who died of adenovirus infection compared with 2 (7%) of 29 other children had high serum levels of adenovirus DNA (identified by polymerase chain reaction at 100-fold or more dilution of the DNA template; $P < .0001$). High serum levels of adenovirus DNA were achieved at a mean of 18 days before death (range, 6-29 days).

Conclusion.—Quantification of serum adenovirus DNA may be useful in diagnosing and monitoring adenovirus infection and disease in immunocompromised children.

▶ Opportunistic infections in the post–bone marrow transplantation setting remain an important cause of morbidity and mortality. One of the most potentially devastating infections in this immunocompromised period is adenovirus. There is still a great deal to be learned about how best to identify early infection and follow the course of the infection and response to therapy as well as the development of more effective treatments. The study by Schilham et al addresses in part the issues of how best to follow the course of an infection as well as how to prognosticate. They examine the utility of performing semiquantitative polymerase chain reaction measurements of adenoviral hexon-encoding sequences in the serum of patients. Their results show that high and persistent serum levels of this adenoviral DNA strongly predicted a significantly worse outcome compared with patients who had a lower serum adenoviral DNA copy number. These results need to be confirmed and expanded to develop and test quantitative approaches to studying such infections as well for identifying early infection, when most current treatments are going to result in improved outcomes.

R. J. Arceci, MD, PhD

6 Adult Lymphoproliferative Disorders

Randomized Comparison of Low-Dose Involved-Field Radiotherapy and No Radiotherapy for Children With Hodgkin's Disease Who Achieve a Complete Response to Chemotherapy

Nachman JB, for the Children's Cancer Group (Univ of Chicago; et al)
J Clin Oncol 20:3765-3771, 2002 6–1

Introduction.—The current standard treatment regimen for children and adolescents with Hodgkin's disease is combination chemotherapy and low-dose involved-field radiation (LD-IFRT). Because radiation may be associated with adverse late effects, the Children's Cancer Group (CCG) examined whether radiation could be excluded in patients who receive a complete response to initial chemotherapy without jeopardizing the excellent outcome achieved with combined-modality therapy.

Methods.—Between January 1995 and December 1998, 829 eligible patients were enrolled in CCG 5942. Of these, 501 who achieved an initial complete response after risk-adapted combination chemotherapy were randomly assigned to treatment with LD-IFRT or no further treatment. Event-free survival (EFS) and overall survival were evaluated from the date of trial entry or the date of randomization, whichever was appropriate.

Results.—The projected overall 3-year EFS from trial entry was 87%. In patients who achieved a complete response to initial therapy, 92% of those who received LD-IFRT were alive and disease-free 3 years after randomization compared with 87% for those randomized to no further therapy (P = .057). By using an "as-treated" analysis, 3-year EFS after randomization for the radiation cohort was 93% compared with 85% for patients in the no further treatment group (P = .0024). Three-year survival estimates for patients who did and did not receive LD-IFRT were 98% and 99%, respectively.

Conclusion.—The 3-year EFS after an initial complete response to risk-adapted chemotherapy was improved with LD-IFRT in children and adolescents with Hodgkin's disease. The 3-year survival rates were not improved with the addition of LD-IFRT.

▶ Reducing adverse sequelae of treatment while improving outcomes for patients with Hodgkin's disease remains an important challenge. To this end, the CCG 5942 study randomized patients with Hodgkin's disease who had achieved a complete remission to either receive radiotherapy or no radiotherapy. When analyzed "as randomized" or "as treated," the results showed that in clinical groups 1, 2 or 3, the EFS was better in the group receiving radiotherapy while no differences were observed in terms of overall survival. Although the incidence of secondary malignancies and other late, adverse sequelae were not reported in detail, previous reports have shown that relapsed disease (and the subsequent treatment) contribute significantly to the incidence of secondary cancers in these patients. Another issue raised by this study is that there are clearly some patients who can be cured without radiotherapy. Unfortunately, this trial did not test any biologic or radiographic surrogates to assess how one might identify the group of patients who might not need or who might require radiotherapy to eradicate their disease during the initial attempt at cure. However, this study does contribute to the conclusion that current standard of care should include combined modality therapy, but that future trials should continue to test for alternative risk-directed therapies and the more refined identification of risk groups.

R. J. Arceci, MD, PhD

Treatment of Unfavorable Childhood Hodgkin's Disease With VEPA and Low-Dose, Involved-Field Radiation

Friedmann AM, Hudson MM, Weinstein HJ, et al (Massachusetts Gen Hosp, Boston; St Jude Children's Research Hosp, Memphis, Tenn; Stanford Univ, Calif)

J Clin Oncol 20:3088-3094, 2002 6–2

Background.—The high incidence of second malignant neoplasms and male infertility among survivors of childhood Hodgkin's disease exposed to high doses of radiation and alkylating agent chemotherapy has been a particular cause of concern. Cardiac and pulmonary toxicity has also been reported with regimens containing radiation plus high cumulative doses of anthracycline-based chemotherapy and bleomycin. The findings of an etoposide-based chemotherapy regimen that eliminated alkylating agents and bleomycin, combined with low-dose, involved-field irradiation in high-risk patients were reported. The goal of this regimen was to reduce cardiopulmonary, gonadal, and neoplastic treatment complications in pediatric patients treated for Hodgkin's disease.

Methods.—From January 1990 to April 1993, 56 children with Hodgkin's disease were treated in a single-arm trial at 3 institutions with a regimen that was designed to maintain a high cure rate while minimizing the potential late effects of treatment. The regimen included 6 cycles of vinblastine, etoposide, prednisone, and doxorubicin (VEPA) chemotherapy and low-dose, involved-field radiation. Unfavorable features included bulky presentations of localized (stage I or II) or advanced (stage III or IV) Hodgkin's disease.

Results.—Unfavorable presentations of stage I/II disease were manifest in 26 (46%) of 56 patients, whereas 30 (54%) patients had advanced (stage III/IV) disease. At a median of 8.9 years after diagnosis, 79% of patients are alive without disease. Nineteen patients had late effects of treatment at a median of 1.5 years from diagnosis, including relapse in 17 patients, 1 death from cardiomyopathy, and 1 death from accidental injuries. For the entire cohort, survival and event-free survival estimates at 5 years were 81.9% and 67.8%, respectively. The 5-year event-free survival by stage was 100% for stage I, 79.2% for stage II, 70% for stage III, and 49.5% for stage IV patients.

Conclusions.—Combined therapy with VEPA chemotherapy and low-dose, involved-field radiation provides adequate disease control in early stage patients with childhood Hodgkin's disease with unfavorable features. However, this regimen may be inferior to other standard regimens in patients with advanced disease.

► An increasing emphasis on reducing short- and long-term treatment-related toxicity while preserving or improving on current outcomes has been the subject of several recent reports for patients with Hodgkin's disease. The study by Friedmann et al represents a 3-institution study of 6 cycles of the VEPA regimen and low-dose, involved-field radiation for patients with unfavorable features and stage I or II Hodgkin's disease or advanced (stage III or IV) disease. The results are similar to those reported previously by other groups in that patients with lower stage disease do reasonably well with such a reduced intensity regimen but that patients with more advanced disease do not do terribly well with a 5-year event-free survival of 70% for stage III and 50% for stage IV patients. In addition, because of the small numbers of patients in this trial, all comparisons are to other studies and historic data, which represents a significant problem in making definitive conclusions. Lastly, while a stated goal of the study was to examine whether adverse sequelae were minimized, very little information is presented except for cardiotoxicity, with 3 events occurring, 1 fatal. This type of study, while important in terms of trying to push the field forward with reduced intensity regimens, needs to be balanced by the lack of a contemporaneous control group and longer follow-up.

R. J. Arceci, MD, PhD

Randomized Comparison of ABVD and MOPP/ABV Hybrid for the Treatment of Advanced Hodgkin's Disease: Report of an Intergroup Trial

Duggan DB, Petroni GR, Johnson JL, et al (State Univ of New York, Syracuse; Univ of Rochester, NY; Duke Univ, Durham, NC; et al)

J Clin Oncol 21:607-614, 2003 6–3

Purpose.—In patients with Hodgkin's disease, research has identified both the combination chemotherapy regimens of doxorubicin, bleomycin, vinblastine, and dacarbazine (ABVD) and mechlorethamine, vincristine, procarbazine, prednisone, doxorubicin, bleomycin, and vinblastine (MOPP/ABV) as effective. Because treatment-related toxicities may not develop for many years after the end of treatment, long-term assessment of the risks and benefits of these regimens is essential. The ABVD and MOPP/ABV regimens were compared as initial chemotherapy for Hodgkin's disease.

Methods.—Eight hundred fifty-six adult patients with advanced Hodgkin's disease, stage III_2A or higher, were randomly assigned to receive ABVD or MOPP/ABV. Responses, survival, and toxic effects were analyzed at a median follow-up of 6 years.

Results.—Response and survival outcomes were similar between the 2 regimens. Complete remission rates were 76% with ABVD and 80% with MOPP/ABV. Five-year failure-free survival was 63% and 66%; overall survival was 82% and 81%, respectively. Patients receiving MOPP/ABV had higher rates of clinically significant acute pulmonary and hematologic toxic effects, whereas cardiac toxicity was similar between groups. Of 24 treatment-related deaths, 9 occurred in the ABVD group and 15 in the MOPP/ABV group. Numbers of second malignancies were 18 and 28, respectively. Eleven of thirteen cases of myelodysplasia or acute leukemia occurred in the MOPP/ABV group. The other 2 patients were initially assigned to ABVD but later received MOPP chemotherapy and radiotherapy.

Conclusions.—The results confirm that both ABVD and MOPP/ABV are effective first-line chemotherapy regimens for Hodgkin's disease. However, MOPP/ABV may carry a higher risk of acute toxic effects, myelodysplasia syndrome, and leukemia. Thus, ABVD is the initial treatment of choice for advanced Hodgkin's disease.

► MOPP was the prototypical combination chemotherapy regimen in medical oncology. Over the past several decades, several randomized trials have strongly evolved to look at improved and less toxic therapy. This trial should finally put to rest this old and faithful battleship. Improvement over ABVD is our next challenge and is discussed well in an accompanying editorial by Dr Volker Diehl.[1]

P. J. Loehrer, Sr, MD

Reference

1. Diehl V: Advanced Hodgkin's disease: ABVD is better, yet is not good enough [editorial]! *J Clin Oncol* 21:583-585, 2003.

High-Dose Therapy and Autologous Stem-Cell Transplantation Versus Conventional Therapy for Patients With Advanced Hodgkin's Lymphoma Responding to Front-Line Therapy

Federico M, for the EBMT/GISL/ANZLG/SFGM/GELA Intergroup HD01 Trial (Universita di Modena e Reggio Emilia, Italy; et al)

J Clin Oncol 21:2320-2325, 2003 6–4

Background.—A variety of combination chemotherapy regimens used to treat advanced Hodgkin's lymphoma (HL) induce high levels of complete remission and prolong long-term survival. However, 5% to 10% of patients do not achieve complete remission, and up to 30% of responders have relapses, necessitating further treatment. Less than one third of patients with early relapses after initial combination chemotherapy are rescued with appropriate salvage treatment. Whether high-dose therapy (HDT) with autologous stem-cell transplantation (ASCT) would be beneficial in the initial consolidative treatment of patients with advanced, unfavorable HL was investigated.

Methods.—One hundred sixty-three patients were enrolled in the study. All had achieved complete or partial remission after 4 initial courses of doxorubicin, bleomycin, vinblastine, and dacarbazine or with other doxorubicin-containing regimens. By random assignment, 83 patients received HDT plus ASCT (group 1), and 80 received 4 courses of conventional chemotherapy (group 2). Lymphoma was considered "unfavorable" if 2 or more poor prognostic indicators were recorded, including high lactate dehydrogenase levels, large mediastinal mass, more than 1 extranodal site, low hematocrit concentrations, and inguinal involvement.

Findings.—At the end of treatment, 92% of the patients in group 1 and 89% in group 2 obtained a complete response. The median follow-up was 48 months. The failure-free survival rates in groups 1 and 2 were 75% and 82%, respectively, at 5 years. The overall survival rates at 5 years were 88% in both groups. The relapse-free survival rates at 5 years were 88% and 94%, respectively, a nonsignificant difference.

Conclusions.—Conventional chemotherapy with 4 courses of a doxorubicin-containing regimen effectively induces complete or partial responses in patients with advanced, unfavorable HL. Early intensification with HDT and ASCT does not appear to confer any advantage.

► The investigators in this trial sought to determine whether the incorporation of HDT as a form of consolidation for patients with HD displaying unfavorable features would be of value. One hundred sixty-three patients with advanced stage HD received 4 cycles of doxorubicin, bleomycin, vinblastine, and dacarbazine or similar chemotherapy. Those attaining complete or partial remission were then randomly assigned to another 4 cycles of standard chemotherapy or a single course of HDT. Assessment of the complete response rate, progression-free and overall survival, and 5-year survival showed absolutely no benefit for HDT. In fact, the trend tended to lean toward standard therapy being less toxic and having a better outcome. As a result, HDT does not have a role in patients responding to chemotherapy. Consideration for its use in patients who are not responding is reasonable since HDT has the ability to convert nonresponding patients into responders with about one third of patients attaining long-term remissions.

M. S. Gordon, MD

Focus on Lymphomas

Staudt LM, Wilson WH (NIH, Bethesda, Md)

Cancer Cell 2:363-366, 2002 6–5

Background.—About 55,000 cases of non-Hodgkin's lymphoma and 7400 cases of Hodgkin's lymphoma are diagnosed each year, making lymphomas the fifth most common cancer type occurring in the United States. The types of lymphoma are diverse, requiring familiarity with the pathogenetic pathways, clinical and molecular characteristics, and treatment options for a successful outcome. The epidemiology, molecular pathogenesis, molecular diagnosis, and treatment advances specific to lymphoma were outlined.

Epidemiology and Pathogenesis.—Risk factors for lymphoma include genetic and acquired immunodeficiencies. Cofactors include Epstein-Barr virus, human herpes virus 8, human T-lymphocytic virus-1, and *Haemophilus pylori*. Autoimmune conditions such as Sjögren's syndrome are also linked to specific subtypes of lymphoma. The alterations at the molecular level characteristic of lymphoma include areas of proliferation promotion, blockage of differentiation, inhibition of cell death, and facilitation of genomic instability (Fig 1).

Chromosomal translocations occur frequently in lymphomas. Anti-apoptotic agents may be overexpressed or apoptosis signaling pathways may be blocked. Gene translocations, specifically that of *BCL-6*, are common, occurring in one sixth of all non-Hodgkin's lymphomas and resulting in cells trapped at the normal germinal center stage of differentiation, where they are exposed to mutagenic effects linked to the Ig somatic hypermutation apparatus. Cell death may be blocked or cell growth and proliferation deregulated in various lymphomas. Genes that monitor genome integrity may have their functions inactivated.

Diagnosis and Treatment.—The clinical outcomes of patients who fall into the same diagnostic category may differ because of molecular differences between tumors. Differing cure rates for diffuse large B-cell lymphoma are noted as a result of molecularly distinct subgroups resulting from different stages of normal B-cell differentiation. Clinical features and biological features also play a role in survival for these patients.

As systemic disorders, lymphomas are generally managed by chemotherapy. Some respond and are potentially curable; others respond but are incurable. The addition of monoclonal antibodies has proved effective in various lymphoma types, the augmentation of immunity against lymphomas (vaccines) shows promise in follicular lymphoma, and the eradication of infec-

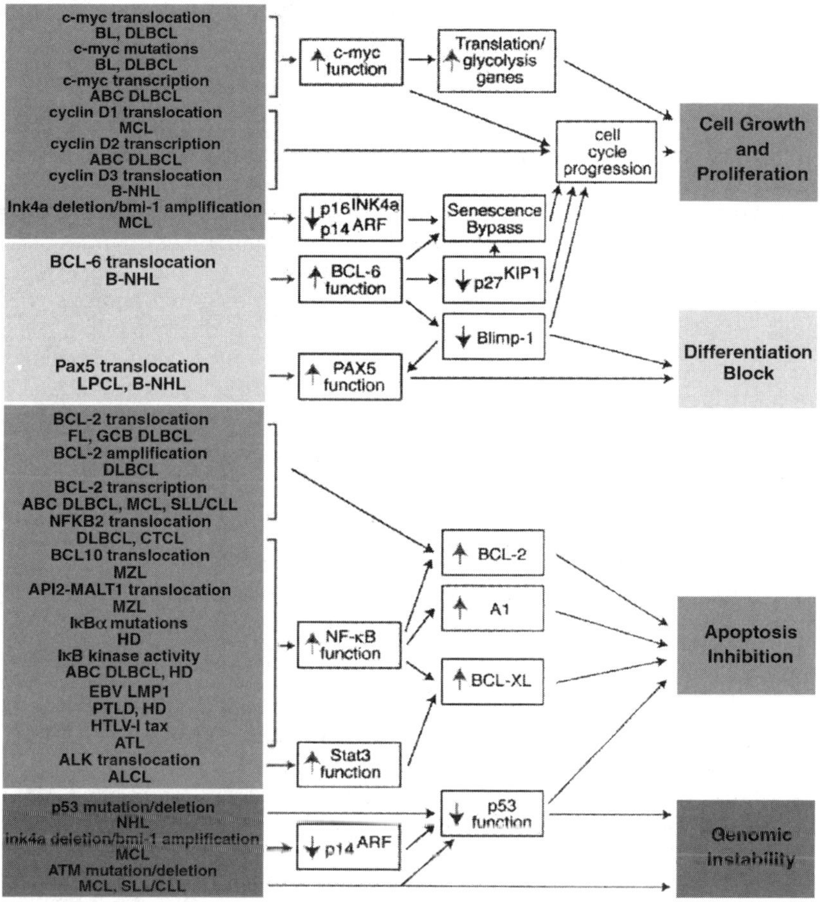

FIGURE 1.—Pathogenic mechanisms in lymphomas. *Arrows* indicate presumptive target genes and pathways affected by oncogenic events in various lymphoma types. An enhanced version of this figure is available as Supplemental Figure S1 at http://www.cancercell.org/cgi/content/full/2/5/363/DC1. *Abbreviations: BL*, Burkitt's lymphoma; *DLBCL*, diffuse large B cell lymphoma; *ABC*, activated B cell; *MCL*, mantle cell lymphoma; *B-NHL*, B cell non Hodgkin's lymphoma; *LPCL*, lymphoplasmacytoid lymphoma; *FL*, follicular lymphoma; *GCB*, germinal center B cell; *SLL*, small lymphocytic lymphoma; *CLL*, chronic lymphocytic leukemia; *CTCL*, cutaneous T cell lymphoma; *MZL*, marginal zone lymphoma; *HD*, Hodgkin's disease; *EBV*, Epstein-Barr virus; *PTLD*, posttransplant lymphoproliferative disorder; *ATL*, adult T cell lymphoma; *ALCL*, anaplastic large cell lymphoma. (Courtesy of Staudt LM, Wilson WH: Focus on lymphoma. *Cancer Cell* 2:363-366, 2002.)

tious agents offers cure in cases of gastric MALT lymphoma or splenic lymphoma with villous lymphocytes.

Conclusion.—Lymphomas present diverse challenges, occurring in a variety of types. Successful therapy depends on a detailed assessment of the pathogenetic pathways involved in the particular lymphoma. Quantitative molecular assays based on gene expression profiling should be used to refine the lymphoma diagnosis for optimal results.

▶ This is a relatively short overview on the biology of non-Hodgkin's lymphomas. A great deal of attention is given to the molecular pathogenesis as well as the molecular diagnosis of lymphomas. There is also a brief discussion of "recent treatment advances." I would certainly not wish to argue with the importance of antibody development, but the other putative advances are less clear to me. Obviously, some of them are still in an evaluation period, but I am not prepared to make a conclusion at this point.

There is no doubt that the answers to the mysteries of lymphomas will be revealed to us by understanding what is going on in the nucleus rather than by assessing surface markers. The latter may be helpful for classification, although I believe that credibility of the REAL (Revised European American Lymphoma) classification rests almost entirely on the recognition of mantle cell lymphoma as a discrete and important entity to recognize. Other than that, it is not clear to me what the REAL classification has added, at least on a quantitative basis. Thus, the attention given to molecular issues is important in the long haul. On the other hand, most of the molecular elements work at more than 1 level. We have dogma evolving about how things are actually going on, and it is not clear to me that we are really proving the dogma with studies of proof of principles.

E. Glatstein, MD

Lymphoma of the Breast: Clinical and Radiologic Features With Pathologic Correlation in 28 Patients

Sabatá JM, Gómez A, Torrubia S, et al (Hosp de Sant Pau, Barcelona; CAP Sant Feliu de Llobregat, Barcelona)

Breast J 8:294-304, 2002 6–6

Background.—Only 0.05% to 0.53% of breast malignancies are primary lymphoma, perhaps because breast lymphoid tissue amounts are small. Primary lymphoma is seldom considered in the differential diagnosis of breast tumors, but secondary forms are slightly more common. Imaging features characteristic of primary or secondary breast lymphoma were assessed to define findings indicative of this diagnosis. Diagnostic methods and clinical values were also assessed and radiologic and clinical results correlated.

Methods.—The medical records of 28 women with breast lymphoma (12 primary and 16 secondary or metastatic disease) were assessed retrospectively.

Results.—For primary lymphoma, the right breast was involved in 58.3% of patients; none had a family history of breast cancer. Half were premenopausal when diagnosed and all had breast symptoms. Three patients had pain, 5 had elevated levels of lactate dehydrogenase, and 2 with high-grade–type disease had B symptoms. Symptoms were noted 1 to 10 months (mean, 2 months) before diagnosis. No skin retraction or nipple discharge was pres-

TABLE 2.—The Radiologic Findings of Lymphoma of the Breast in 28 Patients

Radiologic Patterns of Involvement	Primary Disease (n = 12) Frequency	%	Secondary Disease (n = 16) Frequency	%
Nodular				
Unilateral				
Solitary	7	58.3	2	12.5
Multiple	1	8.3	4	25
Bilateral	0	0	5	31.2
Total	8	66.6	11	68.7
Diffuse				
Unilateral	3	25	5	31.2
Bilateral	1	8.3	0	0
Total	4	33.3	5	31.2

(Courtesy of Sabaté JM, Gómez A, Torrubia S, et al: Lymphoma of the breast: Clinical and radiologic features with pathologic correlation in 28 patients. *Breast J* 8(5):294-304, 2002. Reprinted by permission of Blackwell Publishing.)

ent, but 4 patients had palpable axillary adenopathy. Seven patients had focal masses in the upper outer quadrant. On radiologic assessment, focal masses measured 0.5 to 8 cm (mean, 4.6 cm); 5 had skin thickening, 4 linked to diffuse involvement (Tables 2 and 3).

Ipsilateral axillary lymph node involvement with large, dense, or irregular margins correlated with clinical findings in 4 patients. On US, hypoechoic structure was common. Of 9 patients examined cytologically, 7 were deemed suspicious of malignancy and 2 of breast carcinoma; 7 specimens had lymphoid or related cells. Four patients were misdiagnosed based on axillary dissection and 4 based on frozen section. After surgical intervention, all patients had radiation therapy and/or chemotherapy, with close follow-up for 2 to 24 years.

Nine patients had complete remission for 3 to 16 years; 3 had at least 1 recurrence. One patient died with Burkitt postpartum breast lymphoma 6 months after diagnosis. For patients with secondary or metastatic disease, the right breast, left breast, and both breasts were equally involved. Pathologic diagnosis was based on surgical biopsy (9 patients), biopsy plus cytologic assessment (4 patients), or clear response to chemotherapy (2 patients with widespread metastatic lymphomatous disease).

TABLE 3.—The Radiologic Features of Nodules in Lymphoma of the Breast

Nodular Patterns of Involvement	Primary Disease (n = 8) Frequency	%	Secondary Disease (n = 11) Frequency	%
Well-defined margins	1	12.5	6	54.5
Partially defined margins	3	37.5	3	27.2
Irregular margins	4	50	2	18.1
Total	8	100	11	99.8

(Courtesy of Sabaté JM, Gómez A, Torrubia S, et al: Lymphoma of the breast: Clinical and radiologic features with pathologic correlation in 28 patients. *Breast J* 8(5):294-304, 2002. Reprinted by permission of Blackwell Publishing.)

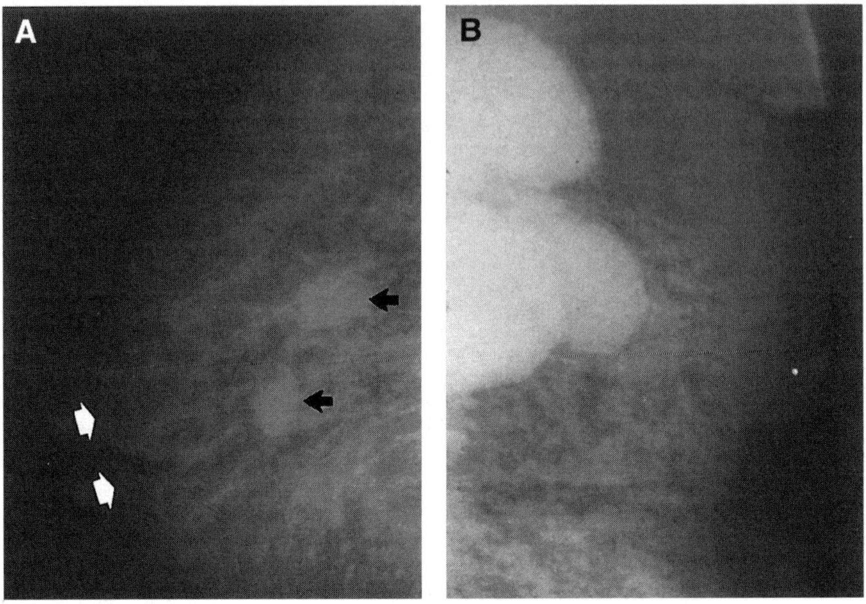

FIGURE 7.—A 55-year-old woman diagnosed with low-grade non-Hodgkin lymphoma who simultaneously presented with left breast involvement. **A**, Mediolateral mammogram shows 2 masses with irregular borders (*black arrows*), skin thickening (*white arrows*), and lymphatic pattern. **B**, Axillary mammographic view demonstrates large and dense lymphomatous nodes. Lymphatic pattern is also noticed and probably related to mechanical blockage. (Courtesy of Sabaté JM, Gómez A, Torrubia S, et al: Lymphoma of the breast: Clinical and radiologic features with pathologic correlation in 28 patients. *Breast J* 8(5):294-304, 2002. Reprinted by permission of Blackwell Publishing.)

Relapse occurred in 6 months to 8 years (mean, 32 months). Nearly 69% of patients had clinically solitary or multiple breast lumps, 4 patients had diffuse breast enlargement, and 2 had diffuse skin edema. Focal masses measured a mean of 2.8 cm (1 to 8 cm) in diameter; nonmasses had calcifications but no spiculated margins. Follicular lymphoma showed a nodular pattern on mammograms. US showed a nodular pattern with hypoechoic texture but no notable posterior enhancement or acoustic shadowing. Clinical findings and axillary involvement correlated well in 10 patients, with 8 having prominent aggressive features; patients with diffuse parenchymal involvement had related unilateral adenopathy (Fig 7). Chemotherapy was performed in all secondary or metastatic cases; most patients had a response exceeding 90%.

Conclusion.—Masses in primary disease were more likely to have less-defined margins and larger diameters than those in secondary disease. In high-grade malignancies, radiologic findings tended to be diffuse, indicating a more aggressive nature. Cytologic evaluation was sufficient for diagnosis in secondary disease.

► This report from Spain evaluates 28 patients who had lymphoma of the breast. Twelve of these patients had primary lymphoma and 16 of them had secondary involvement of the breast. The mammograms are exceptionally clear in this article and for those who are involved in care of patients with breast lesions, this is a useful reference. My only complaint is that the histologic classification does not include the REAL (Revised European American Lymphoma) classification, only the Rappaport classification and the Working Formulation. These are not "wrong," but they have been superceded by the REAL.

E. Glatstein, MD

Lymphoma of the Nasal Cavity and Paranasal Sinuses: Treatment and Outcome of Early-Stage Disease

Proulx GM, Caudra-Garcia I, Ferry J, et al (Harvard Med School, Boston; Roswell Park Cancer Inst, Buffalo, NY)

Am J Clin Oncol 26:6-11, 2003 6–7

Introduction.—The rarity of lymphomas of the nasal cavity and paranasal sinuses and the nonuniformity of treatment make understanding their natural history and treatment outcome difficult. Experience with lymphoma of the nasal cavities and paranasal sinuses was examined to further understand patient outcome for this rare disease.

Methods.—The medical records of 23 patients diagnosed and treated for extranodal non-Hodgkin's lymphoma of the paranasal sinus and nasal cavity were examined retrospectively. Most patients had Ann Arbor stage I disease (10 patients, T1 or T2; 13 patients, T3 or T4). Eight patients had nasal-type natural killer/T cell and 15 had diffuse large B-cell lymphoma (DLBCL). The nasal cavity was predominantly involved in 5 of 8 patients with nasal-type natural killer/T cell. The paranasal sinuses were the primary

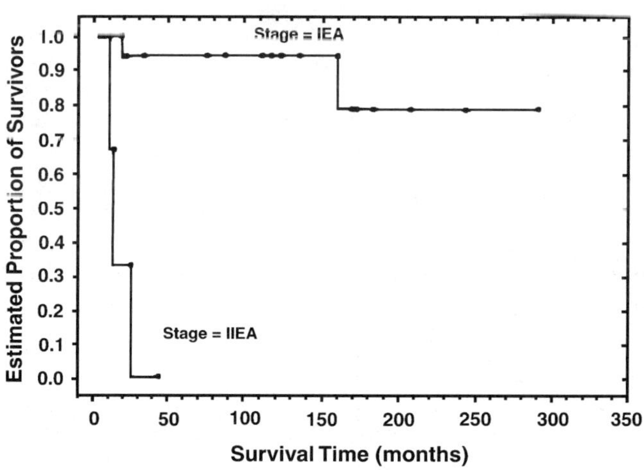

FIGURE 1.—Kaplan-Meier survival plots (overall survival and disease-free survival) for patients with Ann Arbor stage IEA (81 patients) and IIEA (5 patients). The symbols represent patients who died (*vertical drop in curve*) or patients still alive (censored data). (Courtesy of Proulx GM, Caudra-Garcia I, Ferry J, et al: Lymphoma of the nasal cavity and paranasal sinuses: Treatment and outcome of early-stage disease. *Am J Clin Oncol* 26:6-11, 2003.)

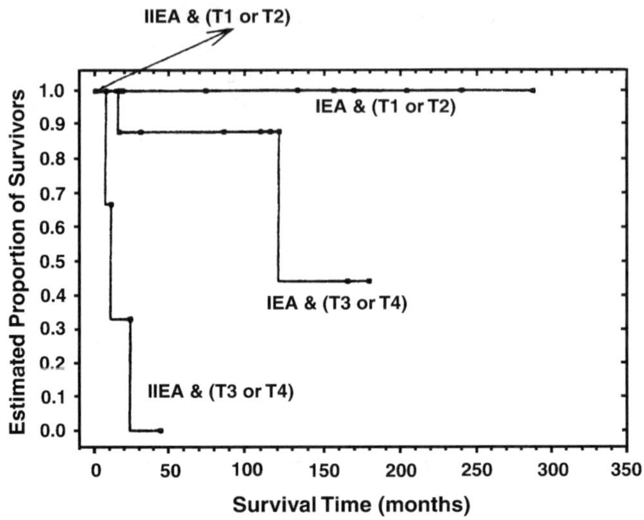

FIGURE 3.—Kaplan-Meier survival plots (overall survival and disease-free survival) for patients with Ann Arbor stage IEA and (T1 or T2) (9 patients); IEA and (T3 or T4) (9 patients); IIEA and (T1 or T2) (1 patient); and IIEA and (T3 or T4) (4 patients). (Courtesy of Proulx GM, Caudra-Garcia I, Ferry J, et al: Lymphoma of the nasal cavity and paranasal sinuses: Treatment and outcome of early-stage disease. *Am J Clin Oncol* 26:6-11, 2003.)

site in 12 of 15 patients with DLBCL. All patients underwent radiotherapy and 3 received chemotherapy as part of the initial therapy for 3 cycles of cyclophosphamide, doxorubicin, vincristine, and prednisone. Patients were followed up for overall survival (OS) and disease-free survival (DFS).

Results.—The estimated OS and DFS rates for 5 and 10 years were the same in all analyses. The year OS was 78% (Fig 1). The combination of stage and T stage was the best predictor of OS and DFS (Fig 3). Significant prognostic factors included Ann Arbor stage IEA versus IIEA (P = .0001) and T stage with T1 or T2 versus T3 or T4 (P = .0243). Combining Ann Arbor stage and T stage produced a highly significant prognostic variable (IEA and [T1 or T2], IEA and [T3 or T4], IIEA and [T1 or T2], IIEA and [T3 or T4]; P = .0001), regardless of site or histology.

Conclusion.—Patients with local-regional disease appeared to be well controlled with radiotherapy alone; distant failure remains problematic. A combined-modality approach with local-regional radiation and systemic chemotherapy is advised.

▶ This is a report from Mass General dealing with extranodal non-Hodgkin's lymphomas involving the paranasal sinus and nasal cavity. It is a modest-sized series of 23 patients, and more than two thirds of them had DLBCL. Most of the DLBCLs were involving the paranasal sinuses. This series was accumulated between 1960 and 1998, and I guess that is why only a few of the patients received chemotherapy, whereas everyone received local radiation treatment.

The authors say that by coincidence the OS and DFS were the same no matter which group of patients was seen at 5 and 10 years. With 23 patients, I am surprised at that. In any event, I have included this because it is not easy to find results for this specific group of patients. Certainly, for more advanced disease, combined modality treatment would appear to be the treatment of choice, and even in the more localized disease, in today's world combined modality treatment would still be the more typical recommendation.

E. Glatstein, MD

CD5+ Follicular Lymphoma: A Clinicopathologic Study of Three Cases

Barry TS, Jaffe ES, Kingma DW, et al (NIH, Bethesda, Md; Univ of Louisville, Ky)
Am J Clin Pathol 118:589-598, 2002 6–8

Background.—Follicular lymphoma (FL) is the most common non-Hodgkin lymphoma in adults in the United States. FL is incurable in most patients, despite their initial responsiveness to a variety of therapeutic approaches. FL is generally regarded as negative for the expression of CD5, a feature that has a critical role in the differential diagnosis of low-grade B-cell malignant neoplasms. The CD5 antigen is expressed on the vast majority of mature T cells and has been shown to have a role in thymocyte development and selection, T-cell activation, and T-cell-antigen–presenting cell interactions. Three cases of FL with unusual expression of CD5 were presented.

Methods.—Three cases of CD5+ FL were obtained from files at the National Cancer Institute, National Institutes of Health. All of the cases manifested histologic features of FL, including effaced nodal architecture, a follicular growth pattern, and a spectrum of grades from 1 to 3 on the World Health Organization criteria.

Results.—Flow cytometric studies in these cases showed a light-chain–restricted, CD19+, CD20+ B-cell population with coexpression of CD10 and low-level CD5. Immunohistochemical studies in these cases demonstrated an identical B-cell expression of CD5 and coexpression of bcl-2 protein as well as CD10 and bcl-6 protein, which are germinal center-associated markers. None of these cases showed expression of CD43, cyclin D1, or IgD. Molecular analysis revealed immunoglobulin heavy-chain gene rearrangements in all 3 cases, and 2 of these cases had a t(14;18) translocation.

Conclusion.—The findings in these 3 rare cases of CD5+ follicular lymphoma demonstrate the difficulty in classifying these lymphomas solely with flow cytometric studies. This report also stresses the importance of recognizing follicular lymphoma in the differential diagnosis of CD5+ B-cell lymphomas.

► FLs are virtually always positive for CD20 and almost always negative for CD5. This group of pathologists reports on 3 cases with an unusual expression of CD5, despite the follicular pattern and CD20 positivity. There is an excellent discussion of CD5 and its functions. This article points out how complex the classification of lymphomas has become. Indeed, I believe there will be some people who will not be happy until every lymphoma case is unique in its antigen expression and in classification.

On the other hand, it is reasonably clear that ultimately the answers to the mysteries of lymphoma will be revealed from activities in the nucleus, as opposed to surface markers. Toward that end, a future classification scheme based on microarray techniques would seem to be inevitable, although the true usefulness of such a classification system remains to be seen at this time. In the meantime, one has to be concerned that morphology receives relatively little attention today. If the surface markers do not fit a predefined pattern, it becomes progressively more difficult to know how to classify the lesions. The emerging principle is that one's confidence in the diagnosis is inversely proportional to the length of the pathology description!

E. Glatstein, MD

Patterns of Outcome and Prognostic Factors in Primary Large-Cell Lymphoma of the Testis in a Survey by the International Extranodal Lymphoma Study Group

Zucca E, Conconi A, Mughal TI, et al (Peter MacCallum Cancer Inst, East Melbourne, Australia; Princess Margaret Hosp, Toronto; British Columbia Cancer Agency, Vancouver, Canada; et al)

J Clin Oncol 21:20-27, 2003 6–9

Background.—Primary testicular lymphoma accounts for 1% to 2% of all non-Hodgkin's lymphomas, and about 85% of the patients are older than 60 years. Lymphomas represent only 1% to 7% of all testicular malignancies, yet they represent the most common testicular tumor in men older than 50 years. Histologically, 80% to 90% of primary testicular lymphomas are of diffuse large cell type with B-cell immunophenotype. Primary testicular lymphoma also manifests a tendency toward systematic dissemination to several extranodal sites, including the contralateral testis, CNS, skin, Waldeyer's ring, lung, pleura, and soft tissues. Clinical features and patterns of outcome of primary testicular diffuse large B-cell lymphomas (DLCL) were determined.

Methods.—This retrospective international survey enrolled 373 patients with primary testicular DLCL. The median age at presentation was 66 years, with a range of 19 to 91 years.

Results.—Most of the patients presented with localized disease (stage I to II), and most of the patients (68%) underwent anthracycline-based chemotherapy. Prophylactic intrathecal chemotherapy was administered to 18% of patients, and 36% of patients received prophylactic scrotal radiotherapy. The median overall survival was 4.8 years, and the median progression-free survival was 4 years. The survival curves showed no clear evidence of a substantial proportion of cured patients. Multivariate analysis identified a favorable international prognostic index, no B-symptoms, the use of anthracyclines, and prophylactic scrotal radiotherapy as significantly associated with longer survival. However, even for patients with stage I disease and good-risk international prognostic index, the outcome appears to be worse than that reported for DLCL at other sites. A total of 195 patients (52%) had relapsed at a median follow-up of 7.6 years. Relapses in the CNS were detected in 15% of patients up to 10 years after presentation. Patients who did not receive scrotal radiotherapy had a continuous risk of recurrence in the contralateral testis.

Conclusions.—Testicular DLCL have a particularly high risk of extranodal relapse, even in patients in whom disease is localized at diagnosis. Outcomes appear to be improved by anthracycline-based chemotherapy, CNS prophylaxis, and contralateral testicular irradiation. The efficacy of these therapies is currently being evaluated in clinical trials.

► Testicular lymphoma is a rare malignancy representing only 1% to 2% of all lymphomas. It does represent the most common form of testicular tumors in men over the age of 50 years. Most of these tumors are diffuse large cell type with a B-cell lineage and have a great propensity to metastasize to extranodal sites, including the other testicle, CNS, Waldeyer's ring, skin, and soft tissues. This is 1 of the largest series (retrospective) published to date. As such, this is a good read and a very good reference.

P. J. Loehrer, Sr, MD

Early Stage Nasal NK/T-Cell Lymphoma: Clinical Outcome, Prognostic Factors, and the Effect of Treatment Modality

Cheung MMC, Chan JKC, Lau W, et al (Queen Elizabeth Hosp, Kowloon, Hong Kong)

Int J Radiat Oncol Biol Phys 54:182-190, 2002 6–10

Background.—Primary nasal lymphomas are uncommon and have a predilection for persons of Asian, Latin, and South American descent. A previous retrospective study of 113 patients found that the most common subtype was natural killer (NK)/T-cell lymphoma with CD56 expression, which carried independent poor prognostic significance. This study sought to determine the clinical outcome, prognostic factors, and effect of adding combination chemotherapy to radiation therapy regarding disease control and survival in early stage (NK)/T-cell lymphoma.

Methods.—A retrospective intention-to-treat analysis was performed on 79 patients consecutively treated with curative intent from 1977 to June 2001. All of the patients had early stage nasal NK/T-cell lymphoma. Combined modality treatment (CMT) was planned for 61 patients, and radiotherapy (RT) alone was planned for 18 patients (Fig 1). Three to 6 cycles of anthracycline-containing regimens were intended for all of the patients scheduled for CMT. The patients selected for RT were, in general, older or were treated in the earlier phase of the study period.

Results.—The overall complete response rate was 68.4%, of whom 44.4% relapsed after a median of 54.9 months of follow-up. The 5-year dis-

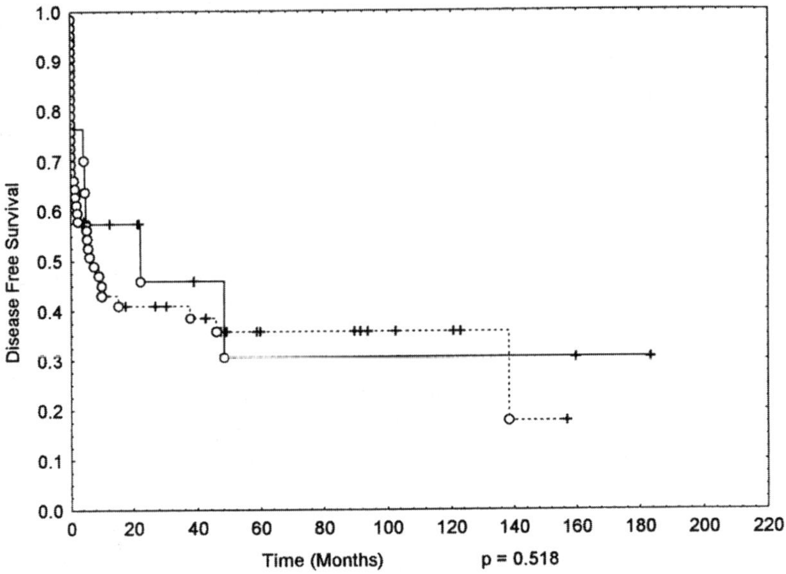

FIGURE 1.—Disease-free survival according to intent to treat. RT = radiation therapy alone (solid line); CMT = combined modality treatment (dashed line). (Reprinted from Cheung MMC, Chan JKC, Lau W, et al: Early stage nasal, NK/T-cell lymphoma: Clinical outcome, prognostic factors, and the effect of treatment modality. *Int J Radiat Oncol Biol Phys* 54:182-190, 2002. Copyright 2002, with permission from Elsevier Science.)

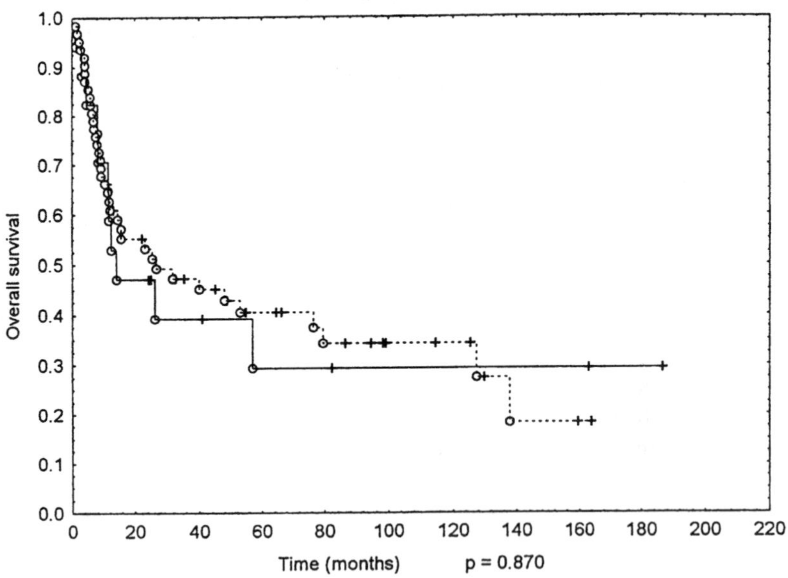

FIGURE 2.—Overall survival according to intent to treat. Radiation therapy alone is indicated by the *solid line*; combined modality treatment, *dashed line*. Radiation therapy alone indicated by *solid line*; combined modality treatment, *dashed line*. (Reprinted from Cheung MMC, Chan JKC, Lau W, et al: Early stage nasal, NK/T-cell lymphoma: Clinical outcome, prognostic factors, and the effect of treatment modality. *Int J Radiat Oncol Biol Phys* 54:182-190, 2002. Copyright 2002, with permission from Elsevier Science.)

ease-free survival (DFS) and overall survival (OS) rates were 35.5% and 37.9%, respectively (Fig 2). Multivariate analysis showed that good performance status (Eastern Cooperative Oncology Group less than 2) was a significant favorable factor for DFS. Good performance status and Ann Arbor stage I_E disease were found to be significant favorable factors for OS.

The type of intended treatment was not a significant factor for DFS or OS, although only 2 of the 16 stage II_E patients were intended for RT alone. Resistance to treatment was common, particularly in patients who received chemotherapy. Of the 61 patients in whom CMT was intended, 31 showed disease progression while undergoing chemotherapy; 17 of these progressed locoregionally. Nine of these 17 patients experienced a complete response to salvage radiotherapy.

Conclusion.—The overall outcome in early stage nasal NK/T-cell lymphoma is poor. Disease-free and overall survival are significantly influenced by performance status and Ann Arbor stage. Stage I_E patients do not appear to gain a survival benefit from the addition of anthracycline-containing chemotherapy to radiotherapy. Radiation therapy remains the standard for treatment of patients with nasal NK/T-cell lymphoma.

► This is a report from a very solid group of investigators from Hong Kong who probably see more nasopharyngeal neoplasm than any other institution around. This particular report is about lymphoma of the nose, of either NK or T-cell origins. The authors report on 79 patients of whom almost 80% have stage I disease. A large majority were planned for CMT with 3 to 6 cycles of multiagent chemotherapy, including anthracyclines.

The RT alone was generally reserved for patients who were older or treated in the early years of the period of interest, starting in 1977. OS and DFS were approximately 35%. In this particular series, the benefit of chemotherapy was hard to determine inasmuch as of 61 patients who were planned for multiagent chemotherapy, 31 progressed during chemotherapy, a particularly high proportion.

These patients are all CD56-positive, which may be a factor in the relatively poor results reported. As might be expected, performance status and stage are the most important prognostic factors. These patients are not particularly common, and an overtly positive CD56 may well represent a negative prognostic factor in and of itself. Nonetheless, these patients are still seen and still require tumor intervention in an effort to control what is clearly a difficult problem.

E. Glatstein, MD

[^{18}F]FDG in Childhood Lymphoma: Clinical Utility and Impact on Management

Montravers F, McNamara D, Land-Parker J, et al (Hôpital Tenon, Paris; Hôpital d'enfants Armand-Trousseau, Paris)

Eur J Nucl Med 29:1155-1165, 2002 6–11

Introduction.—Positron emission tomography (PET) with fluorine-18 fluorodeoxyglucose (FDG) provides unique information regarding the behavior of malignant cells and contributes to more accurate staging of the illness and better assessment of therapy response in adults with lymphoma. The usefulness of FDG PET in childhood lymphoma was compared with conventional imaging methods (CIMs) and clinical data in children with lymphoma.

Methods.—Between July 1998 and August 2001, 42 FDG PET examinations were performed with a dedicated PET system (27 examinations) or a hybrid coincidence PET system (15 examinations) to determine initial tumor staging in 5 patients and restaging or evaluation of response to therapy or residual masses in 20 children with Hodgkin's disease and 7 with non-Hodgkin's lymphoma. The FDG PET findings were compared with those of CIM and clinical examination. Since 2000, a standardized questionnaire has been used to assess the clinical impact of FDG PET on both staging and therapy. Of 16 referring physicians to whom the questionnaire was sent, 13 responded.

Results.—There were no side effects in any children who underwent FDG PET. It was very sensitive (12 of 12) in staging and restaging illness and revealed more lesions than CIMs. The upstaging rate was 50% (6 of 12). The FDG PET was also accurate in monitoring patient response to therapy and in the characterization of residual masses. False-positive findings were seen in 2 patients with non-Hodgkin's lymphoma with thymic uptake and 1 false-negative result was seen in a patient whose non-Hodgkin's lymphoma relapsed 1 month after a negative FDG PET. The questionnaire emphasized the influence of FDG PET on clinical management, which was modified based on FDG PET findings in 23% of patients.

Conclusion.—As demonstrated in the adult population, FDG PET seems to be a very sensitive imaging technique for staging and restaging of lymphoma in children and was very helpful in monitoring therapy response.

► Diagnostic and staging imaging modalities are critical in the evaluation of patients with solid tumors. In lymphoma, the FDG PET scan has rapidly gained acceptance as a sensitive and relatively specific tool for detecting disease. The fact that FDG PET can provide functional information of active disease in addition to simple anatomy adds significantly to its usefulness. There has been much less published on the use of FDG PET scanning in children with cancer. While the article by Montravers et al suffers from relatively small numbers and a nonsystematic approach of prospective evaluation on a single clinical trial, the study represents an attempt at evaluating FDG PET versus CIMs in children with Hodgkin's disease and non-Hodgkin's lymphoma. The data show that FDG PET resulted in upstaging of 50% of the patients evaluated and led to a modification in therapy in close to a quarter of patients. While preliminary, these results should stimulate pediatric radiologists and oncologists to definitively evaluate FDG PET in children with cancer.

R. J. Arceci, MD, PhD

Combination of Fludarabine and Mitoxantrone in Untreated Stages III and IV Low-Grade Lymphoma: S9501

Velasquez WS, Lew D, Grogan TM, et al (Univ of Texas, Galveston; Southwest Oncology Group Statistical Ctr, Seattle; Univ of Arizona, Tucson; et al)

J Clin Oncol 21:1996-2003, 2003 6–12

Background.—Low-grade lymphomas are associated with an indolent clinical course and median survival ranging from 5 to 10 years. Anthracycline-based regimens in the treatment of advanced-stage, low-grade lymphoma have been investigated. The efficacy of combined fludarabine and mitoxantrone was determined in patients with untreated low-grade lymphoma, stages III and IV.

Methods.—Seventy-eight patients were eligible for the phase II trial. The chemotherapeutic regimen, delivered every 4 weeks, consisted of mitoxantrone, 10 mg/m^2, on day 1 and fludarabine, 25 mg/m^2, on days 1, 2, and 3. Six to eight cycles were administered. All underwent *Pneumocystis carinii* prophylaxis.

Findings.—Ninety-four percent of the patients had an objective response. Forty-four percent had complete remission and 50% had partial remission. The median progression-free survival at a median 5.5 years of follow-up was 32 months. The 4-year progression-free survival rate was 38%. The median survival has not been reached to date, with 88% of all patients still alive at 4 years. Overall survival was substantially worse in high-risk groups according to the International Prognostic Index and serologic staging. Mild to severe, reversible myelosuppression occurred, although it was considered to be well tolerated. Other adverse events were rare.

Conclusions.—In patients with advanced-stage, low-grade lymphoma, fludarabine and mitoxantrone appear to be effective and safe. Clinical results were comparable to those of anthracycline-based regimens published previously.

▶ This study from the Southwest Oncology Group assessed the role of this chemotherapy combination in patients with previously untreated low-grade non-Hodgkin's lymphoma. Of 78 patients treated, 94% achieved a clinical response, including 44% who achieved a completed response. The 4-year progression-free survival was 38%; the median survival has not been reached at the time of publication. Similar to other regimens, the patients with the poorest predicted survival did worst. While this regimen provides outstanding responses, its effects are similar to that seen with other anthracycline-containing regimens. Larger randomized trials would have to be performed to define its superiority and, given the evolving role of monoclonal antibodies in this population, these trials or any further combination would have to include these biologic agents.

M. S. Gordon, MD

Prolonged Single-Agent Versus Combination Chemotherapy in Indolent Follicular Lymphomas: A Study of the Cancer and Leukemia Group B

Peterson BA, Petroni GR, Frizzera G, et al (Univ of Minnesota, Minneapolis; Univ of Virginia, Charlottesville; New York Presbyterian-Cornell Univ Med Ctr, NY; et al)

J Clin Oncol 21:5-15, 2003 6–13

Background.—Initial treatment options for follicular small cleaved lymphoma (FSCL) and follicular mixed lymphoma (FML) range from minimal therapy to the use of intensive drug combinations. A single agent and combination chemotherapy capable of curing diffuse aggressive lymphomas were compared in patients with stage III or IV FSCL or FML.

Methods.—Two hundred twenty-eight patients were randomly assigned to cyclophosphamide or the combination of cyclophosphamide, doxorubicin, vincristine, prednisone, and bleomycin (CHOP-B). In responders, treatment was continued for 2 years after maximal response.

Findings.—Overall, 91% of the patients responded to treatment. Sixty-six percent in the cyclophosphamide-only group and 60% in the CHOP-B group showed complete response. The 2 treatments were similar in overall time to failure and survival at 10 years. Twenty-five percent in the cyclophosphamide-only group were free of failure at 10 years compared with 33% in the CHOP-B group. Survival rates were 44% and 46%, respectively. Among the 46 patients with FML, combined therapy had a better failure-free survival rate at 10 years at 48% compared with 9% in the cyclophosphamide-only group. Overall survival rates were 61% and 25%, respectively. However, combination therapy resulted in more acute toxicities. Second malignancies occurred in both treatment groups and may be attributable to treatment.

Conclusions.—The use of the relatively intensive CHOP-B combination therapy appears to have no advantages over single-agent cyclophosphamide in the initial treatment of stage III or IV FSCL. However, the combination therapy may improve disease control and survival in patients with FML.

► This trial assessed the value of single-agent IV cyclophosphamide compared with combination therapy with CHOP-B in patients with previously untreated low-grade follicular non-Hodgkin's lymphoma. There were no differences in response rate, complete response rate, or survival. Specifically, overall survival was no different between the arms. Interestingly, the population of patients with FML had significantly better failure-free and overall survival rates with CHOP-B than with single-agent therapy. This reinforces the fact that FML acts more like an intermediate-grade non-Hodgkin's lymphoma than a low-grade non-Hodgkin's lymphoma and should be treated as such when treatment needs to be instituted. Like studies in the relapsed population of patients, these data need to be assessed in conjunction with emerging data for antibody-based therapy.

M. S. Gordon, MD

Single-Agent Rituximab as First-Line and Maintenance Treatment for Patients With Chronic Lymphocytic Leukemia or Small Lymphocytic Lymphoma: A Phase II Trial of the Minnie Pearl Cancer Research Network

Hainsworth JD, Litchy S, Barton JH, et al (Sarah Cannon Cancer Ctr and Tennessee Oncology, Nashville; Jackson Oncology Associates, Miss; Well Star Health System, Marietta, Ga; et al)

J Clin Oncol 21:1746-1751, 2003 6–14

Background.—Chronic lymphocytic leukemia (CLL), the most common type of leukemia, is histologically and immunologically indistinguishable from small lymphocytic lymphoma (SLL). Treatment for both is palliative. The safety and initial response rate to first-line therapy with rituximab for patients with CLL/SLL were examined in a phase II, multicenter, community-based trial.

Study Design.—The study group consisted of 44 patients with previously untreated CD20+ B-cell CLL or SLL. All patients underwent complete staging evaluation. Initial treatment consisted of rituximab 375 mg/m^2 administered IV once per week for 4 weeks. First evaluation was at 6 weeks. Those with objective response or stable disease were re-treated at 6-month intervals for a maximum of 4 cycles. Patients were reevaluated every 3 months. Actuarial overall and progression free survival (PFS) were calculated by the Kaplan-Meier method. Toxicity and initial response were assessed.

Findings.—Of the 44 patients aged 38 to 85 years enrolled in this study, 39 had CLL and 5 had SLL. All completed the first 4-week treatment course with rituximab. The objective response rate after the first treatment course was 51%, with a 4% complete response rate. Of these 44 patients, 28 received additional courses of rituximab. The overall response rate was 58%, with a 9% complete response rate and 14 patients still receiving maintenance therapy. After a median 20-month follow-up, median PFS was 18.6 months. The 1-year PFS rate was 62% and the 2-year rate was 49%. Treatment was well tolerated, with no cumulative toxicity or opportunistic infections.

Conclusions.—Rituximab was well tolerated as a first-line treatment for CLL/SLL. These findings further suggest that rituximab has activity against these diseases. Rituximab may be beneficial when incorporated into first-line combination regimens for the treatment of CLL/SLL.

► The authors studied the use of rituximab in patients with SLL or CLL. Traditionally, the density of CD20 on the surface of these mature-appearing lymphocytes is low enough that they do not reproducibly respond to antibody therapy. Among the 44 patients treated with standard antibody therapy, responses were seen in 51%, which represents an increase over the percentage of responding patients in the relapsed/refractory setting. Only a small percentage of patients (9%) attain a complete remission. The median PRS was only 18.6 months, which is significantly shorter than that seen in follicular NHL patients. While single-agent rituximab has activity in this setting, it cannot be recommended as aggressively as in the setting of follicular NHL where higher response rates and better durability are seen. Given the activity of this antibody in these patients, however, combinations of rituximab and more effective chemotherapy should be explored.

M. S. Gordon, MD

Randomized Phase III Study of Fludarabine Phosphate Versus Cyclophosphamide, Vincristine, and Prednisone in Patients With Recurrent Low-Grade Non-Hodgkin's Lymphoma Previously Treated With an Alkylating Agent or Alkylator-Containing Regimen

Klasa RJ, Meyer RM, Shustik C, et al (British Columbia Cancer Agency, Vancouver, Canada; Hamilton Regional Cancer Ctr, Ont, Canada; London Regional Cancer Ctr, Ont, Canada; et al)

J Clin Oncol 20:4649-4654, 2002 6–15

Background.—Low-grade non-Hodgkin's lymphoma (NHL) is characterized by a lack of symptoms and advanced stage at presentation. Although all initial treatments available are associated with high overall response rates, the disease inevitably relapses. The median survival ranges from 8 to 10 years. The efficacy and safety of fludarabine compared with that of cyclophosphamide, vincristine, and prednisone (CVP) were investigated in patients with recurrent low-grade NHL.

Methods.—Ninety-one patients were included in the study. All had had a previous response to systemic therapy. By random assignment, patients received IV fludarabine, 25 mg/m^2, on days 1 to 5 every 28 days, or IV cyclophosphamide, 750 mg/m^2, plus vincristine, 1.2 mg/m^2, on day 1 and oral prednisone, 40 mg/m^2, on days 1 to 5, every 21 days.

Findings.—Response rates did not differ between the fludarabine and CVP groups at 64% and 52%, respectively. At a median follow-up of 42 months, fludarabine recipients had a better median progression-free survival and treatment-free survival rate. The median overall survival did not differ between groups. However, 3 fludarabine recipients died of treatment-related toxicity compared with none of the CVP recipients. The CVP regimen was associated more commonly with peripheral neuropathy and alopecia. The only quality of life difference between the groups was a higher social functioning score for the fludarabine recipients.

Conclusions.—Fludarabine therapy in patients with recurrent low-grade lymphoma is associated with better progression-free survival, treatment-free survival, and social function scores compared with CVP. However, fludarabine does not appear to improve overall survival.

► The investigators performed a randomized trial of single agent fludarabine versus standard CVP chemotherapy for patients with recurrent low-grade NHL previously treated with an alkylating agent–based therapy. The study was powered to assess the progression-free survival for the patients treated, and based on the planned analysis, fludarabine therapy produced a statistically significant improvement in progression-free survival and treatment-free survival. There was no difference in overall survival, though this study was severely underpowered to detect this difference. The fludarabine arm had a modestly higher risk of death, though this was balanced by the improvement in quality of life for patients on this arm related to fewer side effects, especially less peripheral neuropathy. While a significantly increased sample size would be required to demonstrate a survival advantage, the treatment-free survival as well as the improvement in quality of life suggest that fludarabine should be considered an effective standard for patients with relapsed low-grade NHL and that the addition of antibodies to this regimen is warranted.

M. S. Gordon, MD

Treatment With Ibritumomab Tiuxetan Radioimmunotherapy in Patients With Rituximab-Refractory Follicular Non-Hodgkin's Lymphoma

Witzig TE, Flinn IW, Gordon LI, et al (Mayo Clinic, Rochester, Minn; Johns Hopkins Oncology Ctr, Baltimore, Md; Northwestern Univ, Chicago; et al)

J Clin Oncol 20:3262-3269, 2002 6–16

Background.—Rituximab (Rituxan) is a chimeric anti-CD20 monoclonal antibody approved for the treatment of relapsed or refractory low-grade or follicular non-Hodgkin's lymphoma (NHL). Ibritumomab tiuxetan consists of the parent murine antibody that rituximab is derived from coupled to a radionuclide for imaging or targeted radiotherapy. The use of ibritumomab was evaluated in patients who did not respond to rituximab.

Study Design.—The study group consisted of 57 adult patients with NHL who had been treated with rituximab and either not responded or progressed within 6 months. The majority of patients had large tumors. Patients received 1 course of outpatient rituximab to deplete peripheral blood B cells followed by IV yttrium-90 ibritumomab on day 8. Radiation dosimetry was performed for the first 28 patients to ensure doses stayed well within tolerated levels. Patients were followed up at 1 month, every 3 months for 2 years, and then every 6 months for 2 more years or until disease progression. Safety and efficacy were evaluated on an intent-to-treat basis.

Findings.—The overall response rate was 74%, of which 15% were complete responses. The Kaplan-Meier estimated time to progression was 6.8 months for all patients and 8.7 months for responders. Adverse events were primarily hematologic. Patients reported satisfaction with treatment and quality of life.

Conclusions.—Patients with NHL can be safely and effectively treated with ibritumomab tiuxetan after prior failure of rituximab therapy. Further research is necessary to optimize the use of ibritumomab radioimmunotherapy in the treatment of B-cell NHL.

▶ This study assesses radioimmunotherapy with ibritumomab tiuxetan in patients refractory to rituximab for treatment of NHL. Critical for this study is the fact that all patients were either rituximab refractory or had a response duration of less than 6 months for this group. Re-treatment with rituximab is not likely to yield treatment benefit. Ibritumomab was well tolerated, with side effects similar to rituximab treatment but with the addition of some myelosuppression. Approximately three fourths of patients treated with this agent responded, including patients with bulky (>10 cm) tumors and those with extensive prior treatment. For patients refractory to rituximab, radioimmunotherapy appears to be effective in inducing responses. Duration of response is modest, with median time to progression of approximately 6 to 9 months, which is felt to be clinically valuable in a patient population so heavily pretreated.

M. S. Gordon, MD

Second Malignant Neoplasms Among Long-term Survivors of Hodgkin's Disease: A Population-Based Evaluation Over 25 Years

Dores GM, Metayer C, Curtis RE, et al (Natl Cancer Inst, Bethesda, Md; Univ of Iowa, Iowa City; Univ of Toronto, Ont; et al)

J Clin Oncol 20:3484-3494, 2002 6–17

Background.—Successful treatment for Hodgkin's disease (HD) has permitted more patients to survive longer and to have second cancers develop. The absolute excess risk and relative site-specific risk for second cancers was investigated among a large group of long-term HD survivors.

Study Design.—This study group consisted of 32,591 HD survivors, of whom 2861 had survived at least 20 years. Cancer registries were searched for second malignant neoplasms that developed at least 1 year after HD diagnosis. The risk of second cancer was stratified by sex, age, elapsed time, and initial treatment.

Findings.—The average age at diagnosis was 37 years. Second malignancies developed in 2153 of these survivors, including 1726 solid tumors. The most common types of cancers in this patient group were lung, digestive tract, and female breast. The actuarial risk of a solid tumor developing was 21.9% after 25 years. The relative risk of a solid neoplasm developing decreased with increasing age at HD diagnosis. Patients aged 51 to 60 years at HD diagnosis had the highest cancer burden. There was a progressive increase in relative risk and absolute excess risk for solid tumors with time after diagnosis until after 25 years, when there appeared to be a decrease. Temporal and treatment group cancer distribution suggested a radiogenic effect.

Conclusions.—Patients who survive HD appear to be at risk for second cancers, especially those of the lung, digestive tract, and breast. This risk is increased with time elapsed since diagnosis for 25 years, after which it appears to decline.

► HD represents one of a number of highly curable malignancies. Even after relapse from initial therapy, salvage with radiation standard to high-dose chemotherapy is associated with significant cure rates. Treatment for HD has traditionally incorporated significant doses of alkylator-based therapy and, hence, the risk of second malignancy in this setting can be significant. Dores et al review more than 32,000 HD patients in long-term follow-up to assess the incidence of second malignancies in this patient population. The study indicates a significantly high risk for second solid tumor malignancy, with common tumors such as lung and breast cancer being particularly prevalent. The risk of solid tumors in radiation therapy ports appeared to be significantly increased, suggesting the increased risk of combined modality therapy. The maximum risk for second tumors appears to be at approximately 15 years, with a decrease beyond 25 years. In addition, the risk of second malignancies was higher in patients diagnosed with HD at a younger age, suggesting that time at risk is an important contributor. Vigilant monitoring of patients with HD after successful treatment is critical for early identification of second tumors. Whether more aggressive screening strategies need to be utilized is not yet defined.

M. S. Gordon, MD

Involved-field Radiotherapy for Advanced Hodgkin's Lymphoma

Aleman BM, for the European Organization for Research and Treatment of Cancer Lymphoma Group (Netherlands Cancer Inst, Amsterdam; et al)

N Engl J Med 348:2396-2406, 2003 6–18

Introduction.—The outcome of treatment in patients with advanced Hodgkin's lymphoma has improved dramatically over the past 2 decades: cure rates are as high as 70% or more with chemotherapy regimens. The use of involved-field radiotherapy after chemotherapy in these patients is controversial. Whether radiotherapy decreases the relapse rate was determined in patients 15 to 70 years of age with untreated stage III or IV Hodgkin's lymphoma in complete remission after 6 to 8 cycles of treatment with mechlor ethamine, vincristine, procarbazine, prednisone, doxorubicin, bleomycin, and vinblastine (MOPP-ABV).

Methods.—Patients were randomly assigned to receive either no further treatment or involved-field radiotherapy, which consisted of 24 Gy to all initially involved nodal areas and 16 to 24 Gy to all initially involved extranodal sites. Patients whose disease was in partial remission underwent treatment with 30 Gy to nodal areas and 18 to 24 Gy to extranodal areas.

Results.—Of 739 patients, 421 had complete remission; 161 were randomly assigned to no further treatment and 172 were assigned to involved-field radiotherapy. The median follow-up was 79 months. The 5-year event-free survival rates were 79% and 84% in the groups that did and did not undergo involved-field radiotherapy, respectively ($P = .35$). The 5-year overall survival rates were 85% and 91% in the groups that did and did not receive radiotherapy, respectively ($P = .07$). Among patients whose disease was in partial remission after chemotherapy, the 5-year event-free and overall survival rates were 87% and 79%, respectively.

Conclusion.—Involved-field radiotherapy did not enhance the outcomes in patients with advanced-stage Hodgkin's lymphoma who had complete remission after undergoing MOPP-ABV chemotherapy. Radiotherapy may be useful in patients with a partial response after chemotherapy.

▶ The use of involved field radiation therapy for patients with Hodgkin's disease is controversial, especially for those patients who achieve a complete response to combination chemotherapy. Traditionally, sites of bulky disease were recognized as being at high risk for relapse. This study addresses the issue of the role of radiation therapy in this setting. Patients with advanced stage (III or IV) Hodgkin's lymphoma in a complete remission were randomly assigned to receive or not receive radiation to their previously involved fields. With a median follow-up of more than 6 years the relapse-free and overall survival times were not statistically significantly different, indicating that radiation therapy in this setting adds no benefit. Of interest will be the fact that patients receiving combined modality therapy tend to be at higher risk for secondary malignancies, which typically do not peak until the second decade. As a result, it is possible that deleterious effects may still be seen for the radiation group. It is interesting to note that all patients who achieved only a partial response to chemotherapy received the same type of radiation therapy and fared similarly to the patients in the complete remission arms. Hence, while radiation therapy cannot be recommended for the patients who achieve a complete remission, those with partial remissions may be benefited and the use of radiation in this setting should be decided on a case-by-case basis.

M. S. Gordon, MD

7 Pediatric Oncology

Is Reexcision in Pediatric Nonrhabdomyosarcoma Soft Tissue Sarcoma Necessary After an Initial Unplanned Resection?

Chui CH, Spunt SL, Liu T, et al (Univ of Tennessee, Memphis; Univ of Toronto, Ont)

J Pediatr Surg 37:1424-1429, 2002 7–1

Background.—Approximately 4% of all pediatric malignancies are nonrhabdomyosarcoma soft tissue sarcomas (NRSTS). These sarcomas often mimic the presentation of a benign mass and in many cases are treated accordingly, with unplanned excision or a shelled-out procedure without consideration of a clear margin of normal tissue around the tumor. Often the adjacent pseudocapsules are infiltrated by tumor. Microscopic residual tumor can lead to local recurrence despite the removal of all gross disease. A common practice at the study center is to perform pretreatment reexcision (PRE), whenever feasible, in all patients after initial unplanned excisions. The importance of PRE in pediatric NRSTS after initial unplanned excision was determined.

Methods.—A retrospective review was conducted of the records of 116 consecutive patients with surgically resected NRSTS treated at 1 institution between February 1978 and September 1999. The majority of patients (81%) had undergone unplanned resections before referral to the study institution for additional therapy. Demographic data, tumor characteristics, type of treatment administered, and outcomes were recorded.

Results.—PRE was performed in 69 (73.4%) of 116 patients at a median interval of 29 days after the initial unplanned resection. In 25 patients, PRE was considered inadvisable because of the proximity to vital neurovascular bundles. Tumors judged to be not feasible for PRE were more likely to be greater than 5 cm and of high grade. Tumor was identified in 33 (47.8%) of the PRE specimens, and 24 of these patients (72.7%) were determined to be disease free after achieving negative surgical margins. Residual tumor was more likely to be identified after PRE in primary tumors of the head and neck than in primary tumors of the trunk wall or extremity. No local failures were observed in the 60 PRE patients who achieved clear margins. The estimated 5-year event-free and 5-year overall survival rates in these patients were 98.3% ± 2.0% and 98.2% ± 2.1%, respectively.

Conclusions.—PRE should be performed whenever feasible in pediatric patients with NRSTS who underwent an initial unplanned resection. There is a high proportion of patients with residual tumor in the PRE specimen, and it is possible to obtain negative microscopic margins after PRE in most patients with residual tumor. In this study population, no local recurrences were seen despite delay in obtaining complete resection. The possibility for NRSTS should be considered in any case in which a soft tissue mass is resected in a pediatric patient. The surgical goal in these patients should be diagnostic incisional biopsy followed by wide local excision with negative microscopic margins.

▶ These authors examine 116 patients over a 21-year period who had NRSTS and an unplanned initial surgical resection. Unplanned resection in this analysis refers to initial surgical incisional biopsies or resections that involved a shelled-out procedure without consideration of a clear margin of normal tissue around the tumor. The results show that of this group of patients, 73.4% had reexcision surgery with a median interval from their initial procedure of 29 days. Of particular interest, residual tumor was identified in close to 50% of these cases and, of those, nearly 73% resulted in negative surgical margins. While surgical approaches could have improved over the long period that this study covers, the conclusions presented by these authors is still an important one. Local control is essential for NRSTS, and complete surgical resection can be an effective modality to accomplish this. When an initial surgical procedure is not optimally performed to achieve a complete resection, the reexcision is warranted if the anatomic position and size of the initial lesion would suggest that complete resection is possible. This study also should sensitize surgeons who see such patients to carefully consider the differential diagnosis and plan their surgical approach accordingly.

R. J. Arceci, MD, PhD

Prognostic Factors and Surgical Treatment Guidelines for Children With Rhabdomyosarcoma of the Perineum or Anus: A Report of Intergroup Rhabdomyosarcoma Studies I Through IV, 1972 Through 1997

Blakely ML, Andrassy RJ, Raney RB, et al (Univ of Texas, Houston)

J Pediatr Surg 38:347-353, 2003 7–2

Background.—Rhabdomyosarcoma (RMS) is the most common soft tissue sarcoma in children. The prognosis for RMS is poor, and these patients are difficult diagnostic and treatment challenges for the pediatric surgeon or oncologist. Outcome in these patients depends primarily on the site of the primary tumor and the extent of disease at presentation. The overall survival rate in children with RMS has improved over the past several decades. RMS of the anus or perineum is a rare sarcoma, and prognosis remains relatively poor. The findings of the Intergroup Rhabdomyosarcoma Study Group (IRSG) studies I through IV were reviewed to identify the determinants of patient outcome and to refine surgical treatment guidelines.

Methods.—This study involved 71 eligible patients treated for RMS of the anus or perineum from 1972 through 1997. The median age of the patients was 6 years. Most of the patients (64%) were at an advanced stage of disease (clinical group III and IV) at initial presentation, and 50% had positive regional lymph node involvement.

Results.—The 5-year failure-free survival rate for all patients was 45%, and the overall survival rate was 49%. A significantly improved survival rate was associated with primary tumor size less than 5 cm, lower clinical group and stage, negative regional lymph node status, and age younger than 10 years. On multivariate analysis, after controlling for the extent of disease, only age younger than 10 years was predictive of an improved outcome. The 5-year overall survival rate for patients younger than 10 years of age was 71% compared with 20% in older patients. Histology and primary site did not have a significant effect on outcome.

Conclusions.—A strategy of routine surgical evaluation of ilioinguinal lymph nodes in all pediatric patients with perineal or anal rhabdomyosarcoma is recommended because of the high incidence of regional lymph node involvement in these patients.

► Although sarcomas involving the perineum or anus are rare in children, they nevertheless represent an important condition. The value of the intergroup RMS studies is shown in the report by Blakely et al in that they were able to analyze prognostic features and outcome in 71 patients with sarcomas of the perineum or anus. Multivariate analysis indicates that age younger than 10 years was associated with a significantly higher 5-year overall survival (71%) compared with patients older than 10 years (20% survival). This significant difference was in contrast to the lack of significance in terms of impact on outcome of histology and primary site (perineal vs anal). Another important point raised by this review is the important recommendation that ilioinguinal lymph node evaluation be performed in these patients because of the relatively high incidence of regional lymph node involvement.

R. J. Arceci, MD, PhD

Treatment of Children With Nonmetastatic Paratesticular Rhabdomyosarcoma: Results of the Malignant Mesenchymal Tumors Studies (MMT 84 and MMT 89) of the International Society of Pediatric Oncology

Stewart RJ, Martelli H, Oberlin O, et al (Queen's Med Ctr, Nottingham, England; Royal Hosp for Children, Bristol, England; Le Kremlin-Bicêtre, Villejuif, France; et al)

J Clin Oncol 21:793-798, 2003 7–3

Background.—Among children and adolescents with rhabdomyosarcoma (RMS), 6% have paratesticular tumors. Most studies of these patients have reported survival rates of more than 90%. The role of lymph node evaluation by lymphadenectomy at diagnosis and the identification of the small number of children who are at risk of treatment failure are controversial. Results from early International Society of Pediatric Oncology (SIOP) studies have showed that para-aortic lymphadenectomy was not required in the treatment of localized paratesticular RMS. Complete surgical resection at diagnosis is frequent in paratesticular RMS, and there have been attempts to decrease the burden of therapy by reducing the intensity and duration of chemotherapy. The results of the Malignant Mesenchymal Tumors studies (MMT 84 and 89) of the SIOP in male patients with nonmetastatic paratesticular RMS were reported.

Methods.—Ninety-six male patients were treated in SIOP protocols from 1984 to 1994. Radical inguinal orchidectomy was recommended, but initial retroperitoneal lymph node dissection was not performed. Disease was staged according to the SIOP tumor node metastasis staging system. Treatment was stratified by age. In the MMT 89 study, patients with completely resected tumors at diagnosis received chemotherapy consisting of vincristine and dactinomycin, whereas patients in the MMT 84 study received ifosfamide, vincristine, and dactinomycin.

Results.—The median age of the patients at diagnosis was 65 months. There were 31 tumors larger than 5 cm, and 13 patients were older than 10 years with a tumor larger than 5 cm. At a median of 7 years of follow-up, 87 of 96 patients were alive, with 79 patients in first complete remission and 8 in second complete remission. Relapse occurred in 16 patients (17%). The overall survival rate at 5 years was 92%, and the event-free survival was 82%. Overall survival and event-free survival were significantly worse for patients with tumors greater than 5 cm and for those older than 10 years at diagnosis.

Conclusions.—Overall, boys with paratesticular rhabdomyosarcomas have an excellent prognosis; the exception is a selected group of patients older than 10 years or who have a tumor larger than 5 cm. In this subgroup of patients, intensified chemotherapy incorporating alkylating agents may be preferred to the use of systematic lymphadenectomy for improvement of survival with minimal burden of therapy.

► The outcome for children with nonmetastatic paratesticular rhabdomyosarcoma has continued to improve such that the overall survival is now greater than 92% and event-free survival is more than 80%. There continues to be some controversy over prognostic factors as well as which subgroups require more intensive therapy or lymphadenectomy. The manuscript by Stewart et al examines the outcome for patients in 2 trials (MMT 84 and MMT 89) of the Malignant Mesenchymal Tumors Study Group of SIOP. Overall and event-free survival rates are comparable to previous studies and show outcomes consistent with greater than 90% and 80%, respectively. Importantly, age greater than 10 years and tumors greater than 5 cm in size represented adverse prognostic factors. This subgroup may thus be appropriate to receive more intensive treatment plans as well as have retroperitoneal lymph node involvement examined by lymphadenectomy.

R. J. Arceci, MD, PhD

Chronic Neuroblastoma: Indolent Stage 4 Disease in Children

Kushner BH, Kramer K, Cheung N-KV (Mem Sloan-Kettering Cancer Ctr, New York)

Cancer 95:1366-1375, 2002 7–4

Introduction.—Indolent, or smoldering metastatic neuroblastoma, has been described in adolescents and adults and is rare in MYCN-amplified disease. This phenomenon was examined in a large series of children who had metastatic neuroblastoma 5 years or more from diagnosis.

Findings.—The median age of 38 children with metastatic disease 5 or more years from diagnosis was 3 years, 10 months. In 2 of 28 patients evaluated, MYCN was amplified. Of 30 children with classic stage 4 neuroblastoma, 9 had a late first recurrence of disease (4.3-13 years from diagnosis). Of 8 patients (1 isolated mandibular lesion, 2 stage 4-N, 5 non-stage 4) with atypical cases at diagnosis, 6 had a late first distant disease recurrence (4 years, 11 months to 38 years, 8 months). Nineteen patients received no therapy for 3 years or more before disease recurred a first or second time. Myeloablative therapy was used to consolidate a first or second response in 27 patients. High-dose conventional therapy was beneficial in achieving a second disease remission in 9 of 20 patients assessable for response to first recurrence. No major responses of second or third relapse were observed in 10 of 11 patients. A combination of anti-G_{D2} immunotherapy and *cis*-retinoic acid, targeted radiotherapy, and multiple cycles of chemotherapy with modest toxicity were useful in prolonging survival. Twelve patients survived at 5 years, 6 months to 19 years, 4 months from diagnosis of lymphoma (median, 6 years, 10 months), including 4 patients with complete disease remission. Of these, 10 underwent anti-G_{D2} immunotherapy after recurrence. The remaining 26 patients died of disease or toxicity (22 and 4 patients, respectively) at 5 years to 41 years, 5 months from diagnosis (median, 6 years, 5 months).

Conclusion.—Smoldering neuroblastoma occurs in children as well as adolescents and adults. The expanding repertoire of anti-neuroblastoma treatments, including biologic therapies and chemotherapy regimens of modest toxicity, can be used to convert childhood neuroblastoma into a chronic disease with prolonged survival after recurrence.

► Instances of very late relapse of neuroblastoma have been known for many years but have largely been considered relatively extreme exceptions. The report by Kushner et al describes a group of 38 patients who had neuroblastoma in their first decade but experienced relapse of their disease 5 years or more from diagnosis. Of importance is that the majority of the patients described had classic stage 4 neuroblastoma, with only 8 having atypical presentations. These cases raise the important issue of whether intensifying treatments changed the course of the disease but did not necessarily result in cures. In addition, if very late relapses occur more frequently in certain subtypes of neuroblastoma, the question arises as to when the proper time is to report outcomes. Further, the development of identifying potential surrogate and early biologic or imaging markers for outcome takes on even greater importance. Last, optimizing a therapeutic approach to patients who develop very late relapses becomes essential. Whether such treatment approaches should be directed at cure or to "reprogramming" or "resetting" the neuroblastoma to a more chronic state remains to be determined.

R. J. Arceci, MD, PhD

Prognostic Value of Tumor Size, Metastases, Extension Into Bone, and Increased Tumor Marker in Children With Malignant Sacrococcygeal Germ Cell Tumors: A Prospective Evaluation of 71 Patients Treated in the German Cooperative Protocols Maligne Keimzelltumoren (MAKEI) 83/86 and MAKEI 89

Calaminus G, Schneider DT, Bökkerink JPM, et al (Univ of Düsseldorf, Germany; Univ of Kiel, Germany; Children's Hosp, Nijmegen, The Netherlands; et al)

J Clin Oncol 21:781-786, 2003 7–5

Background.—Malignant germ cell tumors (GCTs), which represent 3.4% of all malignancies in children, are characterized by heterogeneous histology, localization, and stage. Children with sacrococcygeal tumors are most likely to have tumor extension into the coccyx or sacrum of the spine (in advanced cases). Previous studies have reported spinal involvement and high elevation of alpha-fetoprotein (AFP) as adverse prognostic factors. The prognostic value of metastases, extension into bone, and AFP elevation was evaluated in children with malignant sacrococcygeal GCTs prospectively collected in 2 cooperative Maligne Keimzelltumoren protocols (83/86 and 89).

Methods.—The study group was composed of 76 of 210 patients seen between October 1983 and October 1995 with either pure yolk sac tumor, embryonal carcinoma, or yolk sac tumor and embryonal carcinoma mixed with immature and mature teratoma elements. Stage T1 disease was diagnosed in 15 patients and T2 disease in 61 children. Metastases were present in 41 patients, and 35 children had extension into bone. At diagnosis, 22 children had an AFP elevation of less than 10,000 ng/mL, 36 children had an AFP level between 10,000 and 100,000 ng/mL, and 12 patients had values of greater than 100,000 ng/mL. There were 5 deaths from complications during treatment, and they were excluded from evaluation. The findings were based on analysis of the remaining 71 patients.

Results.—The 5-year relapse-free survival rate was 0.76 ± 0.03 (54 of 71 patients), with a median observation time of 54 months after diagnosis. There was a nonsignificant difference in the relapse-free survival of patients with and without metastases (0.71 vs 0.82). Outcome for patients with and without extension into bone was 0.71 versus 0.80, respectively (relapse-free survival, 5 years). No prognostic significance was noted for above-normal AFP level.

Conclusions.—No prognostic significance was found for the stage, extent of metastasis, extension into bone, and AFP level in children with malignant sacrococcygeal GCTs treated with an intensive, short-interval, platinum-based regimen.

► Approximately two thirds of children with malignant sacrococcygeal tumors have advanced disease. The study by Calaminus et al evaluates the prognostic factors and outcome of this group of children and demonstrates that an intensive, short-interval, platinum-based treatment regimen resulted in a 5-year relapse-free survival (RFS) of 76. Further, while there was a trend toward a worse prognosis in patients with metastases (RFS of 71%) versus those without metastases (RFS of 80%), the differences were not statistically significant. When patients were treated with this regimen, previous prognostic factors, such as stage of disease, extent of metastases including extension into bone, and the AFP level, were not significant. These results are important to consider when determining treatment for such patients as well as counseling families on outcome. The results also provide a good example of improved treatment leading to a reconsideration of past prognostic factors.

R. J. Arceci, MD, PhD

Treatment of Unresectable and Metastatic Hepatoblastoma: A Pediatric Oncology Group Phase II Study

Katzenstein HM, London WB, Douglass EC, et al (Northwestern Univ, Chicago; Univ of Florida, Gainesville; AstraZeneca Pharmaceuticals LP, Wilmington, Del; et al)

J Clin Oncol 20:3438-3444, 2002 7–6

Introduction.—The Pediatric Oncology Group (POG) study 9345 (open May 1993 to February 1995) was designed to increase treatment efficacy and reduce toxicity in children with unresectable and metastatic hepatoblastoma by incorporating carboplatin instead of cisplatin, eliminating doxorubicin, and adding weekly vincristine and continuous infusion of fluorouracil. Patients whose tumors remained unresectable had therapy intensified with high-dose cisplatin and etoposide. Reported is the use of sequential treatment with (1) carboplatin; (2) carboplatin, vincristine, and 5-fluorouracil; and (3) cisplatin and etoposide in children with unresectable and metastatic hepatoblastoma to improve tumor resectability and long-term survival.

Methods.—Thirty-three assessable children with stage III and stage IV (22 and 11 patients, respectively) hepatoblastoma underwent sequential treatment with 1 course of carboplatin (700 mg/m^2), then 3 courses of carboplatin (700 mg/m^2) on day 0; 5-fluorouracil (1000 mg/m^2 per day) by continuous infusion on days 0 to 2; and vincristine (1.5 mg/m^2) on days 0, 7, and 14. Patients whose tumors were resectable underwent surgery, then had 2 additional courses of carboplatin/vincristine/5-fluorouracil. Patients whose tumors remained unresectable after carboplatin/vincristine/5-fluorouracil or who had no response or progressive disease during therapy received 2 courses of high-dose cisplatin (40 mg/m^2) on days 1 to 5 and etoposide (100 mg/m^2 per day) on days 2 to 4.

Results.—The 5-year event-free survival estimates were 59% for 22 patients with stage III hepatoblastoma and 27% for 11 with stage IV hepatoblastoma ($P = .037$). Twenty-seven (82%) children had at least a partial response to chemotherapy; 18 (55%) of 33 responded to carboplatin; 24 (80%) of 30 responded to carboplatin and carboplatin/vincristine/5-fluorouracil; and 9 of 12 (75%) responded to high-dose cisplatin and etoposide. Surgical resection was possible in 19 (58%) of 33 patients, including 15 (86%) of 22 patients with stage III hepatoblastoma and 4 (36%) of 11 with stage IV hepatoblastoma. The 5-year event-free survival in children whose tumors were completely resected was 79%.

Conclusion.—Patients with stage III and stage IV hepatoblastoma treated sequentially with carboplatin, carboplatin/vincristine/5-fluorouracil, and high-dose cisplatin and etoposide had response rates similar to other therapeutic regimens. This regimen is effective in the treatment of localized, unresectable hepatoblastoma and potentially has less toxicity. Novel approaches are required in patients with metastatic disease.

▶ The ability of chemotherapy in patients with initially unresectable hepatoblastoma to produce sufficient tumor responses to allow complete surgical resections has been known since the early 1980s. Of course, one of the problems with such studies in terms of precisely defining what percentage of patients can be converted to surgical resections depends on the definition of unresectability and who is defining it. The current study by Katzenstein et al attempts to use a non–anthracycline- and non–cisplatin-based initial treatment of such advanced-staged patients to determine the disease response rate, the proportion of patients whose tumors can be made resectable, event-free survival, and toxicity. The results, similar to several other studies, suggest that this regimen is potentially as good as anthracycline- and cisplatin-containing regimens. This study still suffers from the potential problem of bias in determining initial resectability. In addition, this regimen may produce few adverse renal toxicities but has not appeared to reduce ototoxicity, although the numbers of patients are small and this is not a randomized trial. Patients with stage IV disease still do poorly. Thus, while this study may provide a small improvement (this needs confirmation in a randomized and larger study), the results remain similar to other studies both in terms of respectability issues and stage IV patients, who clearly need alternative approaches to treatment.

R. J. Arceci, MD, PhD

Relation of Childhood Brain Tumors to Exposure of Parents and Children to Tobacco Smoke: The SEARCH International Case-Control Study

Filippini G, Maisonneuve P, McCredie M, et al (Istituto Nazionale Neurologico "C Besta," Milan, Italy; European Inst of Oncology, Milan, Italy; Univ of Otago, Dunedin, New Zealand; et al)

Int J Cancer 100:206-213, 2002 7–7

Background.—Childhood brain tumors are the second most common malignancy in children younger than 15 years. These tumors are more common in children than in adults, and the central nervous system is more sensitive or accessible to carcinogens early in life. Thus, it is reasonable to consider that exposure to tobacco smoke in the womb or during childhood may increase the risk of development of childhood brain tumors. The association between childhood brain tumors and exposure of parents and children to cigarette smoke was evaluated.

Methods.—This multinational study was conducted as part of the Surveillance of Environmental Aspects Related to Cancer in Humans program of the International Agency for Research on Cancer. A total of 1218 patients with childhood brain cancer (aged 0-19 years) and 2223 population-based control subjects were included in the study, which involved 9 centers in 7 countries. Most maternal interviews were conducted at home, and fathers were interviewed whenever possible. Parents were asked about maternal smoking before and during the index pregnancy, passive exposure to tobacco smoke of the father during the pregnancy, other household members or coworkers, and passive exposure to tobacco smoke during the first year of life. Mothers were also asked about the quantity and type of cigarettes smoked during each trimester and the number of hours per day they were exposed to cigarette smoke from spouses and other household members. Odds ratios were calculated by unconditional logistic regression, adjusted for age, sex, and center, for all types of childhood brain tumor combined, for 4 tumor histotypes and for 5 age groups from each center.

Results.—No association was found between the risk of brain tumors in the child and parental smoking before pregnancy, maternal smoking or regular exposure to others' cigarette smoke during pregnancy at home or at work, or passive smoking by the child during the first year of life. These findings persisted after adjustment for the child's age at diagnosis, histologic type, and center.

Conclusions.—There is no evidence of an increase in the risk of childhood brain tumors associated with maternal or paternal smoking before or during pregnancy or maternal exposure to passive smoke during pregnancy. In the absence of an association with active smoking by the mother, it is unlikely that there could be a relation between childhood brain tumors and passive smoking.

► The etiology of childhood brain tumors remains a challenging and important area of investigative work. While epidemiologic studies are not able to provide mechanistic relationships between cause and effect, they can be quite useful in leading to possible associations as well as pointing laboratory investigators in the right direction. Just as importantly, it is critical for investigators not to be pointed in the incorrect direction. Previous studies have associated prenatal exposure to cigarette smoke with the development of childhood brain tumors. In contrast, this large case-control study by Filippini et al, which includes data from 7 countries, concludes that there is no significant association between maternal or paternal smoking, or prenatal or postnatal exposure, and the development of childhood brain tumors. While such a study should not be used as an endorsement of the safety of cigarette smoking, this type of study should help to at least understand what might not be involved in brain tumor development in children. To that end, this is an important study.

R. J. Arceci, MD, PhD

Induction of Medulloblastomas in Mice by Sonic Hedgehog, Independent of *Gli1*

Weiner HL, Bakst R, Hurlbert MS, et al (New York Univ)
Cancer Res 62:6385-6389, 2002 7–8

Introduction.—The Sonic hedgehog (Shh) signaling pathway has an important role in normal cerebellar development. It has been implicated in medulloblastomas, one of the most common malignant childhood tumors of the cerebellum. To ascertain whether Shh misexpression is adequate for medulloblastoma formation, US biomicroscopy-guided in utero injection of a Shh-expressing retrovirus into the cerebellum was performed in 13.5-day-old mouse embryos to demonstrate that direct activation of the Shh pathway can lead to tumor formation.

Findings.—Medulloblastomas were detected in 76% of animals infected with Shh-expressing retrovirus. Contrary to recent indications that Shh transcriptional target *Gli1* has an important role in Shh-induced tumorigenesis, medulloblastomas formed in *Gli1* null mutant mice.

Conclusion.—An efficient mouse model of medulloblastoma has been developed. When Shh signaling is activated upstream in the pathway, *Gli1* is not necessary for tumorigenesis.

► The development of preclinical models for various cancers holds much potential in terms of increasing our understanding of etiologic mechanisms as well as serving as systems in which to test new treatment approaches. This is particularly true for malignancies that are rare. The study by Weiner et al demonstrates that the overexpression of Shh, a protein that plays an essential role in cerebellum development, in the cerebellum of prenatal mice leads to a high incidence of medulloblastoma. A nice extension of this result shows that the increased incidence of medulloblastoma secondary to Shh overexpression is independent of the *Gli1* pathway. While this type of overexpression may be in part artificial, it represents a clear step forward in the development of potentially important in vivo models for central nervous system tumors.

R. J. Arceci, MD, PhD

High Response Rate to Cisplatin/Etoposide Regimen in Childhood Low-Grade Glioma

Massimino M, Spreafico F, Cefalo G, et al (Istituto Nazionale Tumori, Milan, Italy; Istituto Neurologica Carlo Besta, Milan, Italy; Università Cattolica del Sacro Cuore-Policlinico Gemelli, Rome; et al)

J Clin Oncol 20:4209-4216, 2002 7–9

Background.—Low-grade glioma (LGG) accounts for approximately one third of all childhood brain tumors. Complete surgical removal, when feasible, has been the treatment of choice for LGG, which has provided a cure in the great majority of children. Without additional treatment, tumors that are not completely resectable may progress slowly over years. However, an accelerated rate of growth may occur, particularly in infiltrating lesions or in opticochiasmatic lesions, primarily in children younger than 5 years. The adverse effects of radiotherapy in young children with large tumors make it an undesirable approach in these children. To avoid radiotherapy, an objective response in children with LGG was induced by using a chemotherapy regimen based on cisplatin and etoposide.

Methods.—Thirty-four children (median age, 45 months) with unresectable LGG were treated with 10 monthly cycles of cisplatin (30 mg/m^2 per day on days 1 to 3) and etoposide (150 mg/m^2 per day on days 1 to 2). Origins of the tumor were the visual pathway in 29 patients, the temporal lobe in 2 patients, the frontal lobe in 2 patients, and the spine in 1 patient. MRI and neurologic and functional tests at 3-month intervals were used to obtain objective assessments of tumor response and toxicity.

Results.—An objective response was obtained in 24 (70%) of 34 patients; the remaining 10 patients had stable disease. None of the children was electively irradiated. Overall survival in 31 previously untreated children was 100% and progression-free survival was 78% at 3 years, with a median follow-up of 44 months. The incidence of acute toxicity was unremarkable. A loss of perception of high frequencies was found in 28% of patients evaluated for acoustic neurotoxicity.

Conclusions.—The diagnosis and treatment of LGG is difficult, and little consensus exists regarding treatment guidelines. The results of this study have demonstrated that chemotherapy can modify the natural history of this tumor, inducing high rates of tumor stabilization or regression. Monthly cisplatin and etoposide would appear to be one of the most active regimens in the chemotherapeutic treatment of LGG in children. This regimen makes it possible to avoid the use of radiotherapy and its potential for severe adverse effects in young children.

► The optimal manner used to treat children with LGG has evolved over the years with approaches using surgery, radiotherapy, chemotherapy, or combinations being used. When feasible, complete surgical excision is often considered to be the treatment of choice. However, for tumors that cannot be resected safely and that show progression, treatments have tried to optimize efficacy while reducing toxicity. The study by Massimino et al presents excellent results with a prolonged course of cisplatin and etoposide for children with LGG. Progression-free survival (PFS) was 78% at 3 years and an overall survival of 100%. Approximately one third of patients reveals some degree of high-frequency hearing loss that did not appear to include speech frequencies. No patient received radiotherapy. Of interest, patients with NF1, although small in number, showed a 100% PFS. However, patients older than 1 year represented a higher risk group with only a 33% PFS compared with 87% for the rest of the group. Clearly, this higher risk group requires alternative strategies. In addition, attempts to reduce toxicity from this combination regimen should be considered. While no secondary leukemias were observed in the study, this risk should continue to be assessed.

R. J. Arceci, MD, PhD

Preradiation Chemotherapy in Primary High-Risk Brainstem Tumors: Phase II Study CCG-9941 of the Children's Cancer Group

Jennings MT, Sposto R, Boyett JM, et al (Vanderbilt Cancer Ctr, Nashville, Tenn; Saint Jude's Children's Research Hosp, Memphis, Tenn; Children's Cancer Group, Arcadia, Calif; et al)

J Clin Oncol 20:3431-3437, 2002 7–10

Introduction.—Treatment with hyperfractionated external-beam radiotherapy (HFEBRT) has been disappointing, yet it is worth exploring the various dose relations exhibited between nonproliferating normal tissues and malignant tumor cells. It is also worth determining whether a preradiation response to chemotherapy improves postradiation survival. This Children's Cancer Group group-wide phase II trial (CCG-9941) examined the efficacy and toxicity of 2 chemotherapy arms administered before HFEBRT.

Methods.—Thirty-two children with newly diagnosed brainstem gliomas were randomly assigned to treatment with 3 courses of either regimen A (carboplatin, etoposide, and vincristine) or regimen B (cisplatin, etoposide, cyclophosphamide, and vincristine). Granulocyte colony stimulating factor was included in both treatment arms. Patients underwent MRI after induction chemotherapy and HFEBRT at a dose of 72 Gy.

Results.—Ten percent of patients in the regimen A treatment arm had an objective response to chemotherapy. With combined induction and HFEBRT, 27% improved. The neuroradiographic response rate for the regimen B treatment arm was 19% for chemotherapy and 23% after HFEBRT. There were no significant between-group differences in response rates. Event-free survival was 17% and 6% at 1 year and 2 years, respectively. Survival was significantly longer in patients who had a chemotherapy response ($P < .05$). In patients who underwent regimen A induction, grade 3 and 4 leukopenia occurred in 50% and 65%, respectively; there was 1 toxicity-associated death. In patients who received regimen B, severe leukopenia was observed in 86% and 100%, respectively, with febrile neutropenia in 48% to 60% per course.

Conclusion.—Neither chemotherapy regimen was superior to the other in statistically significant improvement in response rate, event-free survival, or overall survival relative to previous series of patients with brainstem gliomas who underwent radiotherapy with or without chemotherapy.

▶ The outcome for children with brainstem gliomas remains dreadful. Attempts to improve that outcome have involved exposure to radiosensitizers and preradiation chemotherapy. The study by Jennings et al attempts to determine whether 1 of 2 regimens differing in part in their intensity but also in the types of drugs used (carboplatin vs cisplatin or the use of cyclophosphamide in one and not the other) improves objective responses and prolongs survival. The results show that the regimens were similar in their ineffectiveness and not really substantially different than a substantial number of other similar reports. While there is much discussion in this study concerning the Norton-Simon hypothesis and other reasons why these regimens were tested, the basic issue is that we should probably stop doing such trials in patients with brain stem gliomas (none of them work) and focus on truly novel treatment approaches with modern approaches to functional and biologic response imaging. The development of animal models would also be potentially helpful as a system to develop alternative therapeutic approaches.

R. J. Arceci, MD, PhD

Evidence for a Hereditary Neuroblastoma Predisposition Locus at Chromosome 16p12-13

Maris JM, Weiss MJ, Mosse Y, et al (Univ of Pennsylvania, Philadelphia; Northwestern Univ, Chicago)

Cancer Res 62:6651-6658, 2002 7–11

Introduction.—Neuroblastoma is a relatively common cancer of childhood that occurs sporadically and is lethal in more than 40% of the cases. The cell of origin is considered to be an undifferentiated neural crest–derived cell committed to the developing sympathetic nervous system. Hereditary predisposition to the development of neuroblastoma is rare (1%-2%) and segregates as an autosomal dominant Mendelian trait. A linkage analysis was performed on 7 families in which 2 or more first-degree relatives had neuroblastoma to localize a hereditary neuroblastoma predisposition gene.

Findings.—A lone interval at chromosome bands 16p12-13 was the only genomic region consistent with linkage (LOD_{MAX} = 3.30 at *D16S764*. Detection of informative recombination events in linked families defined a 28.0-cm region between *D16S748* and *D16S769* that cosegregate in 5 of 11 familial neuroblastomas and 68 of 336 nonfamilial neuroblastomas (20.2%) at numerous 16p polymorphic loci. A 14.5-cm smallest region of overlap of somatic deletions was observed within the interval defined by linkage analysis (tel-*D16S500-D16S412*-cen).

Conclusion.—Findings from this first genome-wide screen for a predisposition locus in neuroblastoma kindreds indicate that a hereditary neuroblastoma predisposition gene *HNB1*) is located at 16p12-13. Disruption of this gene may contribute to the pathogenesis of nonfamilial neuroblastomas.

▶ Neuroblastoma usually occurs sporadically, although in rare instances it can be familial. In those cases in which hereditary neuroblastoma is observed, investigators have hypothesized that there must be a critical tumor suppressor gene that was mutated, as has been observed in retinoblastoma. Maris et al have studied a group of families in which neuroblastoma has occurred in more than 1 member. Their findings identify a region at chromosome 16p12-13, which shows loss of heterozygosity (a hallmark of tumor suppressor genes) in nearly half of the familial neuroblastoma cases. This locus is further determined to show loss of heterozygosity in about 20% of the sporadic cases of neuroblastoma. Although the approximately 9.1-megabase region could certainly harbor multiple genes, this work takes an important step forward in significantly narrowing this important search.

R. J. Arceci, MD, PhD

Gene Expression Profiling of Favorable Histology Wilms Tumors and Its Correlation With Clinical Features

Takahashi M, Yang XJ, Lavery TT, et al (Van Andel Research Inst, Grand Rapids, Mich; Univ of Tokushima, Japan; Univ of Chicago; et al)

Cancer Res 62:6598-6605, 2002 7–12

Introduction.—Nephroblastoma or Wilms' tumor (WT), the most common cancer of the urinary tract in children under the age of 15 years, can be histologically divided into 2 subtypes: 1 with favorable histology and 1 with anaplasia. The global gene expression profiles of WT were characterized. Genes frequently altered in WT and specific gene sets that correlate with clinical parameters were also examined.

Findings.—Fifteen favorable histology WTs were assessed with microarrays containing 19,968 cDNAs. Commonly altered genes were identified in WT. A total of 267 cDNAs were significantly overexpressed at least 3-fold in all tumor versus noncancerous kidney and contained known WT-associated genes, including *IGF II* and *WTI*. The gene with the highest expression change versus the noncancerous kidney was *topoisomerase IIα*. Hierarchical clustering showed that there was a clear distinction between high-stage and low-stage tumors. Thirty cDNAs were differentially expressed between the high- and low-stage groups. One of the cDNAs, *Stathmin 1*, which is involved in the microtubule system, was highly expressed in high-stage tumors versus low-stage tumors. The present chemotherapy regimens for WT are composed primarily of topoisomerase II inhibitors (ie, actinomycin D, doxorubicin, and etoposide) and antimicrotubule agents (ie, vincristine and paclitaxel). High expression of *topoisomerase IIα* and microtubule-associated genes, including *tubulin* and *Stathmin 1*, may be associated with the high chemosensitivity of WT. In addition, the retinol-associated genes (*CRABP2* and *retinol-binding protein 1* were overexpressed in WT;

CRABP2 was more highly expressed in patients with poor outcome, indicating that retinoid acid may be a potential drug.

Conclusion.—The integration of gene expression data and clinical parameters could be useful in identifying aggressive tumors among favorable histology WT and enhance the discovery of new drugs for WT.

► Favorable histology WT has been of the most curable cancers of children with often relatively minimal chemotherapy treatment. However, in a small percentage of these patients will the disease relapse and prognosis can be poor. Understanding what characterizes the WTs with an excellent compared to a poorer prognosis is therefore important. The article by Takahashi et al compares the microarray RNA expression patterns of close to 20,000 cDNAs from 15 tumor specimens with normal kidney. The results demonstrate a relatively small subset of overexpressed genes in the tumor specimens compared with normal kidney. In addition, a subset of these genes, representing approximately 30 cDNAs, were found to be differentially expressed between high- and low-stage groups. Although these data fall short of determining whether a specific group of patients is at higher risk of relapse, they serve as an important advance in setting a foundation upon which such predictive studies can be done in the future. Furthermore, these studies reveal the increased expression of several intriguing gene products, including *CRABP2* and retinol-binding protein 1, that might predict tumor response to novel agents such as retinoids.

R. J. Arceci, MD, PhD

Human Granulocyte Colony-Stimulating Factor in Children With High-Risk Acute Lymphoblastic Leukemia: A Children's Cancer Group Study

Heath JA, Stienherz PG, Altman A, et al (Mem Sloan-Kettering Cancer Ctr, New York; Children's Natl Med Ctr, Washington, DC; Mayo Clinic, Rochester, Minn; et al)

J Clin Oncol 21:1612-1617, 2003 7–13

Introduction.—The administration of recombinant growth factor granulocyte colony-stimulating factor (G-CSF) to children with acute lymphoblastic leukemia (ALL) has produced conflicting results to date, with no definitive evidence of benefit in several small-scale investigations. The effect of G-CSF on hematopoietic toxicities, supportive care requirements, time to complete intensive therapy, and event-free survival (EFS) and overall survival (OS) in children with high-risk acute lymphoblastic leukemia (HR-ALL) was examined in a large-scale, prospective, open-label, randomized, crossover trial.

Methods.—A total of 287 children with HR-ALL were randomly assigned to an intensive chemotherapy regimen (New York [NY]I or NY II) as part of the Children's Cancer Group (CCG)-1901 protocol. There were 5 drugs in the induction phase: vincristine, prednisone, L-asparaginase, daunorubicin, and cyclophosphamide. Initial consolidation was made up of 6-agent chemotherapy combined with 18 Gy of total-brain irradiation. Participants were randomly assigned to receive G-CSF (5 μg/kg/d) during either induction or initial consolidation. A crossover investigation analysis was performed in the 259 patients who completed both therapy phases.

Results.—The mean time to neutrophil recovery ($\geq$0.5 $\times$ 10^9/L) was decreased with G-CSF (16.7 vs 19.1 days; *P* = .0003). Patients who received G-CSF did not have significantly decreased episodes of febrile neutropenia (149 vs 164; *P* = .41), positive blood cultures (57 vs 51; *P* = .66), or serious infections (75 vs 79; *P* = .62). Hospitalization (14.0 vs 13.9 days; *P* = .87) and induction therapy completion times (NY I, 30.3 vs 31.3 days, *P* = .11; NY II, 33.4 vs 32.3 days, *P* = .40) did not change significantly. No significant differences were observed in 6-year EFS (*P* = .24) or OS (*P* = .54) between patients who did and did not receive G-CSF on CCG-1901, NY I and NY II.

Conclusion.—Children with HR-ALL do not seem to benefit from administration of prophylactic G-CSF.

▶ The use of G-CSF in patients with cancer has been controversial, with some studies showing benefit in terms of reduced hospitalization times, reduced days of neutropenia, and reduced infectious complications. Other studies have not confirmed such findings. Heath et al studied the role of G-CSF in pediatric patients with high-risk acute lymphoblastic leukemia in a randomized crossover-designed trial. Their results demonstrate no significant differences in reduced episodes of febrile neutropenia, hospitalizations, completion times for induction therapy, or, interestingly, even the frequency of positive blood cultures. These are important results in terms of rationally using or not using G-CSF in this patient population as well as in terms of the cost of G-CSF treatment. While such results cannot be extrapolated to other regimens or patients with other cancers, they should serve to help us define the best use of this type of supportive care in high-risk pediatric ALL.

R. J. Arceci, MD, PhD

Intensification of Mercaptopurine/Methotrexate Maintenance Chemotherapy May Increase the Risk of Relapse for Some Children With Acute Lymphoblastic Leukemia

Schmiegelow K, Björk O, Glomstein A, et al (Univ of Copenhagen; Karolinksa Inst, Stockholm; Natl Univ, Oslo, Norway; et al)

J Clin Oncol 21:1332-1339, 2003 7–14

Introduction.—Thioguanine nucleotides (TGNs), which are incorporated into DNA, are the primary mediators of the cytotoxic effect of the antimetabolite mercaptopurine (MP). Methylated MP metabolites (formed by thiopurine methyltransferase [TPMT]) and methotrexate [MTX]) polyglutamates can restrict de novo purine synthesis. Children with acute lymphoblastic leukemia (ALL) were evaluated to ascertain whether dose adjustment of MP and MTX by erythrocyte (E) levels of TGN and MTX (including polyglutamates) could improve patient outcome.

Methods.—The age range of 538 children with ALL participating in the Nordic Society of Pediatric Hematology and Oncology (NOPHO) ALL (acute lymphoblastic leukemia)-92 investigation was 1.0 to 14.9 years. Patients were randomly assigned to have their oral MP/MTX maintenance therapy adjusted by either white blood cell (WBC) counts, E-TGN, and E-MTX (pharmacology group) or WBC only (control group).

Results.—At a median follow-up of 7.8 years, 79 patients had experienced relapse. The risk of relapse was increased in male gender ($P = .00003$), high WBC at diagnosis ($P = .03$), pharmacology arm (6.6 times increased relapse hazard for girls), high TPMT activity ($P = .002$), and high average neutrophil counts during maintenance therapy ($P = .0009$), with a significant interaction between gender and randomization groups ($P = .0007$). For girls, the risk of relapse was 5% and 19% in the control and pharmacology groups ($P = .001$) due to an increased relapse hazard during the first year after cessation of therapy. The TPMT activity was the most significant predictor of relapses among girls in the pharmacology arm ($P < .0001$). Overall, TPMT activity was higher in patients who relapsed after therapy cessation than in those who remained in remission (girls, 19.5 vs 17.4 U/mL, $P = .03$; boys, 19.3 vs 18.0 U/mL, $P = .04$).

Conclusion.—The addition of pharmacologically guided treatment intensification to dose adjustment by blood counts in children with ALL may not be needed in girls, whereas new approaches to optimize maintenance therapy are necessary in boys.

► Although the use of 6-mercaptopurine and methotrexate as maintenance therapy in children with ALL has been standard of care for many years, the optimal way to adjust the dose of these agents remains unclear. In the study by Schmiegelow et al, patients with ALL were randomly assigned to have their dose adjustment of these agents based on either their WBC count alone (standard approach) or on their WBC count and erythrocyte TGN or MTX polyglutamate levels (pharmacologically directed dosing). The findings are intriguing in that girls had a significantly higher relapse rate (19%) when treated according to the pharmacologically directed dosing than with the standard approach (5%). The TPMT, which forms the methylated mercaptopurine metabolite activity, was the most significant predictor of relapse among female patients. Overall, a higher TPMT activity was associated with a higher risk of relapse for girls and boys. These results, while not necessarily expected, reveal that pharmacologic targeting of chemotherapy dosing may be more complicated than commonly believed.

R. J. Arceci, MD, PhD

Results of a Randomized Study of Preradiation Chemotherapy Versus Radiotherapy Alone for Nonmetastatic Medulloblastoma: The International Society of Paediatric Oncology/United Kingdom Children's Cancer Study Group PNET-3 Study

Taylor RE, Bailey CC, Robinson K, et al (Cookridge Hosp, Leeds, England; Univ of Leicester, England; Newcastle Gen Hosp, Newcastle Upon Tyne, England; et al)

J Clin Oncol 21:1581-1591, 2003 7–15

Introduction.—Until about 10 years ago, standard management for medulloblastoma was maximum surgical resection followed by craniospinal radiotherapy (RT) to a dose of 35 to 36 Gy with a boost to the posterior fossa (total dose to the posterior fossa of 55-56 Gy). The 5-year survival rate in patients so treated is 60% to 65%. Children (aged 3-16 years) with histologically confirmed medulloblastoma were evaluated to ascertain whether preradiotherapy chemotherapy would improve outcome for Chang stage MO-1 medulloblastoma versus RT alone.

Methods.—Two hundred seventeen patients were randomly assigned to treatment with either 35 Gy craniospinal RT with a 20 Gy posterior fossa boost or chemotherapy followed by RT. Chemotherapy consisted of vincristine 1.5 mg/m^2 weekly for 10 weeks and 4 cycles of etoposide 100 mg/m^2 daily for 3 days, and carboplatin 500 mg/m^2 daily for 2 days, alternating with cyclophosphamide 1.5 g/m^2.

Results.—Of 217 patients randomly assigned, 179 were eligible for analysis (chemotherapy plus RT, 90 patients; RT alone, 89 patients). The median patient age was 7.67 years, and median follow-up was 5.40 years. The overall survival (OS) rate was 79.5% at 3 years and 70.7% at 5 years. The event-free survival (EFS) rate was 71.6% at 3 years and 67.0% at 5 years. The EFS was significantly better in the chemotherapy plus RT group (P = .0366); 3-year EFS was 78.5% and 5-year EFS was 74.2%. In the RT alone group, EFS at 3 and 5 years, respectively, was 64.8% and 59.8%. No statistically significant difference in 3-year or 5-year OS was observed (P = .0928) in the RT alone group (P = .0928). Multivariate analysis revealed that the use of chemotherapy (P = .0248) and time to complete RT (P = .0100) had a significant effect on EFS.

Conclusion.—This is the first large, multicenter, randomized trial to report improved EFS for chemotherapy with RT versus RT alone. This regimen could decrease toxicity and nephrotoxicity, compared with a cisplatin-containing schedule. The importance of avoiding interruptions to RT has been verified.

► The theoretical advantages of using preradiation chemotherapy in patients with medulloblastoma are many and include the highly vascular tumor bed after surgery and the disruption of the blood-brain/tumor barrier after surgery. Potential disadvantages include delaying RT, which might be associated with disease progression. The study by Taylor et al describes the results of the PNET-3 Study, which randomly assigned patients with Chang stage M0-1 medulloblastoma to received chemotherapy and then radiation or radiation alone. The chemotherapy used included vincristine, etoposide, carboplatin, and cyclophosphamide. The results indicate a statistically improved EFS for patients receiving combination therapy compared with those patients receiving RT alone. Although there was a trend that favored combination therapy to radiation alone in OS, the difference did not reach statistical significance. Another important result of this study was the improved survival for patients who received their RT in less than 50 days versus those who received it in more than 50 days (ie, those who had significant delays in delivery of their radiation). There are several caveats. Of the 217 patients randomly assigned to a treatment modality, 18% were considered ineligible for analysis. Furthermore, the time to follow-up is still relatively short. One must also be careful in extrapolating these results to other stages of medulloblastoma or to other chemotherapy regimens. Nevertheless, the conclusions of this study appear valid and provide important information on how to optimize treatment for this group of patients.

R. J. Arceci, MD, PhD

Correlation of Early Metastatic Response by ^{123}I-Metaiodobenzylguanidine Scintigraphy With Overall Response and Event-Free Survival in Stage IV Neuroblastoma

Matthay KK, Edeline V, Lumbroso J, et al (Univ of California, San Francisco; Inst Gustave Roussy, Paris)

J Clin Oncol 21:2486-2491, 2003 7–16

Background.—Neuroblastoma, which is the most common extracranial childhood tumor, is metastatic in more than 50% of patients at the time of diagnosis. The 5-year survival rate for this tumor, which arises from the sympathetic nervous system, is only 30% to 40%. Tumors resistant to induction therapy occur in approximately 10% to 15% of patients, and 40% of the children who obtain complete or partial remission will relapse, even after myeloablative therapy and treatment of minimal residual disease with 13-*cis*-retinoic acid. At present, it is difficult to identify many of the patients who will eventually progress despite intensive therapy, which hinders the development and testing of new treatments that might improve survival rates. Metaiodobenzylguanidine (MIBG) is specifically taken up in cells of sympathetic origin and provides a highly sensitive and specific indicator for the detection of metastases in patients with neuroblastoma. An effort was made to correlate early response to therapy by MIBG scan with the end induction response and the event-free survival (EFS) rate in stage IV neuroblastoma.

Methods.—A total of 75 children older than 1 year with stage IV neuroblastoma underwent ^{123}I-MIBG scans at diagnosis, after 2 and 4 cycles of induction therapy, and before autologous stem-cell transplantation. A semiquantitative method was used in the reading of the scans by 2 independent observers. Absolute and relative MIBG scores were then correlated with overall pretransplantation response, bone marrow response, and EFS.

Results.—The pretransplantation response rate was 82%, and the 3-year EFS rate was 32%, which is similar to the findings in a concomitant group of 375 stage IV patients. The median relative MIBG scores after 2, 4, and 6 cycles were 0.5, 0.24, and 0.12, respectively. There was a significantly higher probability of complete response or very good partial response before transplantation if the relative score after 2 cycles was 0.5 or less, or if the relative score after 4 cycles was 0.24 or less. Patients with a relative score of 0.5 or less after 2 cycles or a score of 0.24 or less after 4 cycles had an improved EFS rate.

Conclusions.—Semiquantitative MIBG scoring in the early stages of therapy in patients with stage IV neuroblastoma can provide valuable prognostic information in regard to overall response and EFS.

▶ The ability to predict outcome with radiographic, and thus relatively noninvasive, methods is of enormous value in patients with solid tumors. For patients with neuroblastoma, the use of the relatively selective imaging agent, ^{123}I-MIBG, provides a means to measure the extent of disease and thus potentially the response to therapy. The article by Matthay et al pushes this concept further by studying 75 children with stage IV neuroblastoma using ^{123}I-MIBG scintigraphy at diagnosis, at times following chemotherapy and preautologous transplantation. The results show that the MIBG response score was able to distinguish groups of patients with better or worse outcomes. However, the differences are statistically significant only at the $P < .05$ level for MIBG scans after 2 cycles of induction chemotherapy ($P = .045$). Trends are present for other scanning times and for the overall MIBG score. In addition, the EFS in the best group is about 40%, and in the poor-outcome group it is around 11%. While this difference is certainly important, even the best group still experiences more failures than cures. This raises some quite interesting biological questions about resistance mechanisms related to MIBG scanning and the role of N-MYC amplification. This study thus represents an excellent example of a well-done clinical trial leading to hypothesis-driven future questions.

R. J. Arceci, MD, PhD

New Malignancies After Blood or Marrow Stem-Cell Transplantation in Children and Adults: Incidence and Risk Factors

Baker KS, DeFor TE, Burns LJ, et al (Univ of Minnesota, Minneapolis)
J Clin Oncol 21:1352-1358, 2003 7–17

Background.—There is an increasing number of survivors with longer follow- up after successful hematopoietic stem-cell transplant (SCT). In light of this increase, recognition of the types of long-term complications that can occur after SCT, including the development of posttransplant cancers, is becoming increasingly important. The risk factors and incidence of posttransplant cancers have been described, but these studies have had small populations of transplant survivors with 20 or more years of follow-up, and there have been few reports on the unique concerns that arise in the population of patients that have received transplants as children. A study was undertaken to determine the incidence and risk factors for the development of new cancers occurring after SCT in regard to age-specific risks, long-term incidence, and outcome in a cohort of patients at the University of Minnesota.

Methods.—A total of 3732 patients underwent SCT at the University of Minnesota between January 1974 and March 2001. A total of 147 posttransplant cancers in 137 patients were identified and form the basis of this study.

Results.—After exclusion of nonmelanoma skin cancer (19) and carcinoma in situ (5), the remaining 123 cases of posttransplant cancers represented an 8.1-fold increased risk of a posttransplant cancer, for an excess risk of 102.7 cases per 10,000 persons per year (after adjustment for age and sex). Included in this excess risk is a significantly elevated risk of the development of myelodysplastic syndrome (MDS) or acute myeloid leukemia (AML), non-Hodgkin's lymphoma (including posttransplant lymphoproliferative disorder), Hodgkin's disease, or solid tumors overall and specifically mela noma, brain, and tumors of the oral cavity. The cumulative incidence for the development of any posttransplant cancer was 6.9% at 20 years after SCT. For posttransplant lymphoproliferative disorder, the cumulative incidence plateaued at 1.4% by 10 years after SCT. For MDS or AML, the cumulative incidence plateaued at 1.4% by 10 years after SCT. There was no plateauing of the cumulative incidence of development of a solid tumor, which was 3.8% at 20 years after SCT.

Conclusions.—The risk of posttransplant cancers, particularly solid tumors, continues to increase even 20 years after stem-cell transplantation. Long-term close follow-up is therefore required for these patients.

▶ The incidence and outcome of secondary cancers after treatment for children and adults with cancer has become an important concern as more patients are surviving longer with more effective initial treatments. In this report by Baker et al, the incidence and risk factors for developing secondary cancers after hematopoietic stem-cell transplantation are assessed. The cumulative incidence of posttransplant secondary cancers at 20 years was 6.9%. Similar to what has been seen in studies of patients with Hodgkin's disease, the risk of developing solid tumors appears to continue to increase while the risk of developing leukemias plateaus after several years. Another important finding was the influence of age, with children less than 10 years of age having a 60-fold increased risk of developing secondary cancers compared with a 19-fold risk in patients between 10 and 19 years of age when values are compared with age-matched general population values. Although posttransplant lymphoproliferative disorder is significantly more frequent in the younger group of patients, there is still a 33-fold risk of solid tumors in this group. This article is packed with interesting observations that should be carefully examined. The results also bring up the issue of when to do a hematopoietic transplant in patients if alternative (and possibly less toxic) therapies are equally efficacious.

R. J. Arceci, MD, PhD

Deletions in Chromosome Arms 3p and 11q Are New Prognostic Markers in Localized and 4s Neuroblastoma

Spitz R, Hero B, Ernestus K, et al (Univ Children's Hosp, Köln, Germany)

Clin Cancer Res 9:52-58, 2003 7–18

Background.—Alterations in chromosome band 1p36 and amplification of the *MYCN* oncogene are well-known prognostic parameters in neuroblastoma, with strong influence on therapeutic treatment. However, the knowledge regarding these chromosomal aberrations is insufficient for clinical concerns because only 11% of stages 1 to 3 and 13% of stage 4s of good-prognosis neuroblastoma and 29% of those relapsing patients have MNA or 1p36-deleted tumors. An effort was made to find new nonrandom chromosomal changes in neuroblastoma that could be predictive of outcome by investigating alterations in chromosome arms 3p and 11q.

Methods.—The frequency and prognostic potential of 3p and 11q alterations in 144 neuroblastomas were analyzed with interphase fluorescence in situ hybridization with DNA probes for 3p26 and 11q23. Aberrations were defined as deletion (monosomy of a specific region) or imbalance (at least 2 intact and additional 3p26- or 11q23-deleted chromosomes).

Results.—Of the 144 cases evaluated, 42 (29%) demonstrated 11q alterations, including 21% with deletions and 8% with imbalances. In most cases, the aberrations were associated with stage 4 disease (47%), but aberrations were also associated with localized and 4s tumors (16%). Those patients with 11q deletions or imbalance were significantly older at diagnosis. Changes in 3p were detected in 18% of the samples, including 15% with deletions and 3% with imbalances, and these alterations were also associated with stage 4 disease more frequently than with stages 1 to 3 disease (34% vs 7%). The median age was also increased in patients in whom changes in 3p were detected. Aberrations in both chromosomes were highly associated with each other. Amplification of *MYCN* was detected in 10% and 12% of the tumors with 11q and 3p alterations, and changes in 1p36 occurred in 13% of the 3p-aberrant and 26% of the 11q-aberrant tumors. Amplification of *MYCN* and 11q deletion or imbalance tended to demonstrate an inverse correlation as well as 1p and 3p deletion or imbalance. Patients with 3p and 11q abnormalities in localized/4s tumors demonstrated an inferior outcome compared with patients without these alterations, particularly in regard to *MYCN* single copy tumors.

Conclusions.—It was demonstrated in this investigation that alterations in 3p and 11q are frequently occurring nonrandom aberrations in neuroblastoma and thus are representative of a new, high-risk subgroup in *MYCN* single copy stage 1 to 3 and 4s disease.

► Although N-MYC amplification measurement is an enormously important prognostic factor in neuroblastoma, it has not been able to completely account for outcome in all children. For example, some children with low-stage disease and no evidence of N-MYC amplification still relapse. Investigators have thus searched for other prognostic factors. The report by Spitz et al examines the frequency and prognostic significance of chromosome aberrations, especially 3p26 and 11q23 deletions in patients with stages 1 to 3 and in 4s neuroblastoma. Their results indicate that alternations in chromosomes 3q and 11q are relatively frequent and correlate with a worse outcome in these patients in the absence of N-MYC amplification. Whether these are sign posts that predict outcome or involve genetic pathways that lead to altered drug resistance and tumor survival pathways will need to await more definitive identification of the genes involved. Nevertheless, this type of study sheds substantial light on the extent of genetic heterogeneity in neuroblastoma and how it might impact outcome.

R. J. Arceci, MD, PhD

Alterations of the *hSNF5/INI1* Gene in Central Nervous System Atypical Teratoid/Rhabdoid Tumors and Renal and Extrarenal Rhabdoid Tumors

Biegel JA, Tan L, Zhang F, et al (Univ of Pennsylvania, Philadelphia)

Clin Cancer Res 8:3461-3467, 2002 7–19

Background.—Tumors that are partially or totally composed of rhabdoid cells are clinically aggressive and arise predominantly in infants and young children. The CNS and the kidney are the most common locations of rhabdoid tumors, but such tumors can arise in almost any site. The differential diagnosis of these tumors is often challenging because of the presence of overlapping histologic features and complex immunophenotypes among rhabdoid and other embryonal tumors. Germ-line and acquired mutations of the *IhSNF5/INI1* tumor suppressor gene have been reported in rhabdoid tumors arising in the CNS and in renal and soft tissue rhabdoid tumors. The types of IN11 alterations among tumors from a variety of anatomical sites were compared, and mutational "hot spots" were identified.

Methods.—Fluorescence in situ hybridization and polymerase chain reaction (PCR)–based microsatellite, heteroduplex, and sequence analysis were used to characterize chromosome 22 deletions and *INI1* mutations among 100 primary rhabdoid tumors.

Results.—*INI1* deletions and mutations were identified in 75 patients, including 42 children with atypical teratoid/rhabdoid tumors of the brain or spinal cord and 6 children with brain tumors and renal or soft-tissue tumors. The kidney was the origin of 19 tumors, with bilateral location in 1 child, and 8 tumors were extrarenal in origin. Homozygous deletions detected by fluorescence in situ hybridization were most commonly seen in CNS and extrarenal rhabdoid tumors; in contrast, truncating mutations were detected in a high percentage of tumors in the CNS and kidney. The greatest frequency of *INI1* mutations among kidney tumors were found in exons 2, 6, and 7, whereas in tumors of the CNS the highest frequencies of *INI1* mutations were found in exons 5 and 9. Two potential hot-spot mutations for atypical teratoid/rhabdoid tumors of the CNS were noted, including a C-to-T transition in codon 201 in exon 5 and a cytosine deletion in exon 9.

Ten children were found to carry germ-line mutations, including 4 patients with 2 primary tumors.

Conclusions.—The nature and frequencies of *INI1* alterations were evaluated in a large series of rhabdoid tumors from different anatomical sites. Most rhabdoid tumors from all sites contained deletions or mutations of the *INI1* gene. A nonrandom association was observed between specific mutations and anatomical site.

► The genetics of both sporadic and inherited pediatric cancers has had an enormous influence on the understanding of cancer pathogenesis. The initial identification of mutations of the *hSNF5/INI1* factor paved the way for linking a specific genetic aberration in this group of rare but aggressive cancers to the development of animal models of rhabdoid tumors. The report by Biegel et al further extends the analysis of the frequency of *hSNF5/INI1* mutations as well as their heterogeneity. Particularly interesting is the apparent preference of certain mutations to be associated with CNS rather than renal tumors. Such heterogeneity should be important in better understanding the mechanisms leading to mutations in *hSNF5/INI1* as well as in generating more predictive, preclinical animal models.

R. J. Arceci, MD, PhD

Childhood Cancer Patients' Access to Cooperative Group Cancer Programs: A Population-Based Study

Liu L, for the Surveillance, Epidemiology and End Results Childhood Cancer Linkage Group (Univ of Southern California, Los Angeles; et al)

Cancer 97:1339-1345, 2003 7–20

Background.—It has been estimated by the American Cancer Society that 12,400 children aged younger than 20 years were diagnosed with cancer in the United States in 2000, of whom approximately 2300 died of the disease. The Children's Oncology Group (COG) was created by a merger of the Children's Cancer Group (CCG) and the Pediatric Oncology Group (POG) and conducts clinical trials for the treatment of cancer in children. The feasibility of developing a nationwide childhood cancer registry was assessed by determining whether COG could be used as a resource for the identification of all children with cancer.

Methods.—Eleven SEER registries in 10 regions participated in the study. A consolidated file of children aged younger than 20 years who were diagnosed with cancer between 1992 and 1997 and who were registered with either the CCG or POG was linked with records from the participating SEER registries. Age-specific registration rates and age-adjusted registration rates were calculated overall and by year of diagnosis, sex, race/ethnicity, stage of disease at diagnosis, and type of cancer.

Results.—A total of 10,108 children younger than 20 years with cancer were identified by the 11 SEER registries between 1992 and 1997, of whom 5796 were registered with the CCG or POG. The age-adjusted registration rate was 71% for children aged younger than 15 years, 24% for adolescents aged 15 to 19 years, and 57% for children aged less than 20 years. Children with leukemia, hepatic tumors, and renal tumors had the highest registration rates, whereas registration rates were lowest among children with carcinoma and retinoblastoma.

Conclusions.—Not all children with cancer are registered by the cooperative groups. However, it is possible to achieve a national registry program by supplementation of cases identified through the COG with data collected by statewide population-based cancer registries. This collaboration would benefit all parties involved; it would allow the COG to achieve 100% registration of children with cancer while improving the timeliness of case identification and follow-up information for cancer outcomes for statewide cancer registries.

▶ A major challenge for understanding important aspects concerning childhood cancer is to develop a population-based and representative national children's cancer registry. With the recent merger of the CCG and the POG into the COG, the potential for developing such a registry was anticipated. In this interesting analysis by Liu et al, results indicate that only 57% of children with cancer younger than 20 years are likely to be registered with the COG. Thus, the COG database along with statewide and potentially other cancer databases will need to be combined if a truly representative national registry is to be developed.

R. J. Arceci, MD, PhD

Childhood Cancer Survival in Europe and the United States

Gatta G, Capocaccia R, Coleman MP, et al (Istituto Nazionale per lo Studio e la Cura dei Tumori, Milan, Italy; Istituto Superiore di Sanità, Rome; London School of Hygiene and Tropical Medicine; et al)

Cancer 95:1767-1772, 2002 7–21

Background.—The survival rates for most major adult cancers are higher in the United States than in Europe, particularly among the oldest patients. Whether these differences are also present in childhood cancers was determined.

Methods.—A total of 16,148 European patients who were diagnosed with malignant disease at younger than 15 years from 1985 to 1989 were compared with 3476 patients in the United States. The patients were obtained from 34 EUROCARE cancer registries in 17 countries and from 9 SEER registries in the United States. The cancers considered in this review included the major 14 diagnostic categories of the International Classification of Childhood Cancers. In addition, all childhood cancers were compared together to increase the power of comparisons. Actuarial methods were used to calculate observed survival.

Results.—For all cancers combined, northern Europe had the highest 5-year survival rate at 75%; eastern Europe had the lowest survival rate at

55%. The survival rate of 70% for the United States was generally comparable to the survival rates in Italy and other western European nations. Northern Europe also had the highest survival rate for patients with lymphoid leukemias (83%), whereas Germany, Italy, and other western European countries had survival rates similar to the average survival rate of 77% for patients in the United States. For patients with neuroblastoma and Wilms' tumors, the survival rate was 7% to 9% lower in Europe than in the United States. However, for patients with retinoblastoma, the survival rate in Europe was 8% higher than that in the United States. Small, nonsignificant differences in survival rates between the United States and Europe were found for patients with osteosarcoma, ependymoma, and medulloblastoma, with a higher survival rate in the United States, and for acute nonlymphocytic leukemia, with a higher survival rate in Europe. Similar rates between the United States and Europe were observed for other cancers.

Conclusions.—In contrast to the survival of adults with cancer, the survival in European children (with the exception of those in eastern Europe) is quite similar to that in the United States. One explanation for this difference may be that childhood cancers are generally more responsive to therapy than are adult cancers. However, these findings may also be representative of the wide accessibility of these treatments for most patients.

► Although there are established differences in outcomes for adult patients with cancer in Europe compared with the United States, there has been little information on outcomes in children with cancer. The study by Gatta et al report attempts to determine this outcome. The results obtained from 1985 to 1989 suggests that there are significant differences between eastern Europe compared with the rest of Europe and the United States in most disease subtypes. The authors conclude that the lack of differences between Europe and the United States may be due to the overall excellent outcome of more treatment-responsive childhood cancers, while the worse outcome for children from eastern Europe is due to the lack of access to care. While these conclusions may be true, alternative explanations, such as genetic background, should be considered. In addition, the access to care may be an important issue and should be examined more closely for this type of study to be able to lead to changes in care or access to care. Some relatively small but "significant" differences ranging from 7% to 9% were observed. For example, patients with neuroblastoma and Wilms' tumors had a better outcome in the United States while patients with retinoblastoma had a better outcome in Europe. While these differences may be small, they should be more closely examined to determine differences in all variables that could be examined. After all, even small differences, if real, are potentially important when cure rates for some of these disorders are already high.

R. J. Arceci, MD, PhD

8 Lung Cancer

Transcriptional Gene Expression Profiling of Small Cell Lung Cancer Cells
Pedersen N, Mortensen S, Sørensen SB, et al (Natl Univ Hosp, Copenhagen)
Cancer Res 63:1943-1953, 2003 8–1

Background.—Small cell lung cancer (SCLC) is an aggressive disease that initially responds to chemotherapy, but then recurs in a resistant form with a low 5-year survival rate. Global gene expression analysis was undertaken to search for novel potential therapeutic targets for the treatment of patients with SCLC.

Methods.—As it is difficult to obtain adequate SCLC tissue to perform microarray analysis, 21 SCLC cell lines obtained from 5 different laboratories, 8 xenografted tumors derived from these cell lines, and 17 normal tissues were used for the gene expression analysis using oligonucleotide microarrays. The analysis also included expression data from 6 resected, previously published tumors. A 2-dimensional hierarchical cluster analysis of the median levels of expression of genes from these sources was performed.

Results.—Expression of the normal tissues clustered together. The cell lines were distributed into 4 subclasses. One cluster contained only CPH 54 cell lines and was distinct from all other cell lines. The 6 resected tumors clustered together and were closest to normal tissue and to the CPH 54 cell lines. There was a large group of genes expressed by cell lines and xenografts, but not tumors. Expression of these genes is probably not involved in carcinogenesis but in establishing cell lines, and they are not considered potential therapeutic targets. Another gene cluster demonstrates the neuronal or neuroendocrine phenotype of SCLC cells. A final gene cluster is somewhat SCLC specific. Two of the cell line clusters appear to represent the classic type, and another cluster the variant, aggressive phenotype. The neuroendocrine tumor marker ASCL1 was identified as expressed in classic type SCLC cell culture and resected tumors, but not variant type cell cultures and CPH 54 cell lines. It is, therefore, a novel marker for distinguishing classic and variant SCLC cell types. The identification of glutamate receptor expression in SCLC provides a potential novel target for radiotherapy. NPTXR and the apolipoprotein E receptor 2 (LRP8) were also found to be expressed in some SCLC cell lines and may provide novel therapeutic targets. The recently identified oncogene PTTG1 was highly expressed in all SCLC cell lines and tumors. Of the known drug resistance genes, only the ABC C5 multidruug resistance gene was expressed by these cell lines and tumors.

Conclusions.—A global gene expression analysis of SCLC cell lines and xenografts was performed. Comparison with published tumor expression profiles confirmed that cell line and xenograft profiles are similar, although the use of multiple cell lines is necessary to obtain reliable results. The findings indicate that cell lines can be used for expression analysis when insufficient tumor material is available. Microarray analysis was also an effective method of distinguishing between SCLC subclasses. The analysis revealed several potential therapeutic targets, such as ASCL1. Specific expression of genes of unknown function was also detected. As a function is assigned to these genes, more potential therapeutic targets may be identified.

► Gene expression analysis is a technique used to identify genes that are differentially expressed (either overexpressed or underexpressed) in tumors compared with normal tissue. It is hoped that these differential expression profiles can be used to identify subclasses of tumors with different biological behaviors or sensitivities to chemotherapy, or to identify new targets for development of new therapeutic agents. It has been difficult to do these assays on SCLCs, however, because of difficulties in obtaining both the number of specimens and adequate amounts of material, although one analysis of 6 resected SCLC tumors has been reported.[1]

In this study, Pedersen and coworkers performed a global gene expression analysis using oligonucleotide microarrays on SCLC cell lines in cell culture or xenografts, or both, and compared these results with normal tissues and the published literature of 6 SCLC tumors. They were able to group their results into 4 clusters based on their gene effect profile. More importantly, however, from a quality control perspective, they were able to (1) show that all the xenografts clustered closest to the cell lines from which they originated, (2) identify a large group of genes exclusively expressed by the cell lines and xenografts, but not by the tumors, and thus thought to be artifacts of cell culture, and (3) identify clusters highly expressed in normal tissues and SCLC tumors, but not cell lines or xenografts, thought to represent influences of the microenvironment or immune system. Thus, in addition to identifying potential new targets and confirming the expression of known targets, this article also demonstrated that cell lines can be used for expression profiling, although it may be necessary to use many cell lines to obtain reliable results.

J. H. Schiller, MD

Reference

1. Bhattacharjee A, Richards WG, Staunton J, et al: Classification of human lung carcinomas by mRNA expression profiling reveals distinct adenocarcinoma subclasses. *Proc Natl Acad Sci U S A* 98:13790-13795, 2001.

Continued Cigarette Smoking by Patients Receiving Concurrent Chemoradiotherapy for Limited-Stage Small-Cell Lung Cancer Is Associated With Decreased Survival

Videtic GMM, Stitt LW, Dar AR, et al (Harvard Med School, Boston; London Regional Cancer Centre; Kingston Regional Cancer Centre, Ont, Canada; et al)

J Clin Oncol 21:1544-1549, 2003 8–2

Background.—For patients with some types of cancers (eg, stage III/IV head and neck, renal, bladder, and glottic cancers), continuing to smoke during radiotherapy is associated with decreased survival compared with patients who stop smoking during treatment. Whether continuing smoking during concurrent chemotherapy and radiotherapy affects survival in patients with limited-stage small cell lung cancer (SCLC) was retrospectively examined.

Methods.—The participants were 186 patients (112 men and 74 women, most aged ≥60 years) with limited-stage SCLC who underwent chemotherapy (6 cycles of cyclophosphamide, doxorubicin, and vincristine alternating every 3 weeks with etoposide and cisplatin) and radiotherapy (during etoposide and cisplatin therapy). All patients were smokers at the start of the study. Survival was compared between the 79 patents (42.5%) who continued smoking during treatment and the 107 patients (57.5%) who stopped smoking during treatment. The incidence of toxicity (defined as a break during radiotherapy because of hematologic or locoregional toxicity, or both) was also compared between the 2 groups.

Results.—The median follow-up period for the 186 patients was 14.8 months. During radiotherapy, 38 patients (20.5%) experienced toxicity and required a break in treatment (median, 5 days). With respect to causes of death, 71 of 75 deaths (94.9%) in patients who continued smoking during treatment were cancer related, compared with 81 of 96 deaths (84.4%) in patients who quit smoking during treatment. The 5-year actuarial survival was significant better in patients who had stopped smoking during treatment than in patients who continued smoking during treatment (8.9% vs 1%, respectively). The incidence of toxicity did not differ significantly between the 2 groups (42.5% in those who continued smoking vs 57.5% in those who quit). Survival was best in patients who quit smoking and had no treatment breaks (median, 23 months), and worse in patients who continued smoking and who developed toxicity during treatment (median, 13.4 months).

Conclusion.—Patients with limited-stage SCLC who continue to smoke during concurrent chemotherapy and radiotherapy have poorer survival rates than patients who stop smoking during treatment. Smoking status did not affect the incidence of treatment interruptions caused by toxicity. Physicians should urge their patients with limited-stage SCLC who smoke to stop smoking during chemotherapy and radiotherapy.

► Continued smoking has been associated with poorer outcome in patients with a variety of cancers, although results in SCLC have been conflicting. In this study, Videtic and coworkers retrospectively review 186 smokers with limited-stage SCLC treated over 10 years with concurrent chemo-radiotherapy, and conclude that patients who continue to smoke have a poorer survival than patients who quit during treatment. The reasons for this are unclear, but do not appear to be caused by an increase in breaks in radiotherapy because of toxicities or comorbid conditions, such as respiratory or cardiovascular events, in the patients who continue to smoke.

Limitations of the study include the fact that the investigators did not quantitate the amount of cigarette use at the beginning of the study, verify smoking status during treatment, determine how many patients who quit smoking resumed after treatment, or how long they quit. Nevertheless, these findings raise some interesting questions, particularly given the magnitude of the differences in survival observed (a doubling of 5-year survival, from 4% to 8.9%). The magnitude of this difference (a doubling of long-term survival) is better than that observed in most "positive" clinical therapeutic trials. Is the negative impact on survival from smoking caused by an increased resistance to radiotherapy from hypoxia, or would it be observed in patients treated with chemotherapy as well? Is this observation generalizable to non–small cell lung cancer? And if true, should we be stratifying patients with limited SCLC based on smoking status?

J. H. Schiller, MD

Phase II Trial of Gemcitabine in Refractory or Relapsed Small-Cell Lung Cancer: Eastern Cooperative Oncology Group Trial 1597

Masters GA, Declerck L, Blanke C, et al (Evanston Northwestern Healthcare, Ill)

J Clin Oncol 21:1550-1555, 2003 8–3

Background.—Small cell lung cancer (SCLC) usually responds to first-line chemotherapy, yet most patients experience relapse. There is no standard accepted regimen to treat these relapses, but most patients receive either cyclophosphamide, doxorubicin, and vincristine (CAV) or, more recently, topotecan. Each of these treatments has a similar response rate, with a median survival of less than 6 months. Additional treatment modalities would be beneficial for this patient group. Gemcitabine has been used to successfully treat a variety of solid tumors. The activity of gemcitabine as a second-line therapy for patients with relapsed SCLC was examined in a phase 2 trial.

Study Design.—The study group consisted of 42 patients with relapsed SCLC. Patients received gemcitabine IV on days 1, 8, and 15 of a 28-day cycle. Patients were reevaluated after every 2 chemotherapy cycles. The primary objective was to assess the response to gemcitabine in this patient group. Secondary objectives included remission duration, survival, and toxicity. Patients with relapsed SCLC were stratified according to whether their disease was primary refractory or primary sensitive.

Findings.—Overall, an objective response occurred in 12% of patients, including 1 patient with refractory SCLC and 4 patients with sensitive but relapsed SCLC. The overall median survival was 7.1 months. There was no difference in survival between those with refractory and those with sensitive disease. Neutropenia occurred in 27% and thrombocytopenia in 27% of patients. Nonhematologic toxicities included pulmonary toxicity in 9% and neurologic toxicity in 14% of these patients.

Conclusions.—Gemcitabine is well tolerated as a second-line therapy in patients with SCLC. It was modestly active, with an overall response rate of about 12% and a median survival time of about 7 months. Further research is necessary to delineate the role of this agent in the treatment of patients with SCLC.

► Survival for patients with metastatic SCLC has remained disappointingly low over the past several decades, despite the initial sensitivity of the disease to chemotherapy. Effective second-line therapy is also notoriously poor. Topotecan, the topoisomerase inhibitor approved for second-line SCLC in the United States, results in responses in roughly one quarter of patients, with a median survival of less than 6 months—and then only in patients with "sensitive" relapse.[1] For the majority of patients—those who relapse within 3 months of completing first-line therapy—responses with topotecan are even worse.[2]

Given the activity of gemcitabine in other tumor types, it makes sense to test the activity of the drug in SCLC. Although the response rate was low (5.6% in patients with refractory disease and 16.7% in patients with sensitive disease), the median survival was 7.1 months—equivalent to, if not better than, that observed with topotecan. The fact that median survival was the same in both groups, despite the differences in survival, makes one wonder how much patient selection was a factor.

J. H. Schiller, MD

References

1. von Pawel J, Schiller J, Sheperd F, et al: Topotecan versus CAV for the treatment of recurrent small cell lung cancer. *J Clin Oncol* 17:658-667, 1999.
2. Thatcher N: Salvage treatment. *Ann Oncol* 13:4, 2002.

Positron Emission Tomography Scanning With 2-Fluoro-2-Deoxy-D-Glucose as a Predictor of Response of Neoadjuvant Treatment for Non–Small Cell Carcinoma

Cerfolio RJ, Ojha B, Mukherjee S, et al (Univ of Alabama, Birmingham)
J Thorac Cardiovasc Surg 125:938-944, 2003 8–4

Background.—Among patients with non–small cell lung cancer (NSCLC), surgical resection after chemotherapy may be the best strategy only for responders. The abilities of 2-fluoro-2-deoxy-D-glucose positron emission tomography (FDG-PET) and CT to predict this response for the primary tumor and N1 and N2 lymph nodes were determined.

Methods.—Thirty-four patients with NSCLC were prospectively studied. All had had initial FDG-PET scan staging with tissue biopsy, neoadjuvant chemotherapy, repeat FDG-PET scanning, and repeat biopsies.

Findings.—Eleven patients had N2 disease and 7 had N1 disease. Chemotherapy was administered to 27 patients. Seven received chemotherapy plus radiation therapy. Resection was performed in all but 9 patients. In a statistical analysis, FDG-PET scanning was more specific than CT for predicting residual tumor at the primary site. The former also had higher positive and negative predictive values. For paratracheal nodes, FDG-PET scanning was more sensitive and accurate, with greater positive and negative predictive values than CT. In addition, FDG-PET scanning had a greater positive predictive value than CT scanning for the other N2 lymph nodes.

Conclusions.—In patients with NSCLC receiving preoperative chemotherapy, repeat FDG-PET scanning is more specific and has greater positive and negative predictive values than CT scanning. The former is also more sensitive and accurate for paratracheal N2 nodes, though the 2 modalities do not differ significantly in detecting N1 lymph nodes.

► The role of PET scanning in the diagnosis and management of lung cancer has been under considerable scrutiny over the past decade. Numerous studies have shown it to be more specific and sensitive than CT scanning in staging lung cancers. In the study by Cerfolio et al, its use as a predictor of response to neoadjuvant chemotherapy for NSCLS is explored.

Preoperative chemotherapy for patients with N2 disease is also an area of active research based on 2 initial small, randomized studies suggesting that preoperative chemotherapy followed by surgery resulted in improved survival compared with surgery alone.[1,2] However, most surgeons agree that surgery should only be undertaken if the preoperative chemotherapy results in clearing of the nodal disease. Presumably, this could mean 2 diagnostic procedures: a mediastinoscopy at the time of diagnosis to establish N2 disease, and another mediastinoscopy following neoadjuvant chemotherapy. A noninvasive test that could accurately predict who was downstage would therefore be very useful.

In this study, the authors explore the role of PET scanning as a predictor of response. They conclude that PET scanning is indeed more specific, more sensitive, and more accurate, with higher positive predictive and negative predictive values than CT scanning for mediastinal nodes, although not for N1 nodes.

One of the major problems with PET scanning is its false-positive and false-negative rates. However, of note in this study, PET scanning was particularly accurate for paratracheal nodes. Of the 7 nodes that were positive pathologically, all 7 were positive by PET; of the 48 negative pathologic nodes, all 48 were also negative by PET. There were no false-positives or false-negatives for paratracheal nodes.

It should also be noted, however, that this was a relatively small series. Only 11 patients had N2 disease. In addition, it was particularly accurate for N2 paratracheal lymph nodes. It was not as accurate for nodes in other N2 stations, where the authors still recommend biopsies.

If future larger, multicenter trials can corroborate these findings, then perhaps PET scanning may obviate the need for redo mediastinoscopy, which is a difficult and often risky procedure.

J. H. Schiller, MD

References

1. Rosell R, Gomez-Codina J, Camps C, et al: A randomized trial comparing preoperative chemotherapy plus surgery with surgery alone in patients with non-small-cell lung cancer. *N Engl J Med* 330:153-158, 1994.
2. Roth J, Fossella F, Komaki R, et al: A randomized trial comparing perioperative chemotherapy and surgery with surgery alone in resectable stage IIIA non-small-cell lung cancer. *J Natl Cancer Inst* 86:673-680, 1994.

Staging of Non–Small-Cell Lung Cancer With Integrated Positron-Emission Tomography and Computed Tomography

Lardinois D, Weder W, Hany TF, et al (Univ Hosp of Zurich, Switzerland; Univ of Zurich, Switzerland)
N Engl J Med 348:2500-2507, 2003 8–5

Background.—Integrated positron emission CT (PET-CT) scanners have been introduced recently. The accuracy of integrated PET-CT was compared with that of other imaging modalities in staging non–small cell lung cancer (NSCLC).

Methods.—Fifty patients with proved or suspected NSCLC underwent integrated PET-CT scanning. In addition, CT alone, PET alone, and visually correlated PET and CT were done. Tumor-node-metastasis staging was assigned on the basis of image analysis.

TABLE 1.—Comparison of Diagnostic Accuracy of Integrated PET-CT With CT Alone, PET Alone, and Visual Correlation of PET and CT Images

Variable	*P* Value
Tumor stage (n=40)	
PET-CT vs. CT alone	0.001†
PET-CT vs. PET alone	<0.001†
PET-CT vs. visual correlation of PET and CT	0.013†
Node stage (n=37)	
PET-CT vs. CT alone	0.12
PET-CT vs. PET alone	0.013†
PET-CT vs. visual correlation of PET and CT	0.021

The paired sign test was used to calculate *P* values. Stages assigned on the basis of CT alone, PET alone, and PET and CT were assessed by review board A, and stages assigned on the basis of integrated PET-CT were assessed by review board B.

**P* value was significant after Bonferroni's correction.

TABLE 2.—Diagnostic Accuracy of Imaging Methods Regarding Tumor Stage in 40 Patients

Imaging Method	Classification Correct (Score of 3)	Classification Correct but Equivocal (Score of 2)	Classification Incorrect (Score of 0 or 1)
		no. of patients (%)	
CT Alone	23 (58)	8 (20)	9 (22)
PET alone	16 (40)	16 (40)	8 (20)
Visual correlation of PET and CT	26 (65)	5 (12)	9 (22)
Integrated PET-CT	35 (88)	4 (10)	1 (2)

(Reprinted by permission of *The New England Journal of Medicine* from Lardinois D, Weder W, Hany TF, et al: Staging of non–small-cell lung cancer with integrated positron-emission tomography and computed tomography. *N Engl J Med* 348:2500 2507, 2003,)

Findings.—In 41% of the patients, integrated PET-CT provided additional information beyond that available with visual correlation of PET and CT. The diagnostic accuracy of integrated PET-CT was greater than that of the other modalities (Tables 1 and 2). In addition, tumor staging was significantly more accurate with integrated PET-CT than with CT alone, PET alone, or visual PET-CT correlation. Node staging was also significantly more accurate with integrated PET-CT than with PET alone. In 2 of 8 patients undergoing staging of metastasis, integrated PET-CT increased diagnostic certainty.

Conclusions.—When integrated PET-CT becomes more widely available, it will be the preferred modality for determining disease stage in patients with NSCLC. If further research verifies the current findings, integrated PET-CT may become the new standard for imaging lung cancer.

► Accurate staging is the key to appropriate management of lung cancer. Radiologic exams such as CT or PET yield both false-positive and false-negative results. As a result, many clinicians use both to improve diagnostic accuracy. However, whereas CT provides good anatomic detail, it is neither very specific nor sensitive; PET, on the other hand, although more specific and sensitive, is not precise on the exact location of possible abnormalities. Even when PET and CT are visually correlated, the precise location of lesions is sometimes difficult to determine. This study compared the diagnostic accuracy of CT alone, PET alone, and visual correlation of PET and CT with the information obtained with the new PET-CT scanners.

Integrated PET-CT was significantly more accurate in tumor staging than visual PET alone, CT alone, or visual correlation of PET-CT. Integrated PET-CT was also more accurate than visual correlation of PET and CT in staging the mediastinum. PET was more accurate than CT in detecting metastases; integrated PET-CT detected their location in 2 patients where visual correlation could not.

It should be noted, however, that PET or integrated PET-CT is unable to pick up micrometastases; 3 such lesions were missed in this study. Thus, a negative scan does not mean there is no need for mediastinal staging by mediastinoscopy. In addition, false-positives continue to occur, particularly in the mediastinum. One patient classified as having a positive N3 node was found to have inflammatory changes, and 2 patients classified as having N1 disease had hilar extension of the tumor.

Thus, does PET-CT obviate the need for surgical staging of the mediastinum? Apparently not. It does, however, allow for more accurate anatomic location of possible lesions. In addition, PET appears to have a major role in detecting unsuspected extrathoracic metastases (16% in this study). PET detected the location of these in 6 of 8 patients and PET-CT in all 8.

J. H. Schiller, MD

Postinduction Video-Mediastinoscopy Is as Accurate and Safe as Video-Mediastinoscopy in Patients Without Pretreatment for Potentially Operable Non–Small Cell Lung Cancer

Lardinois D, Schallberger A, Betticher D, et al (Inselspital Bern, Switzerland; Centre Hôpitalier Universitaire Vaudois, Lausanne, Switzerland)

Ann Thorac Surg 75:1102-1106, 2003 8–6

Background.—Videomediastinoscopy (VMS) may enable easier identification of lymph nodes requiring biopsy in patients with potentially operable non–small cell lung cancer (NSCLC). The accuracy and safety of VMS were investigated in patients with no pretreatment and after induction therapy.

Methods.—Two hundred nineteen patients underwent VMS at 1 center, including 195 with no pretreatment and 24 who had completed induction therapy. Mediastinal lymph nodes were dissected and biopsied following the American Thoracic Society lymph node mapping and with the use of VMS.

Findings.—In patients without pretreatment, the sensitivity and specificity of VMS was 87% and 100%, respectively, compared with mediastinal lymph node dissection (MLND). The accuracy of VMS was 95.6%. Four percent of the patients experienced procedure-related complication rate. In patients who had completed induction therapy, VMS had an 81% sensitivity, a 100% specificity, and a 91% accuracy compared with MLND. No complications occurred in this group.

Conclusions.—In these patients with NSCLC, VMS is as accurate as MLND. This approach also appears to be safe, resulting in no additional morbidity.

► Recent clinical studies have explored the use of neoadjuvant therapy in patients with N2 disease. These studies have reported that patients with the best prognosis are those whose N2 disease has pathologically cleared after induction therapy. Many surgeons have interpreted these data to reserve resection for patients with pN0 after induction therapy. This, however, necessitates an evaluation of the mediastinum after chemotherapy and/or radiotherapy (a "redo" mediastinoscopy), which may be difficult and associated with increased risk.

In this study, Lardinois and coworkers focused their efforts on patients receiving neoadjuvant chemotherapy. Although they found video-mediastinoscopy safe and accurate, a major limitation of the study is that it was confined to patients who had received preoperative chemotherapy only, since recent studies have suggested patients are more likely to achieve pN0 with chemoradiotherapy.

J. H. Schiller, MD

p53 Mutations and Survival in Stage I Non-Small-Cell Lung Cancer: Results of a Prospective Study

Ahrendt SA, Hu Y, Buta M, et al (Univ of Rochester, NY; Johns Hopkins School of Medicine, Baltimore, Md)

J Natl Cancer Inst 95:961-970, 2003 8–7

Background.—The p53 gene is known to be mutated frequently in non–small cell lung cancer (NSCLC), but the effect of such gene mutations on prognosis are not clear. This prospective study determined the relationship between p53 gene mutations and survival in patients with stage I NSCLC.

Methods.—One hundred eighty-eight patients with operable NSCLC were studied. Tumor samples were collected prospectively and p53 mutations assessed by direct dideoxynucleotide sequencing and p53 GeneChip analysis.

Findings.—Fifty-five percent of the tumors showed p53 mutations. These mutations correlated with nonbronchoalveolar tumors, a history of alcohol consumption, and younger patient age. Patients with p53 mutations had a significantly greater risk of death than did patients with wild-type p53. Factors significantly predicting death in the overall group were tumor stage, the presence of a p53 mutation, and advancing patient age. However, the significant prognostic effect of p53 mutation was observed only in patients with stage I NSCLC. Among patients with stage I disease, actuarial 4-year survival was significantly greater in patients with wild-type p53 than in those with p53 mutations.

Conclusion.—Mutations of p53 independently predict reduced survival in patients with operable NSCLC. However, the prognostic role of p53 appears to be restricted to patients with stage I disease.

► Ahrendt and coworkers examined the frequency of p53 mutations in 188 patients with stage I to III NSCLC and concluded that p53 mutations correlated with poorer survival in stage I NSCLC, but not stage II or III. In addition, p53 mutations were associated with alcohol consumption, younger age, and all nonbronchoalveolar histologic NSCLC. A number of other studies have also looked at p53 mutations, with often conflicting results; many have reported no association with survival, while others have reported that mutations are associated with poorer survival; one study even reported that mutations were associated with better survival.

Why such discrepancies between studies? This study differs from many of the others in that it uses either a GeneChip or direct sequencing analysis, while some of the others used immunohistochemistry or single-strand conformational polymorphism for screening. In addition, most of the other studies were retrospective series, with the inherent selection biases and heterogeneity associated with such studies. The one other prospective study also failed to detect an association with survival in stage II and III NSCLC, although stage I tumors were not assessed in that study.[1]

Thus, these data suggest that p53 mutations may be an early event in lung cancer carcinogenesis and may have a more important impact on outcome before additional mutations accumulate, which are also likely to define behavior. The study also suggests that the presence of p53 mutations in stage I may define a group of high-risk patients for whom adjuvant therapy is warranted, although this remains to be proven in clinical studies.

J. H. Schiller, MD

Reference

1. Schiller J, Adak S, Feins R, et al: Lack of prognostic significance of p53 and K-ras mutations in primary resected non-small cell lung cancer on E4592: A laboratory ancillary study on an Eastern Cooperative Oncology Group prospective randomized trial of postoperative adjuvant therapy. *J Clin Oncol* 19:448-457, 2001.

Randomized Double-blind Placebo-controlled Trial of Bestatin in Patients With Resected Stage I Squamous-Cell Lung Carcinoma

Ichinose Y, for the NK421 Lung Cancer Surgery Group (Natl Kyushu Cancer Ctr, Fukuoka, Japan; et al)

J Natl Cancer Inst 95:605-610, 2003 8–8

Background.—Bestatin, a potent aminopeptidase inhibitor, has been found to have immunostimulant and antitumor activity. Whether postoperative adjuvant treatment with bestatin could prolong the survival of patients with completely resected stage I squamous-cell lung carcinoma was determined.

Methods.—Between July 1992 and March 1995, 402 patients with confirmed, resected stage I squamous-cell lung carcinoma were enrolled in the randomized, double-blind, placebo-controlled trial. Patients received oral bestatin, 30 mg, or placebo daily for 2 years. Surviving patients were followed up for a median 76 months.

Findings.—Overall survival at 5 years was 81% among bestatin recipients and 74% among placebo recipients. Five-year cancer-free survival was 71% and 62%, respectively. Between-group differences in overall and cancer-free survival were statistically significant. Few adverse events occurred in the placebo or active treatment groups.

Conclusions.—Patients with completely resected stage I squamous-cell lung carcinoma treated with bestatin postoperatively had a significantly better survival rate than those given placebo postoperatively. Phase III trials are now needed to verify these findings.

► The role of adjuvant therapy for lung cancer is under intense scrutiny. A meta-analysis published in 1995 showed a 5% benefit to postoperative therapy, which was of borderline statistical significance ($P = .08$).[1] This is a typical case of "beauty is in the eye of the beholder," since many academicians view the meta-analysis as positive, while an equal number have viewed it as negative. Since then, 2 additional trials and 1 abstract have been published that were negative, while a much larger positive trial was presented in the plenary session at the annual ASCO meeting in Chicago in 2003.[2,5]

The study reported by Ichinose et al would seem to support the role of adjuvant therapy. However, bestatin is an immunomodulator, not a classic cytotoxic drug, whose mechanism of action is poorly characterized. This study was limited to stage I squamous cell cancers; its role, if any, cannot be generalized to a broader patient population. Finally, the 5-year survival rate of patients in the placebo group seems high. Thus, the role of bestatin as an adjuvant therapy for lung cancer remains to be defined.

J. H. Schiller, MD

References

1. Chemotherapy in non-small cell lung cancer: A meta-analysis using updated data on individual patients from 52 randomized clinical trials. Non-Small Cell Lung Cancer Collaborative Group. *BMJ* 311:899-909, 1995.
2. Keller S, Adak S, et al: A randomized trial of postoperative adjuvant therapy in patients with completely resected stage II or IIIa non-small-cell lung cancer. *N Engl J Med* 343:1217-1222, 2000.
3. LeChevalier T: Results of the randomized international adjuvant lung cancer trial (IALT): Cisplatin-based chemotherapy (CT) vs no CT in 1867 patients (pts) with resected non-small cell lung cancer (NSCLC). *Proc Am Soc Clin Oncol* 24:6, 2003.
4. Tonato M: Final report of the Adjuvant Lung Project Italy (ALPI): An Italian/EORTC-LCG randomized trial of adjuvant chemotherapy in completely resected non-small cell lung cancer (NSCLC). *Proc Am Soc Clin Oncol* 21:1157, 2002.
5. Waller D, Fairlamb DJ, et al: Big Lung Trial (BLT): Determining the value of cisplatin-based chemotherapy for all patients with non-small cell lung cancer (NSCLC). Preliminary results in the surgical setting. *Proc Am Soc Clin Oncol* 24:2543, 2003.

Interobserver and Intraobserver Variability in Measurement of Non–Small-Cell Carcinoma Lung Lesions: Implications for Assessment of Tumor Response

Erasmus JJ, Gladish GW, Broemeling L, et al (Univ of Texas, Houston)

J Clin Oncol 21:2574-2582, 2003 8–9

Background.—Serial measures of tumor size are usually obtained to determine the response of solid malignancies to treatment. The consistency of measurements obtained by readers assessing lung tumors was evaluated.

Methods.—Thirty-three patients with a total of 40 lung tumors exceeding 1.5 cm were included in the study. Five thoracic radiologists working independently made bidimensional (BD) and unidimensional (UD) measurements on CT scans with World Health Organization (WHO) criteria and the Response Evaluation Criteria in Solid Tumors (RECIST), respectively. These measures were then repeated 5 to 7 days later.

Findings.—The mean tumor size was 4.1 cm, with a range of 1.8 to 8 cm. In an analysis of variance, differences were significant among readers as well as the measured nodules for UD and BD measures. Interobserver misclassification rates were greater than intraobserver misclassification rates. The probability of misclassifying a tumor by the WHO criteria or RECIST was highest with interobserver measures when criteria for progression were used and lowest with intraobserver measures when criteria for response were used. Interobserver misclassification rates were also greater than intraobserver misclassification rates for regular and irregular tumors.

Conclusions.—Lung tumor size measures obtained on CT scans are frequently inconsistent. Such inconsistency can result in incorrect interpretation of tumor response to treatment. When the same reader obtains serial measures in any one patient, consistency can be improved.

▶ Response rate has been the traditional end point for clinically significant antitumor activity in oncology clinical trials for decades. Tumors are measured before and after treatment, either in 1 or 2 dimensions, with standard criteria with precise definitions of response and progression. However, errors in measurements can affect the results of a clinical trial, and the accuracy of tumor measurements has not been well documented. Erasmus et al conducted a study to determine how reproducible these measurements are, both between readers and in the same reader. They report a significant amount of interobserver and intraobserver variability in measurement of non–small cell lung cancer lesions on CT, particularly when the tumor is irregularly shaped, a not uncommon occurrence with speculated lung cancers.

These data serve to underscore some of the problems with the use of response rate as an end point for "clinical benefit" or survival. For example, in 1 randomized lung cancer trial, carboplatin had one of the lowest response rates, but the best survival.[1] Furthermore, some drugs are postulated to be cytostatic rather than cytotoxic in nature, and thus potentially have beneficial clinical activity without shrinking tumors and inducing responses.

J. H. Schiller, MD

Reference

1. Bonomi P, Finkelstein D, Ruckdeschel JC, et al: Combination chemotherapy versus single agents followed by combination chemotherapy in stage IV non-small-cell lung cancer: A study of the Eastern Cooperative Oncology Group. *J Clin Oncol* 7:1602-1613, 1989.

High-Dose Conformal Radiotherapy for Treatment of Stage IIIA/IIIB Non–Small-Cell Lung Cancer: Technical Issues and Results of a Phase I/II Trial

Rosenman JG, Halle JS, Socinski MA, et al (Univ of North Carolina, Chapel Hill; Carolinas Med Ctr, Charlotte, NC)

Int J Radiat Oncol Biol Phys 54:348-356, 2002 8–10

Introduction.—Combined modality therapy (chemotherapy plus radiotherapy) has become the standard of care for good performance status patients who have unresectable stage IIIA/B non–small cell lung cancer (NSCLC). This approach improves both median and long-term survival, yet both local and distant failures remain problematic. Future strategies must address both issues. A phase I/II clinical trial (Lineberger Comprehensive Cancer Center 9603) was performed in which 62 patients with stage IIIA/IIIB inoperable NSCLC were treated with 2 cycles of induction carboplatin/paclitaxel chemotherapy, followed by concurrent weekly carboplatin/paclitaxel with escalating radiation doses of 60 to 74 Gy.

Methods.—Patients were followed up to determine whether 74 Gy of radiation could be safely delivered in this setting and whether it offered a survival benefit. The radiation treatment plans for all 62 patients were reviewed to ascertain the prechemotherapy and postchemotherapy tumor volumes, along with the dose-volume histograms of the normal lung and esophagus.

Results.—Forty-eight patients completed the entire treatment course. The crude survival rate at last follow-up was 32% (20 patients were alive). At a median follow-up of 43 months, the median survival was 24 months (Fig 1).

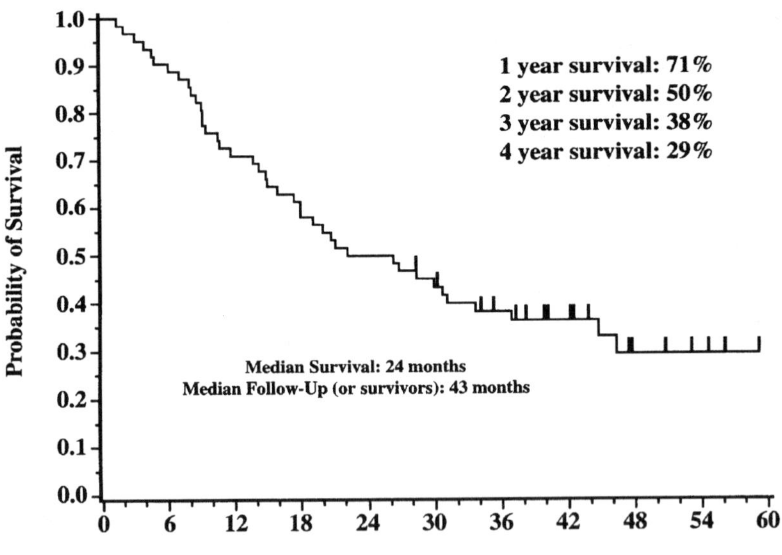

FIGURE 1.—Survival for all 62 patients in Lineberger Comprehensive Cancer Center 9603 (intent to treat). (Reprinted from Rosenman JG, Halle JS, Socinski MA, et al: High-dose conformal radiotherapy for treatment of stage IIIA/IIIB non–small-cell lung cancer: Technical issues and results of a phase I/II trial. *Int J Radiat Oncol Biol Phys* 54:348-356, 2002. Copyright 2002, with permission from Elsevier Science.)

TABLE 2.—Patterns of Initial Failure for 35 Patients With Progression

Failure Site	*n*	%
Locoregional only	13	37
Local + distant	3	9
Distant only†	19	54

*Progression data available for 58 patients, of whom 35 had progression.
†Ten of 19 had brain-only failures.
(Reprinted from Rosenman JG, Halle JS, Socinski MA, et al: High-dose conformal radiotherapy for treatment of stage IIIA/IIIB non–small-cell lung cancer: Technical issues and results of a phase I/II trial. *Int J Radiat Oncol Biol Phys* 54:348-356, 2002. Copyright 2002, with permission from Elsevier Science.)

Survival rates were 50% and 38%, respectively, at 2 and 3 years. Survival was best predicted by whether the patient had received radiotherapy (finished the trial), performance status, disease stage, and log postchemotherapy tumor volume.

Of 35 patients who experienced disease progression, 8 (13%) experienced locoregional relapse as the only site of failure (Table 2). One patient had grade 2 radiation pneumonitis, 5 (8%) had Radiation Therapy Oncology Group grade 3 or 4 esophagitis, and 40 (65%) had a grade 1 or 2 esophagitis. Esophageal toxicity was predicted by the length of esophagus receiving 40 or 60 Gy.

Conclusion.—Radiation doses of 74 Gy, when administered using the guidelines of the Lineberger Comprehensive Cancer Center 9603, seem to be safe and may enhance survival for patients with inoperable stage IIIA/IIIB NSCLC.

▶ These investigators report a series of 62 sequential patients with inoperable stage III NSCLC who were treated with 2 cycles of induction carboplatin and taxol, followed by escalating doses of radiation beginning at 60 Gy and going up to 74 Gy. The results in this study are certainly respectable with essentially 30% of the patients alive at 4 to 5 years later. It is important to recognize that these patients were all in very good condition, with performance status of either 0 or 1. It is also important to note that 14 of the 62 were unable to complete their planned course of treatment for a variety of reasons.

It is unclear that these patients were "improved" by dose escalation or by 3-dimensional treatment planning. I am sure those things did not hurt, but I am not convinced they made for better outcomes. As noted, these patients were well selected for their performance status, and still many of them were not able to complete treatment.

There are individual patients who benefit from dose escalation. However, once the mediastinal nodes are involved, the main issue in terms of defining their survival is a direct reflection of the metastatic potential rather than local control. Even so, local control will remain an important factor that should not be dismissed casually.

E. Glatstein, MD

Pilot Trial of the Epidermal Growth Factor Receptor Tyrosine Kinase Inhibitor Gefitinib Plus Carboplatin and Paclitaxel in Patients With Stage IIIB or IV Non–Small-Cell Lung Cancer

Miller VA, Johnson DH, Krug LM, et al (Mem Sloan-Kettering Cancer Ctr, New York; Cornell Univ, New York; Vanderbilt Univ, New York; et al)

J Clin Oncol 21:2094-2100, 2003 8–11

Background.—Neither advanced nor relapsing lung cancer is curable. It has been hoped that the addition of targeted biologically based therapies to standard chemotherapy regimens would enhance the treatment of lung cancer. The epidermal growth factor receptor (EGFR) is present on most non–small cell lung cancers (NSCLCs) and possesses tyrosine kinase activity. Kinase activation leads to a variety of downstream changes that are characteristic of malignant progression. Gefitinib is an orally active inhibitor of the EGFR tyrosine kinase. Preclinical trials demonstrated activity. Phase 1 and 2 trials demonstrated safety and activity as a single agent. In a pilot trial, gefitinib was combined with carboplatin and paclitaxel to define the toxicities of the combination and assess drug-drug interactions in untreated patients with advanced NSCLC.

Study Design.—The study group consisted of 24 adult patients with stage IIIB, IV, or recurrent NSCLC. In the first part of this trial, patients were randomly assigned to receive 250 or 500 mg of intermittent gefitinib along with chemotherapy. Dose-limiting toxicity was assessed. In the second part, patients received 500 mg of continuous gefitinib along with chemotherapy. Patients were evaluated for both response and toxicity.

Findings.—There were 2 cases of dose-limiting toxicity. One patient had a grade 3 rash and another had prolonged neutropenia develop. The addition of gefitinib did not affect chemotherapy levels, whereas chemotherapy slightly increased exposure to gefitinib. Partial responses to therapy were detected in 5 patients. Overall, the median survival was 8 months.

Conclusions.—Gefitinib in combination with carboplatin and paclitaxel was safe and well tolerated by patients. The number of patients treated was small, but several appeared to respond to this therapeutic regimen. Parallel phase 3 trials are being conducted to assess its efficacy.

▶ Gefitinib is the first in a series of molecules currently being developed to block the tyrosine kinase function of the EGFR. Clinical studies have shown that expression of the EGFR is a poor prognostic factor in a variety of different tumor types. Preclinical studies have demonstrated that inhibition of this pathway can have an antitumor effect, and recently, two phase 2 studies were reported of gefitinib as a single agent in patients with recurrent NSCLC.[1,2] Although the response rates were low in these 2 prior studies (10%-20%), they were often rapid, dramatic, and durable, increasing interest in this pathway and inhibition by EGFR tyrosine kinase inhibitors.

This study by Miller et al is a pilot study of gefitinib plus chemotherapy (carboplatin and paclitaxel) in newly diagnosed patients with stage IIIB or IV NSCLC. The objectives of the trial were to define the toxicities of the combinations and to assess drug-drug interactions in this patient population. The authors concluded that the combination was safe, and gefitinib did not affect exposure to chemotherapy, although chemotherapy did have a modest impact on gefitinib's pharmacokinetics. Of note, the response rate was 21% and the median survival was 8 months. It was based on this trial that 2 subsequent phase 3 trials were conducted of gefitinib plus chemotherapy (INTACT 1 and INTACT 2).

Somewhat surprising to the pharmaceutical industry and clinical investigators, the 2 large randomized trials were negative; there was no difference in outcome or symptom improvement between the chemotherapy arms containing gefitinib and chemotherapy alone.[3,4] In retrospect, however, this should not have been unexpected. This pilot trial had a 21% response rate and median survival of 8 months. Although it was a small trial, this response rate and median survival are exactly the same as one would expect to see with chemotherapy alone. Given that gefitinib has a 10% to 20% response rate as a single agent in patients with recurrent NSCLC and thus is known to be an active drug in this disease, these results are significant in demonstrating that concurrent chemotherapy and gefitinib are not the optimal way to combine these agents. Clearly, additional studies need to be done.

This trial is also significant in that it gives pause to our current thinking regarding how to develop targeted agents. The phase 3 trials were planned and begun before the results of this phase 2 trial were available. Clearly, in the future, investigators will think twice before embarking on large randomized studies without some positive data from the phase 2 studies.

J. H. Schiller, MD

References

1. Fukuoka M, Yano S, Giaccone G: Final results from a phase II trial of ZD1839 (Iressa) for patients with advanced non-small cell lung cancer (IDEAL 1). *Proc Am Soc Clin Oncol* 21:298A, 2002.
2. Kris M, Natale R, Herbst R: A phase II trial of ZD1839 ('Iressa') in advanced non-small cell lung cancer patients who had failed platinum- and docetaxel-based regimens. *Proc Am Soc Clin Oncol* 21:292A, 2002.
3. Johnson D, Herbst R, Giaconne G, et al: ZD1839 ('Iressa') in combination with paclitaxal and carboplatin in chemotherapy-naive patients with advanced non-small-cell lung cancer: Results from a phase III clinical trial (INTACT 2). *Ann Oncol* 13:127S-128S, 2002.
4. Giaccone G, Johnson DH, Manegold C, et al: A phase III clinical trial of ZD1839 ('Iressa') in combination with gemcitabine and cisplatin in chemotherapy-naive patients with advanced non-small-cell lung cancer (INTACT 1). *Ann Oncol* 13:2S, 2002.

Phase III Study Comparing Chemotherapy and Radiotherapy With Preoperative Chemotherapy and Surgical Resection in Patients With Non–Small-Cell Lung Cancer With Spread to Mediastinal Lymph Nodes (N2); Final Report of RTOG 89-01

Johnstone DW, Byhardt RW, Ettinger D, et al (Univ of Rochester, NY; Med College of Wisconsin, Milwaukee; Johns Hopkins Univ, Baltimore, Md; et al)

Int J Radiat Oncol Biol Phys 54:365-369, 2002 8–12

Introduction.—The optimal treatment for stage IIA (N2) non–small cell lung cancer (NSCLC) is uncertain, especially for local control. The outcomes were compared for treatment of mediastinoscopy-confirmed N2 NSCLC with induction chemotherapy followed by either surgery or radiotherapy (RT); both options were followed by consolidation chemotherapy.

Methods.—A randomized phase III trial for stage IIIA (T1-T3N2M0) NSCLC was performed by the Radiation Therapy Oncology Group (RTOG) and Eastern Cooperative Oncology Group between April 1990 and April 1994. After verification of N2 disease via mediastinoscopy or anterior mediastinotomy, patients underwent induction chemotherapy with cisplatin, vinblastine, and mitomycin-C, the last of which was later dropped from the induction regimen. Patients were randomly assigned to surgery or RT (64 Gy in 7 weeks), followed by chemotherapy with cisplatin and vinblastine.

Results.—Of 73 eligible patients, 12 received induction chemotherapy and were not randomly assigned to RT or surgery and 45 were randomly assigned to postinduction RT or surgery. Of analyzable patients, 90% had a Karnofsky performance score of 90 to 100, 18% had weight loss of over 5%, 27% had squamous cell histologic characteristics, and 54% had bulky N2 disease. Distribution of bulky N2 disease was uniform within the treatment arms.

The rate of grade 4 toxicity was 56% in patients who did and 29% in those who did not receive mitomycin-C. One patient in each group had acute nonhematologic toxicity greater than grade 3 (nausea and vomiting) and no patients had acute grade 4 radiation toxicity. The rates of long-term toxicity were equivalent across the treatment arms. There were 3 treatment-associated deaths: 2 patients in the surgical arm (1 late pulmonary toxicity and 1 pulmonary embolus) and 1 patient in the radiation arm (radiation pneumonitis).

Seventy-eight percent of patients completed induction chemotherapy. Of 26 patients who underwent thoracotomy, 73% received a complete resection. Consolidation chemotherapy was completed in 75% of the cohort, with no significant differences among the treatment arms. The overall progression-free survivals were 53% and 17%, respectively, at 1 and 3 years, and the median progression-free survival was 14 months. There were no differences between the surgery and RT groups in 1-year survival (70% vs 66%) or median survival time (19.4 months vs 17.4 months) (Table 2). The median survival for patients who received induction chemotherapy only was 8.9 months. Mitomycin-C had no affect on survival ($P = .75$). No significant

TABLE 2.—Survival of Surgery Plus Chemotherapy Versus Radiation Therapy Plus Chemotherapy

	SURG + CHT		RT + CHT	
Time (mo)	Alive (%)	At Risk (*n*)	Alive (%)	At Risk (*n*)
0	100	29	100	32
12	70	19	66	21
24	48	13	34	11
36	33	9	22	7
48	22	6	22	7
Dead/total (*n*)	21/29		27/32	
Median time (mo)	19.38		17.38	

Note: $P = .4563$ (log-rank test).
Abbreviations: CHT, Chemotherapy; *RT*, radiotherapy.
(Reprinted from Johnstone DW, Byhardt RW, Ettinger D, et al: Phase III study comparing chemotherapy and radiotherapy with preoperative chemotherapy and surgical resection in patients with non–small-cell lung cancer with spread to mediastinal lymph nodes (N2); Final report of RTOG 89-01. *Int J Radiat Oncol Biol Phys* 54:365-369, 2002. Copyright 2002, with permission from Elsevier Science.)

difference was observed in the time to local failure between the surgical and RT treatment arms.

Conclusion.—Patient accrual was closed since a large phase II trial showed the feasibility of preoperative concurrent chemoradiation in this cohort. This made results inconclusive. Histologic verification of N2 disease in the surgical and nonsurgical arms eliminated the usual biases from clinical staging. In this setting, local control and survival were nearly equal between the surgical and RT treatment arms. The 3- and 5-year survival rates for nonsurgical treatment were similar to published surgical trials of N2 disease.

► When it comes to the optimal treatment for patients who have stage IIIA NSCLC, I would argue that there is no standard. There are a variety of treatments that can be offered and the results are not dramatically different, at least as far as I can see, in terms of overall survival. Although many surgeons believe that the IIIAs require surgical resection (especially if they have a good performance status), good evidence to support that is lacking.

The RTOG attempted to look at this in a randomized phase III study, taking patients who had N2 disease and giving them induction chemotherapy followed either by surgery or RT on a randomized basis, followed subsequently by further chemotherapy with cisplatin and vinblastine. Unfortunately, there was relatively poor patient accrual to this trial, presumably due to bias on the part of the various physicians responsible for patient welfare. Nonetheless, they were able to randomize 75 patients, most all of whom were able to be analyzed. Of those that were randomized, there was no obvious trend toward superiority from postchemotherapy surgery versus postchemotherapy radiation.

It is unfortunate that this study could not have been completed as planned because it is an important issue. My view is that if the patient is in good shape and appears to have responded to chemotherapy, a resection is appropriate. A lot depends on the amount of tumor, as well as performance status and pulmonary function. This aborted study offers no supportive data.

E. Glatstein, MD

Induction of p53-Regulated Genes and Tumor Regression in Lung Cancer Patients After Intratumoral Delivery of Adenoviral p53 (INGN 201) and Radiation Therapy

Swisher SG, Roth JA, Komaki R, et al (Univ of Texas, Houston; Introgen Therapeutics Inc, Houston; Aventis, Bridgewater, NJ; et al)

Clin Cancer Res 9:93-101, 2003 8–13

Introduction.—The tumor suppressor gene *p53* is mutated or otherwise altered in more than half of all human cancers, and the finding of altered *p53* often indicates a poor prognosis. In non–small cell lung cancer (NSCLC), conventional radiation and chemoradiation provide poor locoregional control. A prospective phase II study examined the feasibility and mechanisms of apoptosis induction after *Ad-p53 (INGN 201)* gene transfer and radiation therapy in patients with NSCLC.

Methods.—Patients included in the study had histologically proven nonmetastatic NSCLC (stage I-III) and were ineligible for chemoradiation or surgery. The presence of a *p53* mutation in the tumor was not required. Patients received intratumoral injections of *Ad-p53 (INGN 201)* on days 1, 18, and 32 of treatment. Radiation therapy was administered concurrently over 6 weeks, beginning on day 4; a total dose of 60 Gy was directed at the primary tumor and any involved mediastinal lymph nodes. Patients were assessed for overall response, response of the injected tumor, toxic effects, survival duration, and time to progression for metastatic and locoregional disease.

Results.—The patients were 11 men and 8 women (median age, 74 years) who had a median follow-up of 36 months. Seventeen of 19 patients received all planned treatment. There was 1 early death, and 1 patient did not complete the therapy because of tumor progression. The most common adverse effects of therapy were grade 1 or 2 fevers (79%) and chills (53%). Pathologic biopsy specimens of the primary tumor, obtained 3 months after completion of therapy, revealed no viable tumor in 12 patients and viable tumor in 3; 4 patients were not assessed. Overall tumor response was determined by an external review board that considered CT, bronchoscopic, and clinical findings.

One patient achieved a complete response (5%) and 11 had a partial response (58%). Stable disease was found in 3 patients (16%), and progressive disease in 2 (11%); 2 patients were not evaluable. The 4 *p53*-related genes were analyzed by quantitative reverse transcription–polymerase chain reaction, which showed Bak expression to be increased significantly 24 hours after *Ad-p53 (INGN 201)* injection. Levels of *CDKN1A* and *MDM2* expression were increased during the course of therapy.

Conclusion.—In patients with NSCLC, intratumoral injection of *Ad-p53 (INGN 201)* in combination with radiation therapy achieved tumor regression at the primary injected tumor with no dose-limiting toxicity. Findings provide a molecular mechanism for the enhanced antitumoral activity with sequential tumor biopsies and quantitative analysis of *p53*-regulated genes.

► The tumor suppressor gene *p53* is one of the most commonly mutated genes in cancer, including lung cancer. Among other functions, it regulates the progression of cells through the cell cycle via a number of downstream genes, including *p21 (CDKN1A), Fas, BAK,* and *MDM2,* so that damaged or injured cells can be either repaired or undergo apoptosis. In preclinical modes, it can reverse the tumorigenic phenotype. In addition, it makes cells more susceptible to the lethal effects of radiation—perhaps by giving cells injured by radiation therapy the ability to die. Hence, replacing a mutated *p53* with a "normal" or wild-type *p53* plus radiation therapy has aroused considerable interest.

One of the major problems with gene transfer has been getting the gene of interest to the tumor, particularly for patients with metastatic disease; a problem, since most gene vectors are taken up by the reticuloendothelial system. To get around this problem, Swisher and coworkers conducted a clinical study in which patients with local NSCLC received 3 intratumoral injections of an adenoviral vector containing *p53 (Ad-p53).* Patients also received "definitive" radiotherapy of 60 Gy. They observed a pathologic response rate of 63% (a figure that should be taken with caution, given the possibility of false-negative biopsies) and a CT/bronchoscopic response rate of 63%. In addition, upregulation of some of the downstream genes was observed on biopsies taken 24 hours after *p53* injection.

The reported response rate seems high, and median time to locoregional progression had not been reached. Not surprisingly, the majority of patients developed metastatic disease. The investigators plan on building on these results by adding chemotherapy to the regimen.

Although these results are promising, particularly as a "proof-of-principle," it must be kept in mind that this approach is unlikely to be widely used unless a better delivery system can be found. The majority of lung cancer patients present with either bulky, locally advanced disease or metastases, and routine injection and infiltration of large lung lesions with *Ad-p53* will be next to impossible.

J. H. Schiller, MD

Consolidation Docetaxel After Concurrent Chemoradiotherapy in Stage IIIB Non–Small-Cell Lung Cancer: Phase II Southwest Oncology Group Study S9504

Gandara DR, Chansky K, Albain KS, et al (Univ of California, Sacramento; Univ of Washington, Seattle; Loyola Univ, Maywood, Ill; et al)

J Clin Oncol 21:2004-2010, 2003 8–14

Background.—Concurrent chemoradiotherapeutic approaches that integrate radiosensitizing agents and dose levels of chemotherapy effective against micrometastases may be effective in patients with stage IIIB non–small cell lung cancer (NSCLC). This phase II trial assessed the benefits of consolidation docetaxel after concurrent chemoradiotherapy in patients with pathologically proved stage IIIB NSCLC. Outcomes were compared with those of an earlier study with identical eligibility criteria, staging criteria, and treatment except for docetaxel consolidation.

Methods.—Eighty-three patients were eligible. Thirty-one patients had T4N0/1 disease, 22 had T4N2 disease, and 30 had T1-3N3 disease. Treatment consisted of cisplatin, 50 mg/m^2, on days 1, 8, 29, and 36 with etoposide, 50 mg/m^2, on days 1 through 5 and 29 through 33. Thoracic radiotherapy, at a total dose of 61 Gy, was given concurrently. Consolidation docetaxel was begun 4 to 6 weeks after chemoradiotherapy, with an initial dose of 75 mg/m^2.

Findings.—In general, concurrent chemoradiotherapy was well tolerated. However, 2 patients died from probable radiation-related pneumonitis. Neutropenia during consolidation docetaxel occurred at a grade 4 level in 57% of the patients. This adverse effect was most common during dose escalation to 100 mg/m^2. The median progression-free survival was 16 months. The median survival was 26 months. Survivals at 1, 2, and 3 years were 76%, 54%, and 37%, respectively. The most common site of metastasis was the brain. In the earlier study conducted without docetaxel consolidation, median survival was 15 months. Survival rates at 1, 2, and 3 years in that study were 58%, 34%, and 17%, respectively.

Conclusion.—Consolidation docetaxel after concurrent chemoradiotherapy for patients with stage IIIB NSCLC is feasible. However, the current study does not provide definitive evidence of this approach. Further research is needed.

▶ This phase II trial represents the best results for the treatment of stage IIIB NSCLC published to date by a multi-institutional cooperative group. This is perhaps more surprising as it uses the "less than fashionable drugs," cisplatin plus etoposide, in the induction regimen. The results would suggest that docetaxel maintenance therapy contributes to the favorable outcome observed. Two trials will further evaluate this regimen: The Southwest Oncology Group will use this as a standard treatment with or without further gefitinib (Iressa) therapy. The Hoosier Oncology Group will treat all patients with cisplatin and etoposide plus radiotherapy but randomize patients to receive or not receive docetaxel. This latter trial will confirm or refute the role of maintenance docetaxel. These will be important trials to complete to determine the role of consolidative therapy.

P. J. Loehrer, Sr, MD

Efficacy of Gefitinib, an Inhibitor of the Epidermal Growth Factor Receptor Tyrosine Kinase, in Symptomatic Patients With Non–Small Cell Lung Cancer: A Randomized Trial

Kris MG, Natale RB, Herbst RS, et al (Mem Sloan-Kettering Cancer Ctr, New York; Cedars-Sinai Comprehensive Cancer Center, Los Angeles; Univ of Texas, Houston; et al)

JAMA 290:2149-2158, 2003 8–15

Background.—In preclinical studies, oral gefitinib has been found to inhibit the growth of non–small cell lung cancers (NSCLCs) that express the epidermal growth factor receptor, a mediator of cell signaling. In addition, phase I trials of gefitinib have shown that some patients with NSCLC that progresses after chemotherapy have a reduction a lung cancer symptoms and radiographic lesion shrinkage. Differences in symptomatic and radiographic response between recipients of low and high daily doses of gefitinib for NSCLC were evaluated.

Methods.—A total of 221 patients were enrolled in the double-blind, randomized, phase II trial at 30 US centers between November 2000 and April 2001. The patients had stage IIIB or IV NSCLC previously treated by at least 2 chemotherapy regimens. Treatment consisted of daily oral gefitinib, 500 or 250 mg, or matching placebo.

Findings.—Symptoms were improved in 43% of patients given 250 mg of gefitinib and in 35% of those given 500 mg. In 75% of these patients, the benefits occurred within 3 weeks. Partial radiographic responses were observed in 12% of those in the low-dose group and in 9% of those in the high-dose group. Ninety-six percent of patients with partial radiographic responses had improvements in symptoms. Overall 1-year survival was 25%. The high- and low-dose groups did not differ significantly in their rates of symptom improvement, radiographic tumor regression, and projected 1-year survival. The higher dose was more often associated with transient acnelike rash and diarrhea.

Conclusions.—In these patients with NSCLC, gefitinib improved disease-related symptoms persisting after chemotherapy and induced radiographic tumor regressions. The treatment appeared to be well tolerated.

Multi-institutional Randomized Phase II Trial of Gefitinib for Previously Treated Patients With Advanced Non–Small-Cell Lung Cancer

Fukuoka M, Yano S, Giaccone G, et al (Kinki Univ School of Medicine, Japan; Osaka City Univ School of Medicine, Japan; AstraZeneca, Osaka, Japan; et al)

J Clin Oncol 21:2237-2246, 2003 8–16

Background.—Despite advances in lung cancer treatment, survival has improved minimally in the past few decades. Gefitinib is a novel epidermal growth factor receptor tyrosine kinase inhibitor. The efficacy and tolerability of this agent in patients with pretreated advanced non–small cell lung cancer (NSCLC) were reported.

Methods.—A total of 210 patients were enrolled in the randomized, double-blind, multicenter phase II trial. All patients had advanced NSCLC previously treated with 1 or 2 chemotherapy regimens, at least 1 of which contained a platinum drug. By random assignment, patients received 250 or 500 mg oral doses of gefitinib once a day.

Findings.—Treatment efficacies in the 2 dose groups were similar. The objective tumor response rate was 18.4% in the 250-mg group and 19% in the 500-mg group. Symptom rates were 40.3% and 37%, respectively, among the patients who could be evaluated. The median progression-free survival times were 2.7 and 2.8 months, respectively, and medial overall survival times were 7.6 and 8 months, respectively. Among those with a tumor response, symptoms were improved in 69.2% of the 250-mg group and 85.7% of the 500-mg group. In both dose groups, adverse events were generally mild, consisting mostly of skin reactions and diarrhea. The higher dose group more frequently had drug-related toxicities. Drug-related adverse events caused 1.9% of patients in the 250-mg group and 9.4% of those in the 500-mg group to withdraw from the study.

Conclusions.—In this patient series, gefitinib showed clinically meaningful antitumor activity, providing relief of symptoms as second- and third-line treatment. The adverse events profile of the 250 mg/d dose was favorable. Thus, gefitinib at 250 mg/d is an important treatment option for those with advanced NSCLC treated previously.

▶ These 2 articles (Abstracts 8–15 and 8–16) provide the basis for approval of gefitinib by the Food and Drug Administration for treatment of recurrent NSCLC. The study designs are similar as they were both industry sponsored. In both, patients were previously treated and demonstrated a 12% to 18% response rate with gefitinib with a median survival time of around 6 to 8 months. Gefitinib is a novel molecule drug that blocks epidermal growth factor receptor tyrosine kinase. The side effects are generally mild (principally skin rash and diarrhea). Perhaps surprisingly, in previously untreated patients Iressa failed to demonstrate an additive to chemotherapy.[1,2] Whether Iressa is truly antagonistic with chemotherapy or whether a better selection of a population (eg, epidermal growth factor positive) is needed is currently unclear. Future randomized trials of sequential therapy with tissue acquisition are needed to ultimately determine the true importance of this drug in the treatment of lung cancer.

P. J. Loehrer, Sr, MD

References

1. Giaccone G, Johnson DH, Manegold C, et al: A phase III clinical trial of ZD1839 ("Iressa") in combination with gemcitabine and cisplatin in chemotherapy-naive patients with advanced non-small cell lung cancer (INTACT-1). *Ann Oncol* 13 (suppl 5):2, 2002.
2. Johnson DH, Herbst R, Giaccone G, et al: ZD1839 ("Iressa") in combination with paclitaxel and carboplatin in chemotherapy-naive patients with advanced non-small cell lung cancer (NSCLC): Initial results from a phase III trial (INTACT-2). *Ann Oncol* 13(suppl 5):127, 2002.

9 Thoracic Malignancies

Malignant Thymoma in the United States: Demographic Patterns in Incidence and Associations With Subsequent Malignancies

Engels EA, Pfeiffer RM (Natl Cancer Inst, Rockville, Md)

Int J Cancer 105:546-551, 2003 9–1

Background.—The cause of thymoma has not been established. To date, there have been no population-based studies of demographic patterns of thymoma incidence. Previous research has associated thymoma with diverse subsequent malignancies, but these relations remain uncertain. The incidence of malignant thymoma in the United States between 1973 and 1998 was determined.

Methods.—Data were obtained from the Surveillance, Epidemiology and End Results data to determine malignant thymoma incidence by sex, age, and race. These data were also analyzed to compare malignancies after a thymoma diagnosis with those expected in the general population.

Findings.—Overall, the incidence of malignant thymoma was 0.15 per 100,000 person-years. A total of 849 cases were identified. The incidence of thymoma increased by decade of life until the eighth decade, then declined. The incidence was greater in men than women. It was highest in Asians and Pacific Islanders, who had an incidence of 0.49 per 100,000 person-years. Sixty-six malignancies were documented after the diagnosis of thymoma. An excess risk was observed for non-Hodgkin's lymphoma, with a standardized incidence ratio (SIR) of 4.7. An excess was also noted for digestive system cancers, with an SIR of 1.8, and soft tissue sarcomas, with an SIR of 11.1. No other cancers occurred with increased frequency.

Conclusions.—Malignant thymoma is rare. The incidence of this disease appears to peak in late adulthood. The documented variation in incidence by race suggests that genetic factors play a role. There appears to be no broadly increased risk for malignancies after thymoma.

► Thymomas represent a group of interesting, albeit rare, diseases. They are interesting, in part, because of their role in adaptive immunity as the site of maturation for T lymphocytes, and the resultant association with autoimmune conditions such as myasthenia gravis, blood dysplasias, and connective tissue disorders. In addition, prior studies[1,2] have described an increased risk of second malignancies, suggesting that T lymphocyte immune surveillance, thought to be abnormal in thymoma patients, is ineffective in protecting against neoplasms; however, these other studies were primarily case reports. The study by Engels and Pfeiffer is the first to use population-based data to examine demographic patterns of thymoma incidence in the United States.

As expected, they determined that the incidence of malignant thymoma is extremely rare (0.15 per 100,000 per year). It appears to be age related, increases in incidence into the eighth decade, and increased in men and Asian/Pacific Islanders. It is a cancer of middle- or older-age adults.

The only excess risk for subsequent malignancy was for non-Hodgkin's lymphoma (B immunophenotype) and digestive system cancers and soft tissue sarcomas. Of note, there was no significant excess for other cancer types, including lung cancer, or cancers of the urinary or reproductive systems. In addition, there was no increased risk for cancers of solid organs, potentially in the radiation field. There was a risk for acute nonlymphocytic leukemia in irradiated patients.

Questions raised by this summary include the peak in age-specific incidence, suggesting that age-related changes in thymic epithelial cell function affect the probability of neoplastic transformation. Racial differences in thymoma incidence are also unexplained but could suggest genetic factors. The link between thymoma and non-Hodgkin's lymphoma also needs to be explained. It could potentially be due to the abnormal regulation of T lymphocyte proliferation by abnormal T lymphocytes.

J. H. Schiller, MD

References

1. Vogelzang NJ: Emerging insights into the biology and therapy of malignant mesothelioma. *Semin Oncol* 29(6 suppl 18):35-42, 2002.
2. Tomek S, Manegold C: Chemotherapy for malignant pleural mesothelioma. *Curr Opin Oncol* 15:148-156, 2003.

▶ Thymoma is one of the most rare malignancies. Despite this, the association with a variety of paraneoplastic syndromes, including myasthenia gravis, pure red cell aplasia, hypohemoglobinemia, and other autoimmune diseases, makes this a unique tumor. This is an excellent article that highlights one of the other observations associated with thymoma—the association of secondary malignancies. Highest in incidence are non-Hodgkin lymphoma, soft tissue sarcomas, and gastrointestinal cancers. This article only addresses malignancies after the diagnosis of thymoma. As this is an indolent tumor, many cases of malignancies antedate the diagnosis of thymic malignancies. The epidemiologic background of thymoma is well discussed in this article.

P. J. Loehrer, Sr, MD

Using Gene Expression Ratios to Predict Outcome Among Patients With Mesothelioma

Gordon GJ, Jensen RV, Hsiao L-L, et al (Harvard Med School, Boston; Wesleyan Univ, Middletown, Conn; Harvard Med School, Cambridge, Mass)

J Natl Cancer Inst 95:598-605, 2003 9–2

Background.—Recent research has shown the ability of simple ratios of the expression levels of selected genes in tumor samples to distinguish among types of thoracic malignancies. This technique was applied to patients with mesothelioma.

Methods.—Gene expression profiling data collected previously from 17 patients with mesothelioma were analyzed to define 2 outcome-related groups and to develop an expression ratio–based outcome predictor model. A combination of several highly accurate expression ratios and cross-validation methods were used to determine the internal consistency of this predictor model. Quantitative reverse transcription–polymerase chain reaction of tumor RNA was used to verify the microarray data. The model was validated by using Kaplan-Meier survival analysis in an independent set of 29 mesothelioma tumors.

Findings.—The expression-based test developed was able to identify 100% of the 17 samples used to train the model. In cross-validation, the test remained accurate at 88%. A 4-gene expression ratio test significantly predicted treatment-related outcomes independent of the histologic subtype of the tumor.

Conclusions.—Gene expression ratio–based analysis can accurately predict treatment outcomes in patients with mesothelioma. This method enables the preoperative identification of patients with widely varying prognoses.

► Mesothelioma is a highly malignant disease with a poor prognosis; only 40% of patients with a stage I tumor and epithelial histology survive 5 years. These authors chose to use a new molecular biologic technique, ratios of level of expression of genes identified by gene expression profiling with oligonucleotide arrays, to determine if different ratios could predict outcome among patients with mesothelioma.

The authors used previously collected micro array data to identify genes whose expression levels could be used to discriminate among tumors that came from patients with considerably different survival times. Four such genes were identified; a model was constructed to derive different prognostic expression ratios, which was then tested and validated on 29 mesothelioma tumors with a relatively "simple" technique.

This work is important not only because it identified prognostic factors for mesothelioma, but because it is among the first to use gene expression profiling techniques to identify treatment-related prognositc markers for a human cancer that can be used to develop an outcome predictions model, and to validate the model in an independent cohort.

J. H. Schiller, MD

Phase II Study of Pemetrexed With and Without Folic Acid and Vitamin B_{12} as Front-Line Therapy in Malignant Pleural Mesothelioma

Scagliotti GV, Shin D-M, Kindler HL, et al (Univ of Turin, Torino, Italy; Univ of Pittsburgh, Pa; Univ of Chicago; et al)

J Clin Oncol 21:1556-1561, 2003 9–3

Background.—Malignant pleural mesothelioma (MPM) usually presents at an advanced stage and has no accepted therapy. Patients usually receive only supportive care. Pemetrexed is a newer antifolate with broad antitumor acivity. The efficacy of pemetrexed as a treatment for patients with advanced MPM was examined in a multicenter phase II study.

Study Design.—The study group consisted of 64 treatment-naive patients with advanced MPM. Participants received 500 mg/m^2 of pemetrexed IV every 3 weeks. After December 10, 1999, the protocol was changed so that study participants received folic acid and vitamin B_{12} supplementation during their therapy to improve safety. The primary outcome was tumor response. Secondary outcomes included response duration, survival, time to disease progression, time to treatment failure, quality of life, and pulmonary function.

Findings.—A partial response to pemetrexed therapy was observed in 14% of patients. The Kaplan-Meier estimate of median overall survival was 10.7 months. The median overall survival was 13 months for patients who received vitamin supplementation and 8 months for patients without supplementation. Patients who received vitamin supplementation completed more cycles of chemotherapy. Grade 3/4 neutropenia occurred in 23.4% of patients, and grade 3/4 leukopenia occurred in 18.8%. The incidence of toxicity was also lower in supplemented patients.

Conclusions.—Pemetrexed treatment of patients with advanced MPM resulted in a moderate response rate and a median overall survival of 10.7 months. Survival was increased and toxicity reduced in those patients who received folic acid and vitamin B_{12} supplementation. Patients with MPM may be able to benefit from pemetrexed therapy. A recently completed phase III study should help to answer this question.

► Pemetrexed is a new antifolate that attacks multiple enzymatic targets. By unclear mechanisms, folic acid and vitamin B_{12} can help protect against the systemic toxicities of pemetrexed. A theoretic concern with any "chemoprotective" agent that protects against toxicity is the possibility it will also protect against the antitumor effect of the cytotoxic drug, thus reducing efficacy.

In this article, Scagliotti and coworkers report the results of a phase II study of pemetrexed in patients with newly diagnosed mesothelioma. The protocol was changed after 21 patients to add vitamin supplementation. Although the study was not designed to compare the 2 groups, the 2 most commonly reported events (fatigue and febrile neutropenia) were lower in the supplemented group. Response rate, as assessed by an independent reviewer, was 17.1% in the supplemented group and 20% in the nonsupplemented group. The median survival was 13 months and 8 months, respectively.

Thus, this trial illustrates the activity of pemetrexed in a very difficult disease to treat, mesothelioma. It also demonstrates that vitamin supplementation with folic acid and B_{12} can reduce toxicities without reducing efficacy.

J. H. Schiller, MD

► Treatment options for mesothelioma have been limited. For those with localized disease, surgery remains the treatment of choice. Chemotherapy has been largely ineffective with only anecdotal responses reported. Pemetrexed is a new multitargeted antifolate that has at least 3 enzymatic targets, including thymidylate synthase, dihydrofolate reductase, and glycinamide ribonucleotide formyl transferase. Not only did this trial confirm a modest response rate with pemetrexed, but it also demonstrated that supplementation with folic acid and vitamin B_{12} improved the toxicity with an apparent improvement of survival.

P. J. Loehrer, Sr, MD

Lung Cancer Screening With Helical Computed Tomography in Older Adult Smokers: A Decision and Cost-effectiveness Analysis

Mahadevia PJ, Fleisher LA, Frick KD, et al (Johns Hopkins School of Medicine, Baltimore, Md; Johns Hopkins Bloomberg School of Public Health, Baltimore, Md)

JAMA 289:313-322, 2003 9–4

Objective.—Interest exists in the use of helical CT to screen for lung cancer in cigarette smokers. This interest is largely driven by direct marketing to consumers; studies reporting detection of small lung cancers by helical CT have been uncontrolled. Computer simulation models were used to analyze the potential benefits, harms, and cost-effectiveness of helical CT screening for lung cancer among older adult smokers.

Methods.—The analyses included hypothetical cohorts of 100,000 patients (age, 60 years; 55% men) who were current heavy smokers, ex-smokers, or in the process of quitting. In computer simulations, efficacy was simulated by altering the clinical stage of lung cancers (ie, shifting toward fewer advanced cancers and more localized cancers in patients undergoing helical CT screening). The study models considered certain known biases of screening, including lead time, length, and overdiagnosis. Absolute and relative differences in lung cancer–specific deaths were assessed, along with the number of false-positive results. The incremental cost-effectiveness per quality-adjusted life-year (QALY) was assessed as well.

Results.—At a 50% stage shift, helical CT screening would avoid 553 lung cancer deaths among current heavy smokers, which would yield a 13% reduction in lung cancer–specific mortality. However, the number of false-positive invasive procedures was 1186 per 100,000 patients. The incremental cost-effectiveness per QALY gained would be \$116,300 for current smokers, \$558,600 for quitting smokers, and \$2,322,700 for ex-smokers. Besides the extent of stage shift, the performance of helical CT screening would be influenced by a wide range of factors, including screening adherence, extent of length or overdiagnosis bias, quality of life for patients with localized cancers detected by screening, cost of the screening procedure, and level of anxiety about the finding of indeterminate pulmonary nodules. In 1-way sensitivity analyses, none of these factors made screening highly cost-effective for any of the 3 cohorts of older adults. In multiway analyses, achieving highly favorable values for all influential variables would lead to a cost-effectiveness value of $42,500 per QALY gained for current smokers.

Conclusions.—A wide range of barriers must be overcome to make helical CT a cost-effective lung cancer screening technique, even once its efficacy has been established. This test is of unproven benefit, carries potential harm from invasive testing, and carries a high cost. Helical CT is not likely to be highly cost-effective without substantial reductions in mortality, a high adherence rate, a lower rate of overdiagnosis, and reduced costs per screening test.

► Given the extremely guarded prognosis for most lung cancer patients, many smokers are very interested in possible screening techniques, which will allow any lung cancer to be diagnosed at an earlier, hopefully more curable stage. Low-dose, spiral or helical CT has been proposed as one such screening method, as older studies consisting of sputum cytologies or serial chest radiographs did not show a decrease in lung cancer–specific mortality. Helical CTs have the potential benefit in that they are relatively quick (usually can be completed within one held breath), use relatively low doses of radiation, and do not use contrast, thus obviating the need for a physician to be present. However, they are relatively nonspecific, particularly in areas with high rates of granulomatous disease, where up to 50% of the population can have small indeterminate abnormalities, the vast majority of which turn out to be benign. As there is concern regarding the cost to society for workup of these false-positives findings, investigators have conducted cost-effectiveness analysis of this methodology.

Mahadevia and coworkers used a computer-simulated model to compare the potential benefits, harms, and cost-effectiveness of annual screening with helical CT with no-screening. They used hypothetic cohorts consisting of 100,000 current, quitting, and former heavy smokers aged 60 years. Although the current heavy-smoker cohort had a 13% reduction in lung cancer–specific mortality, there were a significant number of false-positive invasive procedures (1186 per 100,000 persons), and the incremental cost effectiveness was $116,300 per QALY gained. These studies depend heavily on the assumptions of the model (anxiety about indeterminate lung nodules, sensitivity and specificity of the screening test, etc); however, even when using the most favorable estimates and modeling, the QALY was still only $42,500 in heavy current smokers. When evaluating former smokers, that cost rose to more than $2 million per QALY. Clearly, more work needs to be done before low-dose helical CT can be routinely recommended.

J. H. Schiller, MD

► In several of the metropolitan areas, entrepreneurial radiologists advertise and advocate lung cancer screening using CT scans. Logic would dictate that if a lung cancer could be caught earlier, the chances for curative resection would be increased. The problem is the time interval between CT scans, identifying the high-risk population, and costs (both financial and physical). Should clinicians be concerned with costs? Heck yes! With increasingly limited health care dollars, efficient use of resources needs to be a priority for today's physicians. Once we can precisely characterize the highest risk population and minimize the costs of imaging, I suspect that the CT scan could be a valuable edge to cancer screening.

P. J. Loehrer, Sr, MD

Lung Cancers Missed at Low-Dose Helical CT Screening in a General Population: Comparison of Clinical, Histopathologic, and Imaging Findings

Li F, Sone S, Abe H, et al (Univ of Chicago; Azumi Gen Hosp, Ikeda, Japan)
Radiology 225:673-683, 2002 9–5

Introduction.—The number of lung cancers missed on CT and reported in the literature has been limited, possibly since it is difficult to identify the missed cases among the many routine CT examinations performed in most medical centers. The clinical, histopathologic, and imaging characteristics of missed lung cancers were examined in patients screened at low-dose CT.

TABLE 2.—Low-Dose CT Findings of 32 Missed Lung Cancers and 73 Detected Lung Cancers

Lesion Characteristic	Missed Lung Cancer (n = 39)*	Detected Lung Cancer (n = 73)†
Mean size (mm)‡	12.2 (6-26)	15.1 (6-47)
Radiologic pattern		
Pure GGO	10	16
Mixed GGO	17	32
Solid nodular opacity	12	25
Subtlety		
Very subtle	9	18
Subtle	16	22
Not subtle	14	33

Note: All data, except those for mean size, are numbers of cancers for the detected lung cancer group but do not equal the numbers of cancers for the missed lung cancer group (because several lung cancers were missed on multiple scans).

*Thirty-two cancers in 16 patients with detection error in 1 year, in 3 patients with detection error with 2 scans, in 10 patients with interpretation error in 1 year, in 1 patient with interpretation error with 2 scans, in 1 patient with interpretation error with 3 scans, and in 1 patient with detection error with the first scan and interpretation error with the second scan.

†Three central cancers were excluded because the tumor size was indeterminate.

‡Numbers in parentheses are size ranges. P = .03 for difference in size between missed and detected cancers.

(Courtesy of Li F, Sone S, Abe H, et al: Lung cancers missed at low-dose helical CT screening in a general population: Comparison of clinical, histopathologic, and imaging findings. *Radiology* 225:673-683, 2002. Radiological Society of North America.)

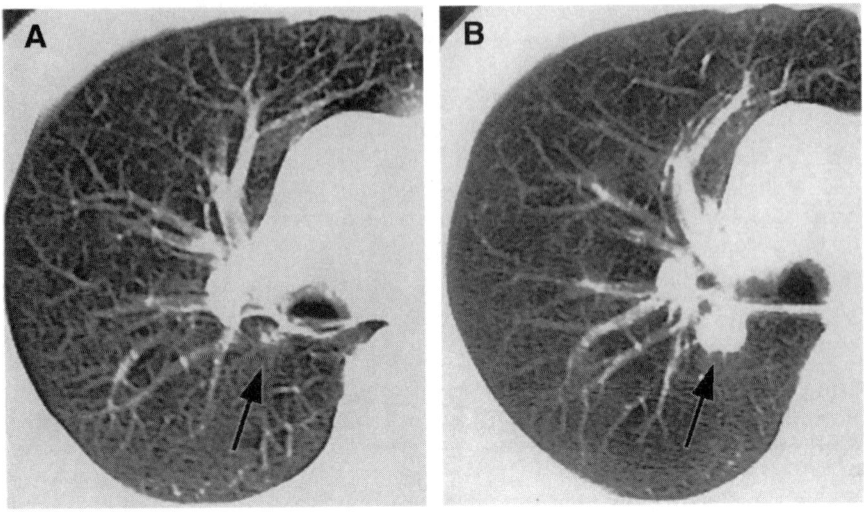

FIGURE 4.—Transverse low-dose CT scans of poorly differentiated stage IIIA adenocarcinoma in a 56-year-old man with a 30-pack year smoking history. **A**, CT scan obtained in August 1996 shows a subtle nodule with mixed ground-glass opacity (*arrows*) behind the right hilum and adjacent to the mediastinum. This lesion was not detected. **B**, CT scan obtained in August 1997, the year the cancer was detected, clearly shows the lesion (*arrow*) increased in size and attenuation. (Courtesy of Li F, Sone S, Abe H, et al: Lung cancers missed at low-dose helical CT screening in a general population: Comparison of clinical, histopathologic, and imaging findings. *Radiology* 225:673-683, 2002. Radiological Society of North America.)

Methods.—Between May 1996 and March 1999, 17,892 examinations were performed in 7847 patients as part of an annual low-dose helical CT screening for lung cancer. Eighty-three primary lung cancers were identified and verified histopathologically at either surgery or biopsy. Thirty-two of these lung cancers were not identified on 39 CT scans. Of these, 23 misses were due to detection errors and 16 were due to interpretation errors. The clinical and CT features and histopathologic findings of these missed lung cancers were examined.

Results.—All missed cancers were intrapulmonary; 28 (88%) were stage IA disease. All 20 detection errors were observed in patients with adenocarcinoma; 17 (85%) were well-differentiated tumors and 11 (55%) were in nonsmoking women. The mean size of cancers missed as a result of detection error was smaller than that of cancers missed due to interpretation errors (9.8 mm vs 15.9 mm; $P < .001$) (Table 2). In the detection error group, the percentage of nodules with ground-glass opacity (91%) or considered to be subtle (91%) (Fig 4) was greater than that of nodules in the interpretation error group (38% and 25%, respectively; $P < .001$). In the detection error group, 83% (19/23) cancers were overlapped with, obscured by (Fig 5), or similar in appearance to normal structures, including pulmonary vessels (Fig 2). On 14 of the 16 CT scans in which there were interpretation errors, the CT findings mimicked benign disease and the patients also had underlying disease (tuberculosis, emphysema, or lung fibrosis) (Table 4).

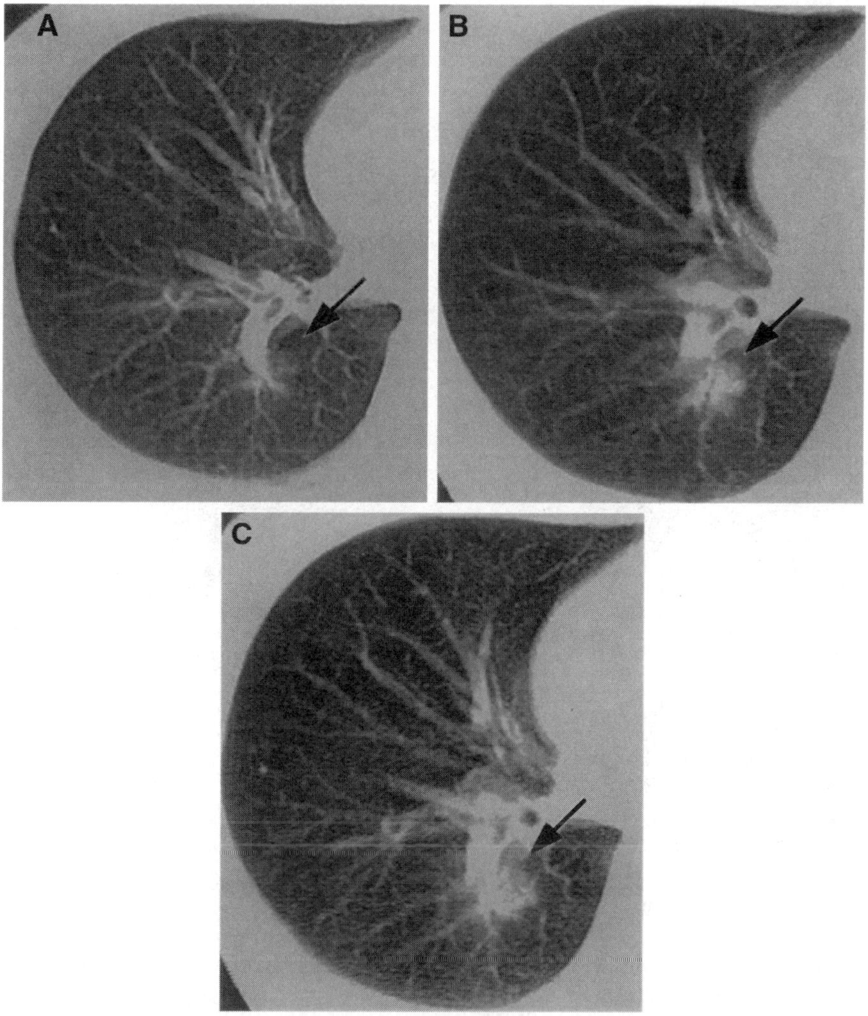

FIGURE 5.—Transverse low-dose CT scans of well-differentiated stage IIA adenocarcinoma in a 53-year-old man with an 80-pack-year smoking history. **A**, CT scan obtained in May 1996 shows a subtle area of pure ground-glass opacity (*arrow*) obscured by the pulmonary vessel branches in the parahilar region; this lesion was not detected. **B**, CT scan obtained in March 1997 clearly shows the lesion (*arrow*) increased in size and attenuation, but it still was not detected. C, On the CT scan obtained in March 1998, the lesion (*arrows*) became more obvious and was detected. (Courtesy of Li F, Sone S, Abe H, et al: Lung cancers missed at low-dose helical CT screening in a general population: Comparison of clinical, histopathologic, and imaging findings. *Radiology* 225:673-683, 2002. Radiological Society of North America.)

Conclusion.—The lung cancers missed on low-dose CT screening in this cohort usually were subtle and appeared as small, faint nodules, overlapping structures, or opacities in a complex background of other disease.

► There has been a tremendous amount of interest—some positive, some negative—with respect to low-dose helical CT screening for lung cancer. The

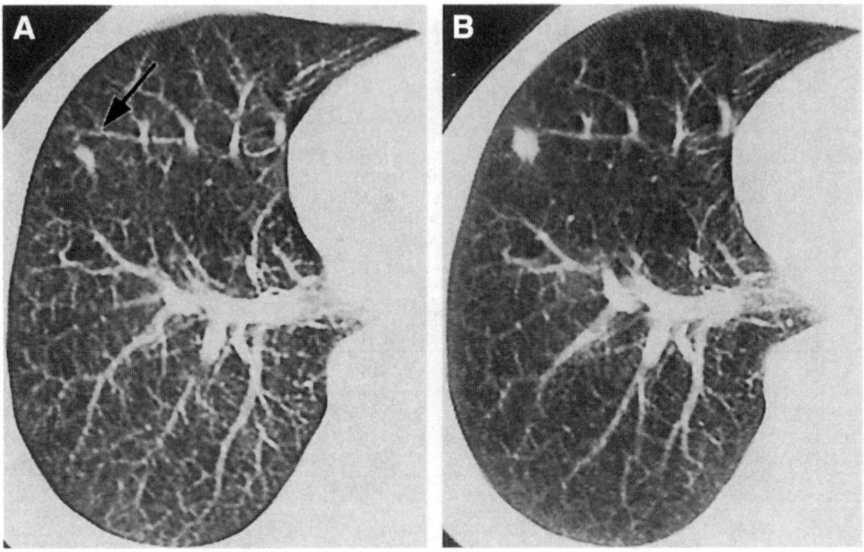

FIGURE 2.—Transverse low-dose CT scans of moderately differentiated stage IA adenocarcinoma in a 64-year-old man with a 30 pack-year history. **A**, CT scan image obtained in May 1996 was considered to be similar to a pulmonary vessel or chronic inflammatory lesion and was not detected. **B**, CT scan obtained in May 1997 depicts the nodule in **A**, which increased in size. (Courtesy of Li F, Sone S, Abe H, et al: Lung cancers missed at low-dose helical CT screening in a general population: Comparison of clinical, histopathologic, and imaging findings. *Radiology* 225:673-683, 2002. Radiological Society of North America.)

National Cancer Institute has responded with a very large (and very expensive) prospective study. I have not seen the formal protocol, but it is my understanding that it is aimed at the issue of detection and not linked to outcome. If true, I hope that can be corrected to permit a meaningful interpretation.

These investigators from the University of Chicago and from Japan have carried out a small study with an annual low-dose CT screening program. They have managed to detect 83 primary lung cancers out of almost 8000 patients who were considered at risk. What is interesting in this study is that of the 83 primary lung cancers, 32 of these cancers (over 30%) were missed on a total of 39 scans. In some instances, these were outright detection errors and in other instances, they were misinterpretations of what was seen. The point is that the detection process is perhaps more subtle than some advocates of this technology would have us believe.

There are other issues of cost in terms of follow-up on nodules, repeat CT scans, or invasive procedures needed to establish a diagnosis. There is another aspect of the cost which I do not believe has received much attention and that is the way the patient (most likely a smoker), will interpret a negative study. From the standpoint of trying to eradicate lung cancer, I am not sure this is a good maneuver. It will cause the majority of patients who will have a negative study to feel they can continue to smoke. In addition, the expense has to take into account the need for repeated studies. While I am anxious to see us improve our detection of lung cancer, I am not sure we as a society can

TABLE 4.—Low-Dose CT Findings in Detection Error and Interpretation Error Groups

Lesion Characteristic	Detection Error ($n = 23$)	Interpretation Error ($n = 16$)
Mean size of missed lesions (mm)*	9.8 (6-17)	15.9 (6-26)
Mean size of detected lesions (mm)*	11.7 (7-19)	18.9 (11-32)
Radiologic pattern*		
Pure GGO	8	2
Mixed GGO	13	4
Solid nodular opacity	2	10
Subtlety*		
Very subtle	7	2
Subtle	14	2
Not subtle	2	12
Lesion appearance relative to that of normal structures†	19	NA
Appearance similar to pulmonary vessel	8	NA
Appearance similar to that of pleural area	2	NA
Lesion overlaps with pulmonary vessels	7	NA
Appearance obscured by hilar structures	5	NA
Lesion features mimic those of benign lesion‡	NA	15
Underlying lung disease‡	NA	14
Focal infectious lesion(s)	NA	14
Emphysema	NA	2
Lung fibrosis	NA	4
Silicosis	NA	1
Asbestosis	NA	3

Note: Unless otherwise noted, data are numbers of CT scans.
*$P < .002$ for difference between the detection error and interpretation error groups.
†Only detection errors occurred in the analysis of this finding.
‡Only interpretation errors occurred in the analysis of this finding.
(Courtesy of Li F, Sone S, Abe H, et al: Lung cancers missed at low-dose helical CT screening in a general population: Comparison of clinical, histopathologic, and imaging findings. *Radiology* 225:673-683, 2002. Radiological Society of North America.)

afford this approach. As a screening technique, it is too expensive. In addition, there is the issue of specificity or lack thereof.

E. Glatstein, MD

Lung Cancer Rates Convergence in Young Men and Women in the United States: Analysis by Birth Cohort and Histologic Type

Jemal A, Travis WD, Tarone RE, et al (American Cancer Society, Atlanta, Ga; Armed Forces Inst of Pathology, Washington, DC; Natl Cancer Inst, Bethesda, Md)

Int J Cancer 105:101-107, 2003 9–6

Background.—Largely because of differences in patterns of cigarette smoking between men and women, age-specific lung cancer rates have been consistently greater for U.S. men than women. In recent birth cohorts, however, these sex differences have decreased. Recent studies suggest that women may be more susceptible to the carcinogenic effects of smoke than men. Population-based incidence and mortality data were analyzed to determine trends in age-specific lung cancer rates by birth cohort according to sex, ethnic group, and histologic findings.

Methods and Findings.—Rates of death from lung cancer were found to converge between men and women born after 1960, especially among whites. Among whites, the male-to-female mortality ratio among 35- to 39-year-olds declined from 3.0 for the 1915 birth cohort to 1.1 in the 1960 birth cohort. Among blacks, it declined from 4.0 in the 1925 birth cohort to 1.5 in the 1960 birth cohort. Incidence rates for white women and men converged rapidly for adenocarcinoma, small cell carcinoma, and large cell carcinoma. Less convergence was seen for squamous cell carcinoma. Cigarette smoking among white men and women aged 24 years was comparable in cohorts born after 1960. However, smoking in these cohorts continued to be greater among black men than among black women.

Conclusions.—Lung cancer death rates have converged among men and women born after 1960. These data suggest that men and women are equally susceptible to lung cancer from a given amount of cigarette smoking.

► A number of studies published in the 1990s suggested that women are more susceptible to the carcinogenic effects of tobacco smoke, even when corrected for amount of nicotine exposure. The authors postulate that if so, lung cancer mortality should be the same between the 2 sexes, particularly since smoking prevalence was about equal in white men and women born after 1960. Using data from the SEER database, they examined trends in age-specific rates of lung cancer by birth cohort. Although there were slight differences in terms of histology (squamous cell carcinoma) and race (black men vs black women), they found that the lung death rate was about equal between young white men and women born after 1960, suggesting that men and women are equally susceptible to the development of lung cancer from a given amount of cigarette smoking.

J. H. Schiller, MD

Lycopene Supplementation Inhibits Lung Squamous Metaplasia and Induces Apoptosis Via Up-regulating Insulin-like Growth Factor-Binding Protein 3 in Cigarette Smoke-Exposed Ferrets

Liu C, Lian F, Smith DE, et al (Tufts Univ, Boston)

Cancer Res 63:3138-3144, 2003 9–7

Background.—Lycopene, an antioxidant found in tomatoes, has been suggested to have anticancer properties. Recent studies have indicated that high dietary lycopene intake is associated with lower circulating levels of insulin-like growth factor I (IGF-I). High levels of circulating IGF-I have been implicated in the development of lung cancer. IGF-binding protein 3 (IGFBP-3) regulates the activity of IGF-I by preventing it from interacting with its receptor. It also inhibits cell growth and induces apoptosis. High dietary intake of tomatoes is also associated with higher circulating levels of IGFBP-3. The effects of lycopene supplementation on cancer pathogenesis were evaluated in a ferret model of smoking-induced lung carcinogenesis.

Methods.—Male adult ferrets were supplemented with 1.1 mg/kg daily of lycopene (low dose) or 4.3 mg/kg daily of lycopene (high dose), with or without exposure to cigarette smoke for 9 weeks. The effect of lycopene supplementation on tissue IGF-I and IGFBP-3 levels, lung histopathology, cell proliferation, and apoptosis was investigated.

Results.—Among ferrets exposed to cigarette smoke, those supplemented with lycopene had significantly higher plasma IGFBP-3 levels and a significantly lower IGF-I/IGFBP-3 ratio than those exposed to smoke without lycopene supplementation. Lycopene supplementation was also associated with inhibition of smoke-induced squamous metaplasia and proliferating cellular nuclear antigen expression in the lungs. Exposure to cigarette smoke significantly increased phosphorylation of BAD, reducing its apoptotic effects, but phosphorylation was inhibited by lycopene supplementation. Lycopene levels increased in a dose-dependent manner in the plasma and lungs of all ferrets supplemented with lycopene, but cigarette smoke reduced this increase.

Conclusions.—Lycopene supplementation inhibited many of the antiapoptotic actions of cigarette smoke in the lung. The protective effects of lycopene may be mediated through upregulation of IGFBP-3 and decreased phosphorylation of BAD, which promote apoptosis and inhibit cell proliferation.

► Lycopene is an antioxidant found in tomatoes that has a number of pleiotropic effects in preclinical models. Epidemiologic and murine studies suggest that it may have a chemopreventive effect, although the exact mechanism is unknown. In this study, Liu and coworkers seek to determine whether one mechanism is through modulation of IGF. IGFs are mitogens that have been implicated in lung carcinogenesis by increasing cell survival by phosphorylation of BAD. BAD is a member of the Bcl-2 family and is part of the downstream pathway of the IGF-I receptor PI3K/Akt/protein kinase B pathway. Nonphosphorylated BAD is localized to the mitochondria and binds to Bcl-xL, promoting its apoptotic effect, whereas phosphorylated BAD is found in the cytosol, binds to proteins other than Bcl-xL, and does not induce cell death. Low blood levels of the IGF-binding protein, IGFBP-3, and high IGF-I concentrations and IGF-I/IGFBP-3 ratios have been implicated in a variety of cancers, including lung cancer, and it is postulated that one mechanism by which cigarette smoke may induce lung cancer is by affecting normal IGF-I signaling, cell proliferation, and apoptosis.

Although no changes in plasma IGF-I concentrations were found in ferrets exposed to smoke, Liu and colleagues observed elevated IGFBP-3 concentrations and lowered IGF-I/IGFBP-3 ratios in ferrets with lycopene supplementation. In addition, smoke induced phosphorylation of BAD and downregulated apoptosis, which was inhibited by lycopene supplementation, as was the development of lung squamous metaplasia. These results suggest that lycopene may mediate its protective effects against smoke-induced lung carcinogenesis in ferrets through upregulation of IGFBP-3 and downregulation of BAD, thus inhibiting cell proliferation and promoting apoptosis.

The authors have used this model to demonstrate that high-dose β-carotene supplementation in smokers may be detrimental, based on production and accumulation of undesirable oxidative metabolites in lung tissue. Those findings were borne out in clinical studies, which showed either no beneficial effect or a possible harmful effect among smokers receiving β-carotene supplementation.[1,2] Thus, this current work suggests that this might be a clinically relevant model for future chemoprevention studies in lung cancer.

J. H. Schiller, MD

References

1. Hennekens CH, Buring JE, Manson JE, et al: Lack of effect of long-term supplementation with β-carotene on the incidence of malignant neoplasms and cardiovascular disease. *N Engl J Med* 334:1145-1149, 1996.
2. Omenn GS, Goodman GE, Thornquist MD, et al: Effects of a combination of β-carotene and vitamin A on lung cancer and cardiovascular disease. *N Engl J Med* 334:1150-1155, 1996.

Gene Promoter Hypermethylation in Tumors and Lymph Nodes of Stage I Lung Cancer Patients

Harden SV, Tokumaru Y, Westra WH, et al (Johns Hopkins Univ, Baltimore, Md; Univ of Rochester, NY)
Clin Cancer Res 9:1370-1375, 2003 9–8

Background.—Promoter hypermethylation, an important pathway for repressing gene transcription in cancer cells, is also a promising marker for detecting cancer. Five gene promoters were tested by real-time methylation-specific polymerase chain reaction in primary lung tumors for aberrant DNA methylation.

Methods.—Ninety patients with stage I lung cancer were assessed. The presence of tumor methylation was then used as a marker to determine the presence of occult metastasis in corresponding histologically negative lymph nodes.

Findings.—Eighty-one percent of the primary tumors had promoter hypermethylation in at least 1 of the genes studied. Seventeen percent had promoter hypermethylation at the gene promoters p16, 16% at O^6-methylguanine-DNA-methyltransferase, 8% at glutathione *S*-transferase P1 (*GSTP1*), 72% at adenomatous polyposis coli (APC), and 17% at death-associated protein kinase. Squamous histology predicted lower overall survival rates. Nonsquamous histology correlated with APC and *GSTP1* methylation in the primary tumor. The finding of both APC and death-associated protein kinase methylation in the primary tumor predicted worse outcomes, with 54% of the patients in this group dying compared with 27% in the group without methylation in both genes. In 15% of cases, the same methylation pattern was found in DNA from at least 1 of the corresponding lymph nodes. Forty-five percent of patients with occult metastasis on methylation analysis died compared with 27% of those with negative lymph nodes, though survival analysis was not statistically significant.

Conclusions.—Promoter hypermethylation is common in lung cancer. It is also a promising marker for molecular staging of patients with this disease. A larger prospective study is now needed to better understand the ability of methylation analysis to detect occult metastasis.

► In addition to allelic deletion, another method of silencing tumor suppressor genes is hypermethylation of CpG islands within promoter regions of cancer-associated genes. Aberrant methylation of these genes results in a transcriptional block and loss of the protein. A number of genes have been found to have hypermethylated promoters in non–small cell lung cancer, and this phenomenon has been thought to play a role in carcinogenesis.

In addition, detection of aberrantly methylated tumor cells in blood or sputum is being explored as a mechanism for detecting occult metastasis. Harden et al used a panel of 5 gene promoters to assess both tumor and corresponding "negative" lymph nodes in 90 stage I patients. Gene methylation was found in about 80% of tumors and was detected in "normal" lymph nodes in 15% of cases. A trend toward worse survival was observed in patients with occult metastasis by mutation analysis and in patients whose tumor was methylated for both APC and *GSTP1*. These results need to be confirmed on a much larger scale but suggest that this method may be important in detecting occult metastases and in predicting prognosis.

J. H. Schiller, MD

Association Between Self-Reported Environmental Tobacco Smoke Exposure and Lung Cancer: Modification by *GSTP1* Polymorphism

Miller DP, De Vivo I, Neuberg D, et al (Harvard School of Public Health, Boston; Harvard Med School, Boston)

Int J Cancer 104:758-763, 2003 9–9

Background.—Research has shown an association between lung cancer risk and exposure to environmental tobacco smoke (ETS), which contains a greater concentration of tobacco smoke carcinogens than mainstream smoke. Investigators have studied polymorphisms in genes that metabolize tobacco smoke carcinogens as effect modifiers of the relation between active smoking and lung cancer risk. The association between ETS and lung cancer risk as well as the modification of this relation by the *GSTP1* polymorphism were determined.

Methods.—The case-control study included 1041 patients with lung cancer and 1159 control subjects. All participants were genotyped for *GSTP1* with PCR-RFLP methods. The relation between ETS exposure and lung cancer risk was assessed in different strata on the basis of smoking habits. The effect of the *GSTP1* polymorphism on lung cancer risk was determined by considering the joint effect of having both ETS exposure and the *GSTP1 GG* genotype compared with no ETS exposure and the *GSTP1 AA* genotype.

Findings.—In all strata analyzed, ETS exposure was consistently associated with greater lung cancer risk. Among nonsmokers, the adjusted odds ratio (OR) for ETS exposure was 1.38; among ex-smokers, 1.66; and among current smokers, 1.56. Among ex-smokers, the ORs were 2.64 for those who had quit for 19 years or longer, 1.16 for those who had quit for 10 to 19 years, and 1.45 for those who had quit for 10 years or less. The ETS-related lung cancer risk was greater among those with the *GSTP1 GG* genotype than among those with the *GSTP1 AA* genotype. Among those with the *GSTP1 GG* phenotype, nonsmokers had an OR of 7.85; ex-smokers, 2.32; current smokers, 1.75; and persons with less than 15 pack-years and nonsmokers, 1.93.

Conclusions.—Exposure to ETS is associated with an increased risk of lung cancer. The presence of the *GSTP1 GG* genotype apparently increases the magnitude of this association. Further research involving larger numbers of participants will be needed to verify these preliminary findings.

▶ Similar to the article by Harden et al (Abstract 9–8), this paper also seeks to explore possible mechanisms by which some smokers get lung cancer and others do not. Instead of looking at polymorphisms in DNA repair enzymes, Miller et al evaluated polymorphisms in the carcinogen detoxifying enzyme glutathione S-transferase (GSTπ), and correlated these with passive smoking exposure. GSTπ is encoded by a polymorphic gene, *GSTP1*, and is one of the main detoxifiers of benzopyrene, a major carcinogen in tobacco smoke. A single base pair substitution results in lower enzymatic activity and higher levels of PAH-DNA adducts in human lymphocytes (PAH-DNA adducts are associated with smoking, as are cotinine and 4-ABP-hemoglobin adducts).

Unlike the Harden article, this paper looks at environmental tobacco exposure by passive smoking exposure. They found that ETS was associated with lung cancer risk in all smoking groups, although not statistically significantly. Nonsmokers, light smokers, and smokers who had quit for a long time were more likely to be affected by environmental tobacco because the exposure effect of active smoking was greatly reduced in these groups. The presence of the *GSTP1 GG* phenotype increased the lung cancer risk.

The risk associated with ETS has been controversial due to issues of sample size, recall bias, and estimation of ETS exposure. The authors attempt to address these issues. Sample size is typically an issue because of the small number of nonsmokers who get lung cancer; in this study, the investigators included different subgroups of smokers. To control for recall bias, they include friends or non-blood-related family members of cases. To try to improve the accuracy of ETS exposure estimation, the investigators collected information on both frequency and location of exposure. Despite these attempts to address these issues, however, the authors conclude that further research and larger sample sizes will be needed to evaluate the statistical significance of the interaction between *GSTP*, polymorphism, and ETS.

J. H. Schiller, MD

Cyclin D1 Overexpression in Bronchial Epithelia of Patients With Lung Cancer Is Associated With Smoking and Predicts Survival

Ratschiller D, Heighway J, Gugger M, et al (Univ of Bern, Switzerland; Roy Castle Centre, Liverpool, England)

J Clin Oncol 21:2085-2093, 2003 9–10

Background.—The majority of lung cancers are caused by smoking. These investigators have previously found that deregulation of cyclin D1 expression, especially imbalanced expression primarily from one allele, is a characteristic of non–small cell lung cancer (NSCLC). Cyclin D1 expression was examined in tumor-free bronchial epithelia from patients with resectable NSCLC.

Study Design.—Tumor and bronchial samples were collected prospectively from 37 men and 11 women, aged 30 to 80 years, who had resection of NSCLC at the University Hospital of Berne. DNA was isolated and ampli-

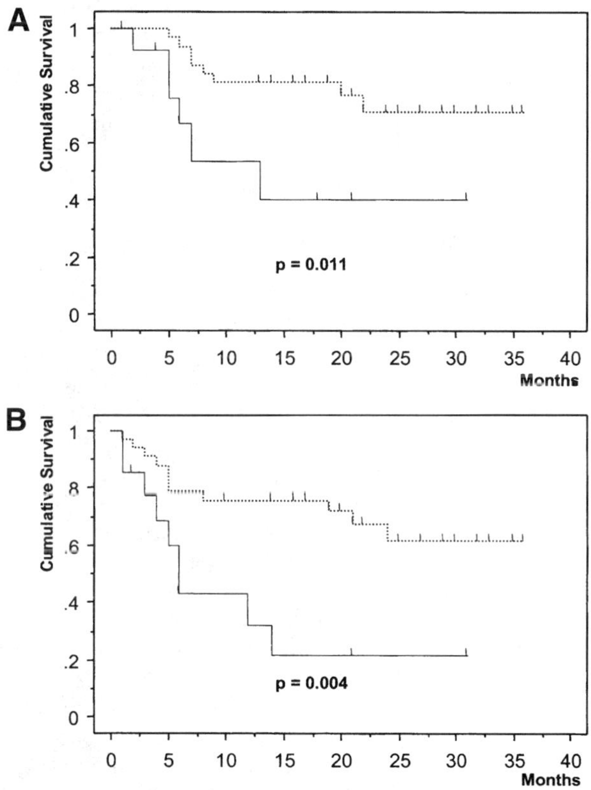

FIGURE 5.—Overall survival (**A**) and remission duration (**B**) of patients with nuclear cyclin D1 overexpression (*solid line*) as compared with patients with no detectable nuclear cyclin D1 in the bronchial epithelium (*dotted line*); log-rank test, (**A**) *P* = .011; (**B**) *P* = .004. (Courtesy of Ratschiller D, Heighway J, Gugger M, et al: Cyclin D1 overexpression in bronchial epithelia of patients with lung cancer is associated with smoking and predicts survival. *J Clin Oncol* 21:2085-2093, 2003. Reprinted with permission from the American Society of Clinical Oncology.)

fied by polymerase chain reaction (PCR). RNA was also extracted and amplified by reverse transciptase–PCR to quantitate cyclin D1 expression. Immunohistochemistry was used to identify the cyclin D1 protein and to localize it. Expression was compared with smoking habits.

Findings.—Cyclin D1 was overexpressed at 58% of all bronchial sites assayed. Cytoplasmic localization of the D1 product was detected in more than half of all samples. Nuclear overexpression was more common at premalignant sites. Allele-specific expression imbalance was detected in about half of all sites. For about 60% of patients, the degree and balance of expression were consistent at all sites, whereas it varied for other patients. Nuclear cyclin D1 expression was associated with heavy smoking and decreased overall survival (Fig 5).

Conclusions.—This study of bronchial epithelia of patients with resectable NSCLC is the first to demonstrate that (1) cyclin D1 is often overexpressed, and the protein is mainly located in the cytoplasm; (2) nuclear localization of cyclin D1 is associated with premalignant transformation; (3) the distribution of similar allelically imbalanced expression, in conjunction with cyclin D1 overexpression, is consistent with the concept of the clonal dispersion of a malignant or premalignant cell across the lung; and (4) bronchial epithelia with nuclear cyclin D1 staining occurs especially in heavy smokers and is predictive of poor outcome. These findings suggest that cyclin D1 might provide a novel therapeutic target in patients with NSCLC. It also may serve as a molecular marker for patients who are at high risk.

► Considerable evidence exists to suggest that cancer is the result of a stepwise accumulation of multiple genetic alterations, that lung cancer is related to tobacco exposure, and that the entire tracheobronchial tree of a smoker is at risk for development of lung cancer. This last process, called field cancerization, explains the diffuse mucosal changes of the tracheobronchial tree often found in smokers. Of significant interest is identification of preneoplastic lesions that predict for development of lung cancer and survival. A number of studies are ongoing looking at different potential markers that may describe an early step in the neoplastic transformation of bronchial epithelia. Many of these look at sputum cytology; others involve bronchoscopy and serial biopsies. Markers that have been assessed include KI-67, and hypermethylation of oncogenes or tumor suppressor genes.

This study differs somewhat in that it is a retrospective series examining tumor samples and "normal" bronchial epithelia distant to the tumor for abnormalities in the G1 restriction point control element. Cyclin D1 controls movement of cells out of G1 into S phase; overexpression of cyclin D1 has been observed in primary non–small cell lung tumors. In this study, the investigators looked at cyclin D1 expression in microdissected bronchial epithelial cells at 6 different sites distant from the primary cancer. In addition to looking at protein expression, they also examine RNA and DNA (*CCND1*, the cyclin D1 allele).

Cyclin D1 overexpression was associated with premalignant lesions, heavy smoking, and decreased survival. These results suggest that deregulation of the cyclin D1 gene is not only important in the neoplastic transformation of bronchial epithelial cells, but it is also probably related to smoking. Thus, cyclin D1 expression may be an early step in the neoplastic transformation of bronchial epithelium, and this may be caused by changes at the *CCND1* allele, suggesting genetic mutations in this area.

In addition, in some patients, similar allelically imbalanced expression and cyclin D1 overexpression were also observed in normal bronchial epithelium, suggesting the spread of premalignant clones across the bronchial epithelium.

Why are these data important? First, they suggest that cyclin D1 may be an early step in the neoplastic transformation of bronchial epithelia. They also suggest that the theory of field cancerization may not be true in all smokers, and that premalignant clones do spread within the tracheobronchial tree. Lastly, they suggest that cyclin D1 may be an appropriate target for chemoprevention or lung cancer therapeutic trials.

J. H. Schiller, MD

Glutathione *S*-transferase M1, T1, and P1 Polymorphisms and Survival Among Lung Cancer Patients

Sweeney C, Nazar-Stewart V, Stapleton PL, et al (Univ of Minnesota, Minneapolis; Oregon Health and Science Univ, Portland; Univ of Washington, Seattle; et al)

Cancer Epidemiol Biomarkers Prev 12:527-533, 2003 9–11

Background.—Glutathione *S*-transferase (GST) enzymes detoxify drugs and reactive oxidants. Therefore, GST polymorphisms could influence cancer survival. The relationship between survival and 3 common GST polymorphisms was examined in a population-based cohort of men with lung cancer.

Study Design.—The study group consisted of 274 primarily white men, aged 18 to 74 years, with a first diagnosis of primary lung cancer. Each study participant provided a blood sample for genotyping. GST genotypes were determined by polymerase chain reaction of DNA extracted from lymphocytes. Survival analysis was performed to investigate the influence of GST phenotype on survival.

Findings.—Lung cancer patients with the *GSTM1* null genotype had shorter survival times than those with the *GSTM1* present genotype. The relative risk of death associated with the *GSTM1* null genotype was 1.36. There were no associations between either the *GSTT1* or the *GSTP1* genotypes and survival in this population.

Conclusions.—Men with primary lung cancer who had the *GSTM1* null phenotype had shorter overall survival than men who did not have this genotype. Perhaps the *GSTM1* genotype should be considered in future studies and in future treatment regimens for patients with lung cancer.

► Whereas the article by Miller et al (Abstract 9–9) looked at the correlation between GST polymorphisms and lung cancer risk, this report by Sweeney et al examines the relationships between GST polymorphisms and survival in lung cancer patients. GST polymorphisms may influence survival by 1 of 2 mechanisms: (1) several chemotherapeutic agents and cellular byproducts of reactive oxygen damage are substrates for GST-catalyzed glutathione conjugations, possibly resulting in differences in response rates to chemotherapy or radiotherapy; and (2) certain genetic changes have been associated with GST genotypes, and thus GST genotypes may serve as markers of these somatic changes and any associated survival differences.

In the study by Sweeney and coworkers, one GST polymorphism—*GSTM1* null genotype—negatively correlated with survival. The *GSTM1*-survival association correlated with radiotherapy, but not chemotherapy, although details of the types of drugs used were not collected. Reduced capacity for GST-mediated detoxification may be expected to cause increased therapy-related toxicity; this information was not available.

Although it may not be clear as to how one can use these data to treat lung cancer patients, it does illustrate the importance that genetic polymorphisms may play in prognosis.

J. H. Schiller, MD

Polymorphisms in the DNA Repair Genes *XRCC1* and *ERCC2*, Smoking, and Lung Cancer Risk

Zhou W, Liu G, Miller DP, et al (Harvard School of Public Health, Boston; Harvard Med School, Boston)

Cancer Epidemiol Biomarkers Prev 12:359-365, 2003 9–12

Background.—The carcinogens and reactive oxygen species in tobacco smoke can damage DNA by a variety of mechanisms. Some evidence suggests certain polymorphisms in 2 major DNA repair proteins—the *Arg399Gln* polymorphism in excision repair cross-complementing group 2 (ERCC2) and the *Asp312Asn* and *Lys751Gln* polymorphisms in x-ray cross-complementing group 1 (XRCC1)—are associated with altered DNA repair capacity and increased cancer risk. The interaction between these 3 polymorphisms and smoking in the development of lung cancer was examined in a case-control study.

Methods. XRCC1 and *ERCC2* genotyping was performed in 1091 patients with lung cancer (53.6% men; mean age, 64.9 years) and 1240 controls (45.6% men; mean age, 58.5 years). All participants were white. Frequencies of the *ERCC2 Arg/Gln* and the *XRCC1 Asp/Asn* and *Lys/Gln* polymorphisms were examined according to smoking status (nonsmoker, ex-smoker, current smoker), pack-years of smoking (light, moderate, heavy), and years since smoking cessation. Data were analyzed by logistic regression after adjusting for relevant confounding variables.

Results.—Compared with the *XRCC1 Arg/Arg* genotype, the adjusted odds ratios (aORs) in lung cancer were 1.0 for the *Arg/Gln* genotype and 1.3 for the *Gln/Gln* genotype (borderline significant). In analyses stratified by pack-years of smoking, having the *Gln/Gln* genotype was a significant risk factor for lung cancer in nonsmokers (aOR, 2.4) and light smokers (<25 pack-years; aOR, 1.3), but actually protected against lung cancer in heavy smokers (>55 pack-years; aOR, 0.5). When all 3 polymorphisms were considered together, nonsmokers had an aOR of 5.2 for having 5 or 6 variant alleles (vs 0 variant alleles), and light smokers had an aOR for 5 or 6 variants of 2.2. In contrast, heavy smokers had an aOR of 0.3 for having 5 or 6 variant alleles. Similar gene-smoking interactions were seen when pack-years of smoking (or smoking duration and smoking intensity) was entered as a continuous variable, and when different subgroups were analyzed by age, sex, histologic cell type, or clinical stage.

Conclusion.—There is a significant interaction between the 3 polymorphisms examined and cumulative cigarette smoking in lung cancer risk. This interaction depends on cumulative smoking exposure, and at high smoking exposure, the positive association between these 3 polymorphisms and lung cancer risk is reversed compared with little or no smoking history. Exactly how cigarette smoking changes the DNA repair capacity (DRC) of each of these repair protein polymorphisms is not clear. It is possible that heavy smoking overwhelms different DRCs of different genotypes. It is also possible that smoking stimulates DRC in response to the DNA damage caused by the carcinogens in tobacco. Also, because heavy smokers tended to be older than nonsmokers or light smokers, the lower risk of the variant alleles in the former may reflect a prolonged survival for patients who have lung cancer develop. Further research is needed to understand the impact of DNA repair polymorphisms on survival in patients with lung cancer.

► It has been postulated that lung cancer is caused, in part, by the inability of the cell to repair DNA damage caused by carcinogens found in tobacco smoke. Two such DNA repair pathways exist: base-excision repair (involved in repair of DNA base damage and single-strand breaks) and nucleotide-excision repair (NER), involved in repair of bulky mono adducts, cross-links, and oxidative damage. *XRCC1* and *ERCC2* are 2 major DNA repair proteins involved in base-excision repair and NER, respectively.

Polymorphisms are variant alleles of genes found in more than 5% of the population. In this study, Zhou et al examine the relationship of smoking, specific polymorphisms of *XRCC1* and *ERCC2*, and lung cancer risk. They found that smoking and nicotine exposure result in a high level of carcinogen-DNA adducts, but somewhat surprisingly, that only nonsmokers or patients with a "light smoking history" with polymorphisms were more likely to get lung cancer. Heavy smokers with polymorphisms were not at increased risk. The authors postulate a variety of possible reasons for this unexpected finding.

J. H. Schiller, MD

Local Particle Deposition Patterns May Play a Key Role in the Development of Lung Cancer

Balásházy I, Hofmann W, Heistracher T (KFKI Atomic Energy Research Inst, Budapest, Hungary; Univ of Salzburg, Austria; Polytechnical Univ of Salzburg, Austria)
J Appl Physiol 94:1719-1725, 2003 9–13

Introduction.—Ambient particles ranging in diameter from 1 nm to 20 μm can be deposited in human lungs on inspiration and are available for interactions with pulmonary surfaces. Many diseases of the respiratory tract may be directly linked to inhaled materials, including cigarette smoke and toxic occupational or environmental aerosols. The regional pattern of deposition of inhaled particles may be a determinant of pathogenic potential. Three-dimensional particle deposition patterns in lobar-segmental airway bifurcations were computed. The resulting inhomogeneous deposition patterns were determined.

Methods.—A recently developed numerical particle deposition model was used to analyze local deposition patterns in airway bifurcations. Only symmetric branching was used to characterize the most general relationships of the local deposition patterns. Aerosol particles in the model are randomly selected at the inlet cross section. Particle trajectories are calculated by using an earlier numerical particle deposition model that assumes inertial impaction, gravitational sedimentation, Brownian diffusion, and interception operate simultaneously. The whole surface of the bifurcation was scanned via a prespecified surface element for the quantification of the inhomogeneity of predicted deposition patterns.

Results.—A small fraction of epithelial cells located at carinal ridges can receive massive doses that may be a few hundred times higher than the average dose for the entire airway.

Conclusion.—The distribution of deposition enhancement factors shows that the extent of inhomogeneity of particle deposition in bronchial airway bifurcations is rather high for all particle sizes, even for nanometer-sized ultrafine particles. Cells located in the vicinity of the dividing spur may receive doses that are a few hundred times higher than the average dose for the whole airway.

▶ Cigarette smoke contains small particles with adsorbed carcinogens. In this article, the authors demonstrate that these particles tend to get "hung up" around the carina and sites of bronchial airway bifurcations. In fact, epithelial cells at the carina often had deposition patterns several hundred times higher than the average dose for the whole airway. This may explain why neoplastic lesions predominate at the bifurcation of central airways.

J. H. Schiller, MD

Hypermethylation of *RASSF1A* Promoter Is Associated With the Age at Starting Smoking and a Poor Prognosis in Primary Non-Small Cell Lung Cancer

Kim D-H, Kim JS, Ji Y-I, et al (Sungkyunkwan Univ, Seoul, Korea; Sungkyunkwan Univ, Suwon, Korea)

Cancer Res 63:3743-3746, 2003 9–14

Background.—The risk of lung cancer is greatest among persons who started smoking early in life and continued throughout their lives. However, the molecular mechanisms underlying lung cancer susceptibility in young smokers are unclear. The association between age at smoking initiation and hypermethylation of *p14*, *p16*, and *RASSF1A* promoters was investigated.

Methods and Findings.—Two hundred four patients with primary non–small cell lung cancer (NSCLC) were included in the study. Methylation rates were 9% for *p14*, 27% for *p16*, and 32% for *RASSF1A*. Hypermethylation of *p14* and *p16* was unrelated to age at initiation of smoking. However, hypermethylation of the *RASSF1A* promoter correlated significantly with age at smoking initiation. The methylation status of the *RASSF1A* promoter was unassociated with other smoking variables, such as pack-years, smoking status, and smoking duration. The mean age at which smoking was started was 19 years in patients with hypermethylation of *RASSF1A* and 25 years in persons without *RASSF1A* promoter hypermethylation. Patients who started smoking before 19 years of age were 4.23 times more likely to have *RASSF1A* promoter hypermethylation than patients starting after age 19 years. Hypermethylation of the *RASSF1A* promoter was also associated with a poor prognosis among patients with stages 1 and 2 NSCLC.

Conclusion.—Starting cigarette smoking at an early age appears to be associated with hypermethylation of the *RASSF1A* promoter. Hypermethylation of this promoter may be an independent prognostic factor among patients with primary NSCLC.

▶ More important than the number of packs smoked per day is how long a smoker has been smoking. Thus, individuals who start in their early teenage years are at particular risk for the development of lung cancer. In this study, Kim and coworkers report that the Ras Association Domain Family 1A (*RASSF1A*) gene is more commonly inactivated via aberrant methylation of CpG islands in the promoter region, although the reason for this increased susceptibility in young smokers is not clear. In addition, methylation of this promoter was also associated with a poorer survival.

J. H. Schiller, MD

10 Head and Neck Cancer

The Impact of Second Opinion Surgical Pathology on the Practice of Head and Neck Surgery: A Decade Experience at a Large Referral Hospital

Westra WH, Kronz JD, Eisele DW (Johns Hopkins Med Insts, Baltimore, Md; Univ of California, San Francisco)

Head Neck 24:684-693, 2002 10–1

Background.—Second-opinion surgical pathology reveals discrepancies in diagnosis in major organ systems and significantly alters management and prognosis in many cases. It is important to identify sites especially susceptible to varying interpretations, as well as pathologic conditions often linked to diagnostic error, so that policy decisions are based on accurate information. Technical advances in surgical procedures, chemotherapy, radiation protocols, and genetically based therapies require precise, specific characterizations for patients with head and neck cancer. Even the most competent and experienced general surgical pathologist may be led astray by the diversity and complexity of head and neck pathologic processes. The frequency with which aberrant diagnoses are made, the specific anatomic sites or pathologic specimens that are most often involved, and the clinical impact that second-opinion surgical pathology has on the management and prognosis for these patients were explored.

Methods.—The pathologic reports for all patients (total of 814 surgical pathology cases) referred to The Johns Hopkins Hospital Department of Otolaryngology–Head and Neck Surgery from January 1, 1990, to January 1, 2000, were reviewed, comparing the outside diagnoses with those of the referral hospital. Discrepancies were noted as anything significantly changing therapy or prognosis. Three types of alterations were not considered major diagnostic changes: (1) those only altering histologic tumor grade, (2) differences in quantifying the severity of squamous dysplasia, and (3) changes in T staging by the conventional TNM staging format.

Results.—Cases were separated by anatomic site or type of specimen. For 7% of cases, the second-opinion diagnosis differed significantly from the outside diagnosis; rates of discrepancy varied with site. Twenty-two percent involved the thyroid and only 1% the oral cavity. However, no specific site had a statistically significant greater chance of having a changed diagnosis than the group as a whole. Treatment modifications were required in 87% of the 54 changed diagnoses. Thirty percent of these cases were improvements, 56% were worse diagnoses, and 15% did not affect the prognosis. Twenty-four percent of the cases involved a change from an overtly benign diagnosis to an overtly malignant diagnosis; 15% showed the opposite. For 80% of the changed diagnoses, follow-up information allowed confirmation. A total of 95% of the second-opinion diagnoses were upheld, but in 5% of the cases both diagnoses were wrong.

Conclusions.—Histopathologic diagnoses can be imprecise, with a 7% major change in diagnosis rate in this evaluation. Many diagnostic errors occurred in high-grade tumors that did not exhibit specific differentiation on light microscopy, leading to their classification as a poorly differentiated carcinoma. Another difficult situation was thc papillary ncoplasm of the upper respiratory tract that was dismissed as squamous papilloma. A third area was the basaloid neoplasm, which, in the head and neck, may be confused with the basaloid morphology of cutaneous, mucosal, and salivary gland tumors. The final area was squamous atypia of the surface epithelium, in which a reactive atypia was not clearly different from a premalignant dysplasia.

► This report is part of an increasing body of literature that emphasizes the importance of review of surgical pathology material before formulating a therapeutic plan (involving surgery, radiotherapy, or systemic treatment) if the diagnosis has been made at another institution. The 7% diagnostic discrepancy rate reported here includes only changes from benign to malignant or vice versa, as well as changes in tumor type. It is an estimate of the minimum benefit that can be obtained from a second review of a pathology specimen. Additional information that may alter therapy, such as a change in margin status or changes in grade, may also be obtained from second-opinion reviews.

It is not clear whether there is any organ site for which pathology review can be safely avoided. Similar results have been reported for neuropathology and gynecologic specimen review.[1,2] We reviewed the results of 346 second-opinion consultations for a diagnosis of invasive and intraductal breast cancer, extremely common clinical problems, and found a 7.8% major diagnostic discrepancy rate.[3] The reported rates of diagnostic discrepancy are certainly greater than the thresholds used to determine that a therapy has a worthwhile clinical benefit, emphasizing that pathology review is a cost-effective procedure that should be a routine practice.

M. Morrow, MD

References

1. Scott CB, Nelson JS, Farnam NC, et al: Central pathology review in clinical trials for patients with malignant gliomas. A report of Radiation Therapy Oncology Group 83-02. *Cancer* 76:307-313, 1995.
2. Selman AE, Nieman TH, Fowler JM, et al: Quality assurance of second opinion pathology in gynecologic oncology. *Obstet Gynecol* 94:302-306, 1999.
3. Staradub VL, Messenger KA, Hao N, et al: Changes in breast cancer therapy due to pathology second opinion. *Ann Surg Oncol* 9:982-987, 2002.

An Intergroup Phase III Comparison of Standard Radiation Therapy and Two Schedules of Concurrent Chemoradiotherapy in Patients With Unresectable Squamous Cell Head and Neck Cancer

Adelstein DJ, Li Y, Adams GL, et al (Cleveland Clinic Found, Ohio; Arthur G James Cancer Hosp, Columbus, Ohio; Dana-Farber Cancer Inst, Boston; et al)

J Clin Oncol 21:92-98, 2003 10–2

Background.—Radiation therapy has been standard care for patients with unresectable squamous cell head and neck cancer. Unfortunately, overall survival after radiation has been less than 25%. The Head and Neck Intergroup reported a phase III randomized study of the benefits of adding chemotherapy to radiation in this patient population.

Methods.—Two hundred ninety-five patients were enrolled in the trial between 1992 and 1999. Patients were assigned randomly to 1 of 3 arms (Fig 1). Arm A, the control group, received single daily fractionated radiation at 70 Gy at 2 Gy/d. Arm B received identical radiation therapy with concurrent bolus cisplatin on days 1, 22, and 43. Arm C received a split course of single daily fractionated radiation plus 3 cycles of a concurrent infusional fluorouracil and bolus cisplatin chemotherapy, 30 Gy administered with the first cycle and 30 to 40 Gy given with the third cycle (Fig 2). Surgical resection was done if possible after the second chemotherapy cycle in patients assigned to arm C. If necessary, salvage therapy was performed in all groups.

Findings.—Toxicity of grade 3 or higher occurred in 52% of patients in arm A, 89% of those in arm B, and 77% of those in arm C. The median follow-up was 41 months. The 3-year projected overall survival rate for arm A patients was 23%, compared with 37% for arm B patients. The projected overall survival rate for arm C patients was 27%, not significantly different from that for arm A.

Conclusion.—Concurrent high-dose, single-agent cisplatin with conventional single daily fractionated radiation increases toxicity but also significantly improves survival. Splitting the radiation course resulted in a loss of efficacy that was not offset by multiagent chemotherapy or the possibility of midcourse surgery.

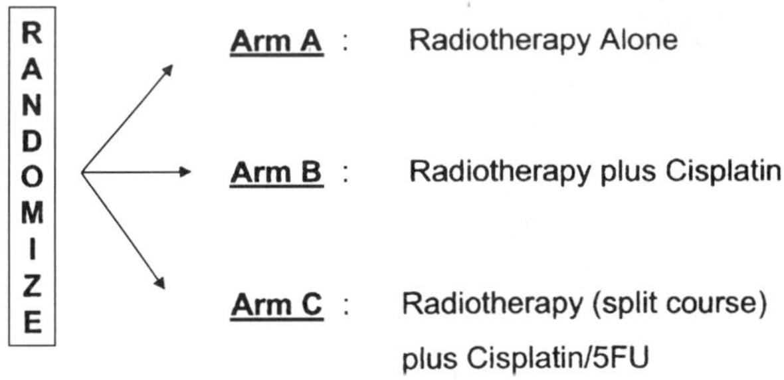
RANDOMIZE
Arm A : Radiotherapy Alone
Arm B : Radiotherapy plus Cisplatin
Arm C : Radiotherapy (split course)
plus Cisplatin/5FU

FIGURE 1.—Treatment schema. (Courtesy of Adelstein DJ, Li Y, Adams GL, et al: An intergroup phase III comparison of standard radiation therapy and two schedules of concurrent chemoradiotherapy in patients with unresectable squamous cell head and neck cancer. *Abbreviation: FU*, Fluorouracil. *J Clin Oncol* 21(1): 92-98, 2003. Reprinted with permission from the American Society of Clinical Oncology.)

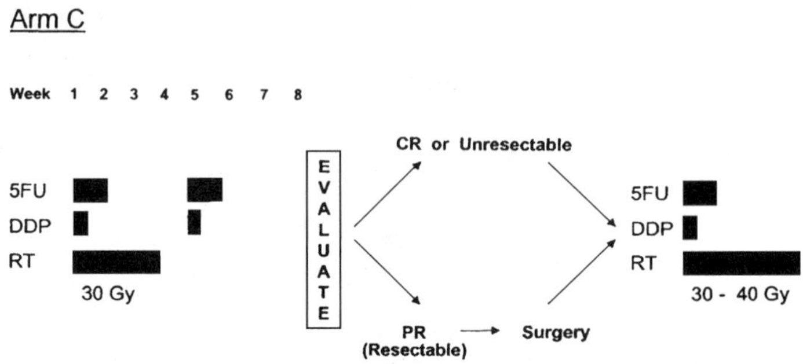

FIGURE 2.—Detail of treatment schema for arm C. *Abbreviations: FU*, Fluorouracil; *DDP*, cisplatin; *RT*, radiation therapy; *CR*, complete response; *PR*, partial response. (Courtesy of Adelstein DJ, Li Y, Adams GL, et al: An intergroup phase III comparison of standard radiation therapy and two schedules of concurrent chemoradiotherapy in patients with unresectable squamous cell head and neck cancer. *J Clin Oncol* 21(1): 92-98, 2003. Reprinted with permission from the American Society of Clinical Oncology.)

▶ Head and neck cancer is one of the most challenging diseases to treat. It clearly represents one of the models for multimodality therapy with surgery, radiation, and chemotherapy. The optimal treatment for unresected squamous cell carcinoma of the head and neck has been poorly defined. It has been suggested that cisplatin-based chemotherapy plus concurrent radiation therapy was superior to radiation therapy alone, but this has not been proven through phase III studies.

This is a nicely performed phase III trial evaluating 3 popular approaches for the treatment of stage III or IV (without evidence of distant hematogenous metastases) disease. Cisplatin plus radiotherapy, though more toxic, was associated with the best 3-year overall survival and disease-specific survival. Arm C of the study actually had 2 variables (the addition of 5-FU and use of split course radiotherapy) but was no better than the other 2 arms. Debate may continue regarding the role of fluoropyrimidine therapy, but, as of now, cisplatin plus radiation appears to be the optimal therapy.

P. J. Loehrer, Sr, MD

11 Malignant Melanoma

Granulocyte-Macrophage–Colony-Stimulating Factor Added to a Multi-peptide Vaccine for Resected Stage II Melanoma

Weber J, Sondak VK, Scotland R, et al (Univ of Southern California, Los Angeles; Univ of Michigan, Ann Arbor; Upstate Group, Inc, Charlottesville, Va; et al)

Cancer 97:186-200, 2003 11–1

Background.—Many studies have used peptides, DNA plasmids, and antigen-fusion constructs—alone, pulsed onto antigen-presenting dendritic cells, or with adjuvants—to augment antigen-specific immune responses in patients with cancer. Two melanoma antigen peptides recognized by T cells were given and immune responses assayed in patients with resected melanoma in stages IIA or IIB.

Methods.—Forty-eight patients were immunized with 2 tumor antigen epitope peptides derived from $gp100_{209\text{-}217}$ (210M) and $tyrosinase_{368\text{-}376}$ (370D) emulsified with incomplete Freund's adjuvant (IFA). By random assignment, patients received peptides and IFA alone or with 250 μm of granulocyte macrophage–colony stimulating factor (GM-CSF) subcutaneously every day for 5 days. Immune responses were assessed by release of interferon γ in an enzyme-linked immunosorbent assay (ELISA) by effector cells in the presence of peptide-pulsed antigen-presenting cells; by cytokine release of interferon-γ, GM-CSF, and tumor necrosis factor-α in a Luminex assay; or by an antigen-specific tetramer flow cytometry assay.

Findings.—Grade 1 or 2 toxicities included local pain and granuloma formation, fever, and lethargy. Transient vaccine-related grade 3 toxicity was also observed, but no grade 4 toxicity. Of the 40 patients undergoing post-treatment skin testing, 17 had a positive skin test response to the gp100 peptide. However, only 1 of 40 patients had a positive skin test response to tyrosinase. Of the 39 patients for whom the ELISA data were performed, 34 showed an immune response after vaccination. This was also documented in 37 of 42 patients by tetramer assay. The GM-CSF/peptide/IFA group had higher ELISA, Luminex, and tetramer responses than did the peptide/IFA group. In 10 patients epitope spreading to the MART-1/MelanA 27-35 and 26-35 (27L) epitopes were identified by tetramer assay. Disease recurred in 7 of the 48 patients at a median of 24 months. Two patients in this intermediate- to high-risk group have died.

Conclusions.—A significant number of patients with resected melanoma have an antigen-specific immune response against a peptide vaccine. A trend toward GM-CSF to modestly increase the immune response was noted. These data further support the development of GM-CSF as a vaccine adjuvant.

► Vaccine strategies for melanoma have been the focus of clinical development for many years. Unfortunately there has not been a way to improve on the type or significance of the immune response seen. The authors explored the ability of GM-CSF to improve the immune response in patients with resected stage IV melanoma to a peptide vaccine. The study reveals that a significant number of patients will develop an immune response without any adjuvant and that GM-CSF has the ability to enhance this immune response modestly. Of the 48 patients reported on, 7 had had relapse. This study suggests that peptide vaccines with superior adjuvants may have the ability to enhance the immune response and should still be considered as adjuvants for patients with melanoma. The optimal combination remains to be determined, though a large randomized trial should be considered if one can be identified.

M. S. Gordon, MD

Tumor Lymphangiogenesis: A Novel Prognostic Indicator for Cutaneous Melanoma Metastasis and Survival

Dadras SS, Paul T, Bertoncini J, et al (Harvard Med School, Boston; John Radcliffe Hosp, Headington, England; Univ of Tübingen, Germany)

Am J Pathol 162:1951-1960, 2003 11–2

Background.—Malignant skin melanoma has a propensity for early metastatic spread through lymphatic vessels to regional lymph nodes. Lymph node metastasis is a major determinant of disease staging and clinical management. The significance of tumor-induced lymphangiogenesis for lymphatic melanoma spread is still not clear. Whether tumor lymphangiogenesis occurs in human malignant skin melanomas and whether the degree of tumor lymphangiogenesis may be associated with the risk for lymph node metastasis and patient survival were determined.

Methods.—Tumor samples were obtained from 18 cases of primary melanomas with early lymph node metastasis and 19 cases of nonmetastatic melanomas. The samples were closely matched clinically and histologically. Double immunostains for the novel lymphatic endothelial marker LYVE-1 and for the panvascular marker CD31 were used.

Findings.—A large number of melanomas showed hot spots of proliferating intratumoral and peritumoral lymphatic vessels. The incidence of intratumoral lymphatics was significantly greater in metastatic melanomas. This incidence was associated with low disease-free survival. Metastatic melanomas had significantly more and larger tumor-related lymphatic vessels. A relative lymphatic vessel area of more than 1.5% correlated significantly with poor disease-free and overall survival. However, there was no difference in the density of tumor-related blood vessels. In both groups, an equal minority of patients showed vascular endothelial growth factor and vascular endothelial growth factor-C expression.

Conclusions.—This study has demonstrated the presence of intratumoral and peritumoral lymphangiogenesis in primary human cutaneous melanomas. The extent of tumor lymphangiogenesis may be associated with the risk of lymph node metastasis as well as patient survival. Peritumoral lymphatic vascular density may be a novel prognostic indicator for the risk of lymph node metastasis of cutaneous melanomas.

► The authors investigated whether the presence of tumor lymphatic vessels in primary melanomas was associated with the risk of relapse in lymph nodes. A group of primary melanoma specimens from patients without lymph node metastases was compared with a group of primary melanoma samples from patients with early lymph node metastases. The group with lymph node involvement had a significantly greater number of stainable lymphatic vessels compared with the primary tumors without involvement. When the relapse-free and overall survival rates of these groups of patients were assessed, tumors with the greatest lymphatic area were associated with the poorest survival. Importantly, microvessel density and vascularization were not associated with any survival end point or lymph node involvement. This suggests that like in many other tumors lymphatic invasion may be an important predictor of relapse and that consideration should be given to retrospectively assessing lymphatic volume in previous trials of adjuvant therapy. The possible incorporation of lymphatic volume as an independent prognostic factor needs to be assessed prospectively but may have the ability to differentiate patients who would benefit from aggressive adjuvant therapy or who should be targeted for sentinel node biopsies.

M. S. Gordon, MD

12 Sarcoma

Sarcoma Tumor FDG Uptake Measured by PET and Patient Outcome: A Retrospective Analysis

Eary JF, O'Sullivan F, Powitan Y, et al (Univ of Washington, Seattle; Univ College, Cork, Ireland)

Eur J Nucl Med 29:1149-1154, 2002 12–1

Background.—Treatment planning for patients with sarcoma tumor is based on several methods of assessment of tumor biological aggressiveness, including histologic tumor grade assessment by biopsy and also by proliferation markers and flow cytometry. However, there is still a need for better methods for predicting tumor behavior in patients with sarcoma. Previously acquired fluorodeoxyglucose positron emission tomography (FDG PET) data showed a relationship between tumor uptake and histopathologic markers of tumor aggressiveness or metastatic potential. The ability of tu-

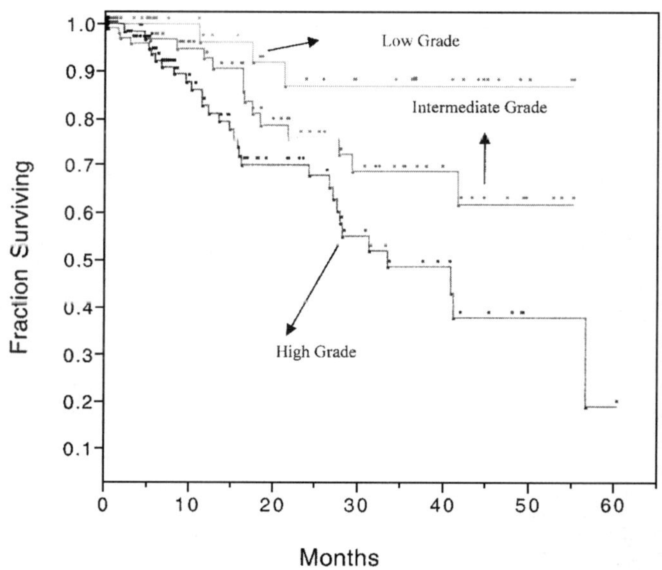

FIGURE 1.—Overall survival by tumor grade. (Courtesy of Eary JF, O'Sullivan F, Powitan Y, et al: Sarcoma tumor FDG uptake measured by PET and patient outcome: A retrospective analysis. *Eur J Nucl Med* 29:1149-1154, 2002. Copyright Springer-Verlag.)

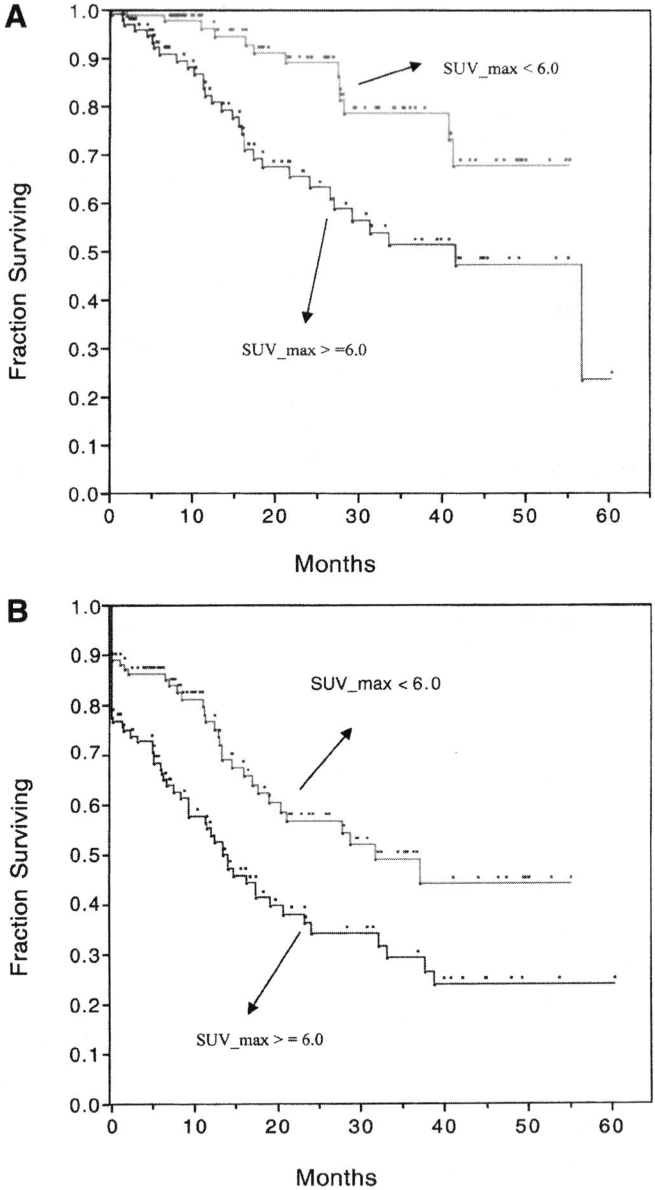

FIGURE 2.—**A**, Overall survival for all sarcoma patients using the baseline maximum standard uptake value (SUV_{max}) median = 6.0. **B**, Disease-free survival for all sarcoma patients using baseline SUV_{max} median = 6.0. (Courtesy of Eary JF, O'Sullivan F, Powitan Y, et al: Sarcoma tumor FDG uptake measured by PET and patient outcome: A retrospective analysis. *Eur J Nucl Med* 29:1149-1154, 2002. Copyright Springer-Verlag.)

TABLE 5.—Multivariate Analysis Results: Disease-Free Survival (192 Patients, 73 Events)

	Hazard Ratio	Lower Confidence Interval	Upper Confidence Interval	*P* Value
Tumor grade (low vs intermediate or intermediate vs high)	1.91	1.31	2.80	0.001
Tumor type				
Cartilage vs bone	1.64	0.94	2.86	0.082
Soft tissue vs bone	0.99	0.84	1.19	0.92
Age	1.00	0.98	1.02	0.90
Sex				
Female vs male	1.06	0.84	1.33	0.62
Baseline SUV_{max}	1.24*	0.96	1.61	0.11

*Relative hazards for a doubling of standard uptake value (*SUV*).

(Courtesy of Eary JF, O'Sullivan F, Powitan Y, et al: Sarcoma tumor FDG uptake measured by PET and patient outcome: A retrospective analysis. *Eur J Nucl Med* 29:1149-1154, 2002. Copyright Springer-Verlag.)

mor maximum FDG uptake to predict survival and disease progression was investigated in sarcoma patients who underwent FDG PET imaging.

Methods.—A total of 209 patients with sarcoma were imaged with FDG PET before treatment with neoadjuvant chemotherapy or resection. Tumor FDG uptake, which was expressed as maximum standard uptake value (SUV_{max}), was compared with disease-free and overall survival. Multivariate Cox regression analysis was used to investigate the role of SUV_{max} in predicting time to death or disease progression after adjustment for standard clinical prognostic factors.

Results.—Of the 209 patients included in this review, baseline tumor SUV_{max} ranged from 1.4 to 60 and corresponded to tumor grade medians as previously reported. The mean follow-up was 19 months, with 47 deaths reported during that period (Fig 1). There were 38 cases of local tumor recurrence and 53 cases of distant metastases. Multivariate Cox regression analysis showed that the SUV_{max} data are a statistically significant independent predictor of patient survival (Fig 2). The prognosis is significantly poorer for patients with tumors with greater SUV_{max} values (Table 5).

Conclusion.—These findings demonstrate that the SUV_{max} of a sarcoma as determined by FDG PET can be used as an independent predictor of survival and disease progression.

► These investigators from the University of Washington conclude that the uptake of FDG on PET scans is an independent predictor of survival and disease progression in patients with sarcomas. They include 209 patients of relative heterogeneity in the sense that cartilaginous, bony, and soft tissue sarcomas are all included and they really do not discuss the locations in which these tumors occurred.

It is not clear to me that you can conclude that PET is an independent predictor. My interpretation of their data is that the tumor grade is the major issue, and they do not discuss the impact of tumor grade on uptake of FDG. Based on what they do include in Table 5, I do not really believe you can link the outcome to the scan as much as you can scan to the grade, which really does predict for outcome.

E. Glatstein, MD

Neoadjuvant Chemotherapy and Local Radiotherapy for High-Grade Osteosarcoma of the Extremities

Machak GN, Tkachev SI, Solovyev YN, et al (NN Blokhin Cancer Research Ctr of AMS, Moscow)

Mayo Clin Proc 78:147-155, 2003 12–2

Introduction.—Osteosarcoma has traditionally been viewed as a radiation-resistant neoplasm. As a single modality, radiotherapy (RT) is not successful in either controlling the primary tumor or preventing the appearance of lung metastases. The effectiveness of RT for local control of nonmetastatic osteosarcoma of the extremities after induction chemotherapy was examined.

Methods.—Between January 1986 and February 1999, a protocol of preoperative intra-arterial monodrug chemotherapy, surgery, and response-adapted adjuvant chemotherapy was used for treatment of nonmetastatic osteosarcoma. In March 1999, a new protocol with more aggressive chemotherapy and surgical local control was initiated. Twenty-seven of 157 patients from the first protocol and 4 of 30 from the second protocol refused recommended surgery for the primary tumor and underwent standard, fractionated external beam RT for local control. The median dose of RT was 60 Gy (range, 40-68 Gy). Medical records were examined through April 2002. Radiologic and biochemical response, local control, limb function, and survival were assessed. The end point included local progression-free, metastasis-free, and overall survival.

Results.—The mean overall, local progression-free, and metastasis-free survival at 5 years were 61%, 56%, and 62%, respectively. Outcome was significantly associated with patient imaging and biochemical response. In patients with a pronounced response, the overall and metastasis-free survival at 5 years were 90% and 91%, respectively; they were only 35% and 42%, respectively, for nonresponders ($P = .005$ and $P = .005$, respectively). Local control was not associated with response after induction chemotherapy.

None of the 11 patients with both good imaging and a good biochemical response experienced a local relapse at a median follow-up of 67 months. The mean estimated local progression-free survival rates were 31% and 0% at 3 and 5 years, respectively. Of 22 patients who survived without local disease progression, 19 (86%) had excellent limb function (Enneking score between 90% and 100%) at the time of the most recent examination.

Conclusion.—When used after effective induction chemotherapy for osteosarcoma of the extremities, RT can be a reliable modality for controlling local disease and preserving limb function.

► This report from Russia consists of 31 patients with extremity osteosarcoma without metastases who refused surgery and underwent RT along with neoadjuvant chemotherapy. Their overall survival and progression-free survival and metastasis-free survival appear quite comparable to any surgical series.

The textbooks have said that osteogenic sarcoma is "radio-resistant." I think what they mean is that it does not shrink, which means that it is radio-unresponsive. Most bone tumors other than Ewing's are. Some of the reason for this is the extensive matrix that is involved. Killing the tumor cells will not make the matrix go away. This is true with a lot of sarcomas. Radio-sensitive or radio-resistant refers to the quantitative cell killing that takes place with specific doses of radiation in a relatively short time frame. Cell killing is a different concept than measurable regression. When there is extensive matrix involved, those terms cannot be synonymous with each other.

I have not treated primary extremity osteosarcoma, but I have treated a moderate number of patients who have had osteosarcoma of the spine or sacrum which could not be resected. I have 3 such patients with unresectable osteosarcoma who are long-term survivors. They are part of reference 29 in this report.[1] In all 3 patients, the tumor masses did not regress at all. Because they received IV halogenated pyrimidines as a radiosensitizer, they did not receive adjuvant chemotherapy since the tumor was not resected and there was no adjuvant setting. These patients did not metastasize and have remained under control for over a decade. Perhaps positron emission tomography might have been helpful at showing that the masses were functionally sterilized.

The cells of osteogenic sarcoma are not resistant. It takes a pretty good dose to control them, but it is possible and it is incorrect to assume that these tumors are "resistant."

E. Glatstein, MD

Reference

1. Kinsella TJ, Glatstein E: Clinical experience with intravenous radiosensitizers in unresectable sarcomas. *Cancer* 59:908-915, 1987.

Whole Abdominopelvic Radiotherapy for Desmoplastic Small Round-Cell Tumor

Goodman KA, Wolden SL, La Quaglia MP, et al (Mem Sloan-Kettering Cancer Ctr, New York)

Int J Radiat Oncol Biol Phys 54:170-176, 2002 12–3

Background.—Desmoplastic small round-cell tumor (DSRCT) is a rare aggressive neoplasm with unique clinical, histologic, and biological features and is primarily found in adolescent boys. Most patients are seen with a bulky intra-abdominal or pelvic, peritoneal-based mass, and extraserosal primary sites have also been reported recently. These tumors have an extremely poor prognosis. Clinicopathologic studies and case reports have demonstrated rapid disease progression and a poor response to conventional chemotherapeutic agents. Surgical debulking is limited by the diffuse na-

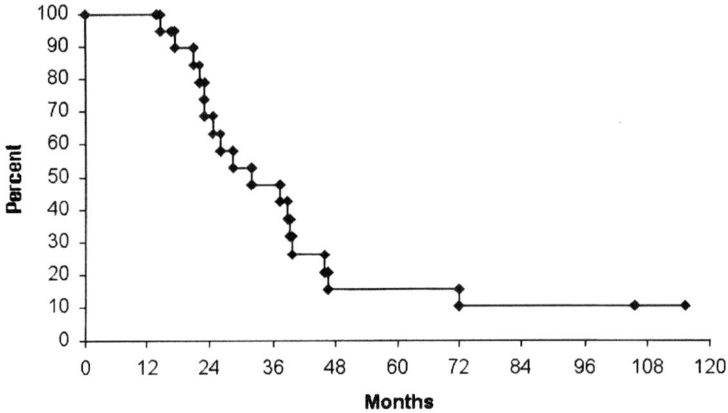

FIGURE 3.—Overall survival. (Reprinted from Goodman KA, Wolden SL, La Quaglia MP, et al: Whole abdominopelvic radiotherapy for desmoplastic small round-cell tumor. *Int J Radiat Oncol Biol Phys* 54:170-176, 2002. Copyright 2002, with permission from Elsevier Science.)

ture of the peritoneal disease and direct visceral organ invasion. The pattern of spread in DSRCT is similar to that of ovarian cancer, with dissemination throughout the serosal surfaces of the abdomen and pelvis. The feasibility and outcome of whole abdominopelvic irradiation (WAPI) as part of a combined modality protocol for patients with DSRCT were evaluated.

Methods.—This retrospective review included 21 patients who underwent WAPI for the treatment of DSRCT. All of the patients were treated on an institutional protocol with 7 cycles of an alkylator-based chemotherapy. The patients underwent surgical debulking and were then treated with external beam radiotherapy to the whole abdomen and pelvis to a dose of 30 Gy.

Results.—The patients were followed up for a median of 28 months. The overall survival and relapse-free survival rates at 3 years were 48% and 19%, respectively (Fig 3). The median survival was 32 months, and the median time to relapse was 19 months; most of the relapses were intraperitoneal or hepatic (Table 1). Acute toxicities included Radiation Therapy Oncology Group grade 2 upper and lower gastrointestinal toxicity in 81% and 71% of patients, respectively. All of the patients experienced some acute hematologic toxicity, with grade 4 thrombocytopenia in 76%, leukopenia in

TABLE 1.—Initial Sites of Failure

Location	*n*
Abdomen and pelvis	5
Liver	4
Mediastinum	1
Liver and abdomen	6

(Reprinted from Goodman KA, Wolden SL, La Quaglia MP, et al: Whole abdominopelvic radiotherapy for desmoplastic small round-cell tumor. *Int J Radiat Oncol Biol Phys* 54:170-176, 2002. Copyright 2002, with permission from Elsevier Science.)

29%, and anemia in 33%. The most significant long-term toxicity was small-bowel obstruction, which occurred in 7 patients (33%) after surgery and WAPI.

Conclusion.—WAPI is feasible, in conjunction with intensive chemotherapy and surgery, for the treatment of DSRCT. Hematologic and gastrointestinal toxicities do occur but can be managed with diligent supportive care. However, the long-term efficacy of WAPI has thus far been disappointing, and novel approaches are being explored.

► This team of investigators at Memorial Sloan-Kettering reports on the results of WAPI for DSRCT. This is an intraperitoneal neoplasm occurring mostly in young males. The authors report 21 patients treated with an intensive multidisciplinary approach, including chemotherapy, maximal surgical debulking, and then WAPI to approximately 30 Gy. These patients tend to have fairly bulky disease, and the prognosis is poor despite the aggressive approach. Toxicity is also significant.

On the other hand, the poor outcome would appear to justify this approach. Although the authors describe the dose to the whole abdomen as being 30 Gy, they have shielded the liver and kidneys, as necessary. That significantly reduces a major portion of that volume to doses which are probably not tumoricidal. They report significant hematologic toxicity, and one third of the patients also developed small-bowel obstruction.

This is a somewhat sobering report, and it suggests that we desperately need a better strategy. Because the disease is rare, it will probably be difficult to identify a molecular target, but that is probably the best long-term strategy, if it can be done.

E. Glatstein, MD

Soft Tissue Tumours: Intensive Chemotherapy for Children and Young Adults With Metastatic Primitive Neuroectodermal Tumors of the Soft Tissue

Bisogno G, Carli M, Stevens M, et al (Hematology/Oncology Division, Padova, Italy; Birmingham Children's Hosp, England; Institut Gustave Roussy, Villejuif, France; et al)

Bone Marrow Transplant 30:297-302, 2002 12–4

Introduction.—Peripheral neuroectodermal tumor (PNET) and Ewing sarcoma are histologically similar. They share the same chromosomal translocation t(11;22) and are therefore grouped with the Ewing family of tumors. In 1989, a collaborative investigation, the MMT4 for patients with metastatic soft tissue sarcoma, was initiated by 3 European groups (International Society of Pediatric Oncology, International Co-operative Group on Childhood Soft Tissue Sarcoma, and German Co-operative Soft Tissue Study). The protocol was amended in 1991 to examine the role of high-dose chemotherapy with stem cell rescue. The outcome of patients with extraosseous PNET included in the MMT4 protocols are reported.

Methods.—Of 31 patients with PNET treated between 1989 and 1995, 11 were treated according to MMT4-89 and 20 according to MMT4-91. There were 4 CEVAIE cycles in the chemotherapy protocol, each including 3-week courses: CEV (carboplatin 500 mg/m^2, epirubicin 150 mg/m^2, vincristine 1.5 mg/m^2), IVA (ifosfamide 9 g/m^2, actinomycin 1.5 mg/m^2), and IVE (ifosfamide 9 g/m^2, etoposide 600 mg/m^2, vincristine 1.5 mg/m^2). In the MMT4 protocol, the fourth CEVAIE was replaced with melphalan 200 mg/m^2 with stem cell rescue. The CEV combination was assessed as a window study. Surgery was performed after the second cycle. Radiotherapy was administered in the presence of postoperative residual disease.

Results.—The response rate was 55% after CEV and increased to 80% after the initial CEVAIE. Complete remission was observed in 25 patients. Local control was observed in 77% of irradiated patients compared with 45% of those who were not irradiated. The overall event-free survival was 22.6%: 36.4% and 15%, respectively, for patients treated according to the MMT4-89 and MMT4-91 protocols ($P = .3$). Age older than 10 years was linked with significantly poorer outcome ($P = .04$).

Conclusion.—Even in the presence of a high complete remission rate, intensive chemotherapy with or without high-dose melphalan seemed to have little impact on survival rate among patients with metastatic extraosseous PNET.

▶ The outcome for patients with metastatic primitive neuroectodermal tumors remains extremely poor. The study by Bisogno et al attempts to improve this poor prognosis by intensifying therapy, including a melphalan-based autologous bone marrow transplantation. While their study had only a single arm, the outcome for their 31 patients does not appear significantly different than that reported by other studies using more conventional chemotherapeutic regimens. Of some interest, however, is the apparent difference in outcome according to age, with patients younger than 10 years doing significantly better than those older than 10 years. Thus, we remain at a standstill in terms of advances in the effective treatment of such patients. Alternatives are needed and should probably best focus on augmenting currently used chemotherapies to obtain minimal residual disease states rather than escalating conventional chemotherapeutic approaches.

R. J. Arceci, MD, PhD

External Beam Radiotherapy for Primary and Adjuvant Management of Aggressive Fibromatosis

Zlotecki RA, Scarborough MT, Morris CG, et al (Univ of Florida, Gainesville)
Int J Radiat Oncol Biol Phys 54:177-181, 2002 12–5

Background.—Aggressive fibromatosis usually appears to be a benign tumor process, but its locally aggressive character and diffusely spreading margins require effective treatment to avoid immediate local, as well as marginal or regional, recurrence. The experience of the University of Florida in handling aggressive fibromatosis is instructive, providing support for the use of external beam radiotherapy (EBRT) as postoperative adjuvant therapy and as primary therapy when definitive surgery is not the best option.

Methods.—A total of 72 patients were treated with EBRT for aggressive fibromatosis that had been confirmed pathologically. Thirty cases were primary and 42 were locoregional recurrences. All patients received megavoltage irradiation with ^{60}Co to 20 MV photons or electron therapy, most after complete surgical resection had been attempted, although 16 patients had only pretreatment biopsy. The prescribed treatment in 42 cases was 1.8 Gy daily fractions; in 23 cases, it was 1.2 Gy fractions twice a day. The median prescribed dose was 54 Gy. A median of 6 years' follow-up was available for 65 patients (minimum, 2 years).

Results.—One patient died from complications of regional recurrence followed by diffuse progression of aggressive fibromatosis, but 52 of the 65 cases achieved locoregional control, with absolute survival of 100% for this group at 5 years. Eleven patients had local failure (2 in the radiotherapy fields and 9 at a margin of the irradiated field), and 2 had regional failure. These recurrences all developed in patients with primary tumors of an extremity. The actuarial recurrence-free locoregional control rate at 5 years was 83%. Surgical salvage worked in 11 patients with locoregional recurrence. The actuarial locoregional control rate at 5 years for patients treated for a primary occurrence was 96%, and that for patients treated for recurrent disease was 75% (Fig 1). Patients who had gross total resection before radiotherapy had an actuarial locoregional control rate of 100%, while that for control of gross tumor at primary presentation was 95%.

Patients with recurrent fibromatosis derived no benefit from gross total resection in terms of locoregional control, with rates of 72% at 5 years without irradiation and 77% with irradiation. Mild to moderate extremity lymphedema was the late effect seen most often, requiring conservative management of symptoms. Three patients had late pathologic fracture develop; all had bone involvement by fibromatosis.

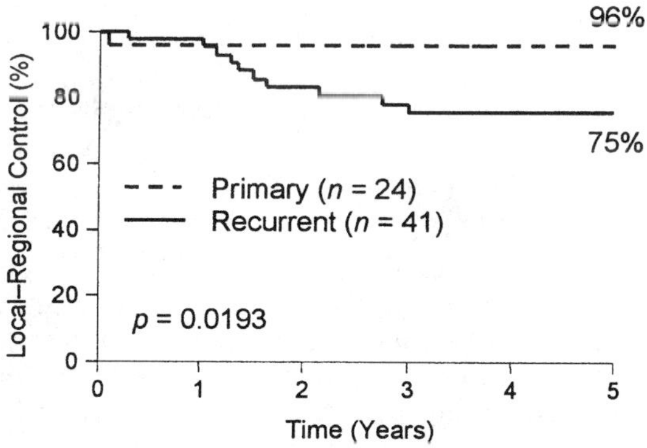

FIGURE 1.—Actuarial locoregional control by primary versus recurrent presentation. (Reprinted from Zlotecki RA, Scarborough MT, Morris CG, et al: External beam radiotherapy for primary and adjuvant management of aggressive fibromatosis. *Int J Radiat Oncol Biol Phys* 54:177-181, 2002. Copyright 2002, with permission from Elsevier Science.)

Conclusion.—Aggressive fibromatosis responds well to EBRT. Locoregional control is less likely with multiple previous recurrences. Thus, the size of the irradiation ports should allow coverage of the tumor bed and all operative fields so that potential fibromatosis infiltration is included. Careful attention should be paid to anatomical and functional relationships between the tumor and operative and/or irradiation fields to ensure that a sufficient margin exists.

► This article represents the experience of a very strong group of investigators from the University of Florida with unusual expertise in soft tissue tumors. Here they report 72 patients treated for a diagnosis of aggressive fibromatosis or desmoid. This is a relatively unfavorable group of patients with this diagnosis inasmuch as a majority of the patients (42) treated for recurrent disease and only 12 of the entire population had a gross surgical resection. Despite these relatively unfavorable characteristics, EBRT appears to have been effective treatment in achieving local control in 96% of the initial presentations and in three fourths of the patients with recurrent disease.

These are excellent figures and certainly are results that we need to emulate. These lesions tend to be undertreated. Typically, the surgeon does a resection which is not big enough from the standpoint of margins, and, typically, the radiation oncologist does not use big enough volumes to target. The result is that when recurrences occur, they tend to be at the edges of the field, resection or radiation. That has certainly been my own experience and that is the experience that they report here, with only 2 patients recurring within the radiation field and the others representing marginal recurrences.

These kinds of lesions do not metastasize but tend to occur locally only. Even though they do not metastasize, that does not mean they are necessarily easy to deal with as many of these lesions occur in very awkward locations, and the typical lesion tends to be large. The authors furnish a good bibliography for the reader who wants additional information.

E. Glatstein, MD

Esthesioneuroblastoma: Irradiation Alone and Surgery Alone Are Not Enough

Gruber G, Laedrach K, Baumert B, et al (Univ of Berne, Switzerland; Univ Hosp Zurich, Switzerland)

Int J Radiat Oncol Biol Phys 54:486-491, 2002 12–6

Background.—Esthesioneuroblastoma (ENB), or olfactory neuroblastoma, is a rare malignancy of the upper nasal cavity and accounts for approximately 3% of all intranasal tumors. There is controversy regarding the optimal treatment in relation to tumor stage, and there are few reports in the literature regarding treatment of ENB with definitive radiotherapy (RT). Nearly one half of the recurrences of ENB occur more than 5 years after diagnosis, so long-term observation is required for a more precise diagnosis.

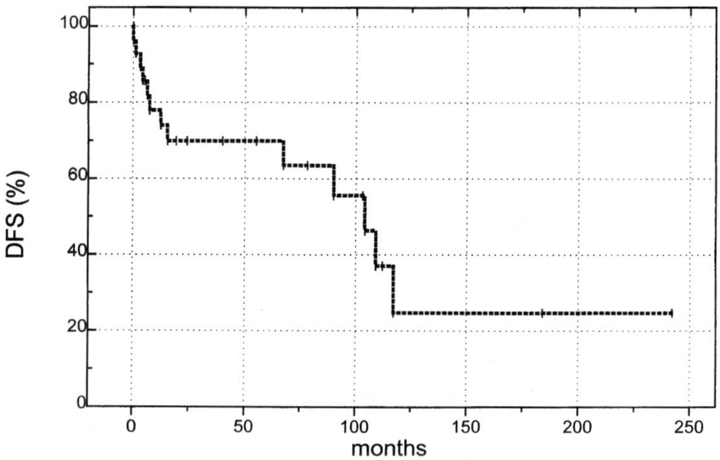

FIGURE 1.—Disease-free survival rate in 28 patients with esthesioneuroblastoma. *Abbreviation: DSF*, Disease-free survival. (Reprinted from Gruber G, Laedrach K, Baumert B, et al: Esthesioneuroblastoma: Irradiation alone and surgery alone are not enough. *Int J Radiat Oncol Biol Phys* 54:486-491, 2002. Copyright 2002, with permission from Elsevier Science.)

The long-term outcome of patients with ENB with neoadjuvant or definitive RT was evaluated.

Methods.—RT was administered from 1980 to 2001 at a median dose of 60 Gy to a total of 28 patients with histologically confirmed ENB. The patients ranged in age from 16 to 85 years (median age, 58 years). On the Kadish classification, 4 patients had stage A tumors, 8 had stage B tumors, and 16 had stage C tumors. Radical resection was performed in 13 patients (9 before RT and 4 after RT) because of stable or progressive disease. The

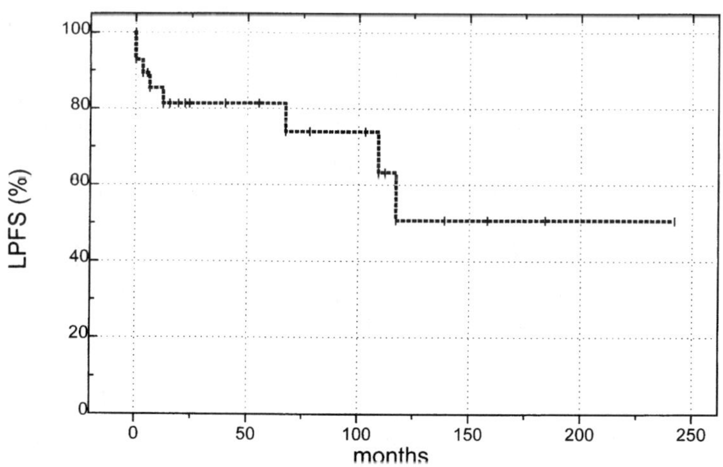

FIGURE 2.—Local progression-free survival rate in 28 patients with esthesioneuroblastoma. *Abbreviation: LPFS*, Local progression-free survival. (Reprinted from Gruber G, Laedrach K, Baumert B, et al: Esthesioneuroblastoma: Irradiation alone and surgery alone are not enough. *Int J Radiat Oncol Biol Phys* 54:486-491, 2002. Copyright 2002, with permission from Elsevier Science.)

main outcome measures were median age, Kadish stage, skull-base penetration, intraorbital extension, resection status, and total dose (60 Gy or less vs more than 60 Gy).

Results.—Fifty-four percent of patients were free of tumor progression at a mean follow-up of 68 months. The 5-year and 10-year disease-free survival rates were 70% and 25%, respectively (Fig 1). The 5-year and 10-year local progression-free survival rates were 81% and 51%, respectively (Fig 2). Of the 10 deaths, 4 were intercurrent, resulting in cause-specific survival rates of 77% and 69% at 5 and 10 years, respectively. Radical resection provided significantly better local progression-free survival and disease-free survival. The most important factors in impaired disease-free survival were skull-base penetration, infraorbital extension, and Kadish C stage.

Conclusion.—Radical RT, even at doses up to 73 Gy, cannot replace radical resection. A radical strategy including resection, high-dose RT, and simultaneous chemotherapy is recommended because of the biology and high rates of late recurrence in ENB.

► ENBs are lesions that are very difficult to control long-term. These Swiss investigators report a goodly sized series of 28 patients. Approximately half of them have had a complete resection, either before or after RT. The median dose was 60 Gy. That means that roughly half the patients had less than that, and less than 60 is probably an inadequate dose, at least for long-term local control. The fact that the series goes back to 1980 implies strongly that some of the patients may not have been treated with CT planning, which is probably critical in terms of defining the full extent of the tumor.

The authors conclude that "radical" RT cannot replace radical resection. I do not think that is entirely clear, but long-term data from other institutions may help in that regard. Certainly, it is important to have 10-year follow-up as a minimum to really understand whether the primary has been controlled or not.

E. Glatstein, MD

Outcome of Primary Soft Tissue Sarcoma of the Knee and Elbow

Alektiar KM, McKee AB, Jacobs JM, et al (Mem Sloan-Kettering Cancer Ctr, New York)

Int J Radiat Oncol Biol Phys 54:163-169, 2002 12–7

Background.—Local management of soft tissue sarcoma of the elbow and knee is difficult to treat. The proximity of many of these tumors to adjacent neurovascular structures makes wide local excision more difficult, and the lack of expandable tissue makes primary wound closure more difficult in some patients, leading to tissue transfer. For the radiation oncologist, concern centers on the tolerance of irradiation over a joint space. The risk of relapse and the potential complications of limb-sparing surgery with and without adjuvant radiotherapy (RT) for patients with knee or elbow soft tissue sarcoma was investigated.

Methods.—This retrospective review identified 86 adult patients with primary soft tissue sarcoma of the knee (65 patients) or elbow (21 patients) treated with limb-sparing surgery from June 1982 to December 1999. The tumors had high-grade histologic features in 72% of patients and measured more than 5 cm in 48% of patients. Adjuvant RT was administered to 46 (54%) patients. It was delivered as postoperative external beam RT to 63% of patients and as brachytherapy to 37% of patients. Of the 46 patients who received RT, 85% had deep tumors, 78% had high-grade tumors, and 54% had tumors measuring more than 5 cm. The complications assessed for this study were wound complications requiring repeated surgery, bone fracture, nerve damage, and joint stiffness.

Results.—The 5-year actuarial rates for local control, distant control, and overall survival were 75%, 82%, and 81%, respectively, with a median follow-up of 48 months. The 5-year local control rate for patients who received RT was 80% compared with 71% for patients who did not receive RT. The rate of local control was not significantly affected by the type of RT. External beam RT had a 5-year local control rate of 84% compared with 73% for patients treated with brachytherapy.

Multivariate analysis showed that tumor size greater than 5 cm remained a significant independent predictor of poor local control. In addition, high-grade histologic features were found to be an independent predictor of local recurrence (Table 2). There were no statistically significant differences between the RT and non-RT groups in terms of the 5-year actuarial rate of wound reoperation, bone fracture, or nerve damage. The RT group had a significantly higher rate of joint stiffness (24% vs 0%), but this stiffness was moderate to severe in only 2 patients.

TABLE 2.—Local Control

	Local Recurrence (*n*)	5-y LC (%)	*P*	95% CI
Size (cm)				
≤5	7/45	84	0.03	72-96
>5	13/41	66		50-83
Depth				
Superficial	5/18	76	0.9	56-97
Deep	15/68	74		62-87
Site				
Elbow	7/21	71	0.3	50-93
Knee	13/65	76		65-88
Grade				
Low	2/24	90	0.07	78-100
High	18/62	70		58-83
Margin				
Negative	14/69	76	0.2	65-88
Positive	6/17	70		48-93
RT				
No	11/40	71	0.3	55-87
Yes	9/46	80		67-93

Abbreviations: LC, Local control; *CI,* confidence interval; *RT,* radiotherapy.

(Reprinted from Alektiar KM, McKee AB, Jacobs JM, et al: Outcome of primary soft tissue sarcoma of the knee and elbow. *In J Radiat Oncol Biol Phys* 54:163-169, 2002.

Conclusion.—Adjuvant RT for the treatment of primary soft tissue sarcoma of the knee and elbow is relatively well tolerated despite inclusion of a portion of the joint space in the irradiation portal. Joint stiffness occurred more frequently with adjuvant RT, but this stiffness was moderate to severe in a small proportion of patients.

▶ When irradiating patients who have lesions that approach a joint, there are always concerns about long-term effects and decreased functional results. This experienced team of investigators from Memorial Sloan-Kettering reports on the outcome of patients receiving treatment for soft tissue sarcomas of the knee and elbow regions. They have 86 patients and a majority represent high-grade lesions and lesions larger than 5 cm. Forty-six of the 86 received postoperative RT and the local control was similar with or without RT. Because the RT was presumably given to the patients who had larger lesions, positive margins, and higher grade lesions, I think it demonstrates that the investigators picked the right patients to receive postoperative RT.

When the elbow or the knee is involved, it is almost always necessary to include some of the joint. A trick includes trying to spare as much joint as you think you can, and shrinking the field after about 45 Gy. At Sloan-Kettering, they frequently treat with brachytherapy alone, which is excellent in their hands. The consideration of brachytherapy is individualized, but the point is that one has to be prepared to do it at the time of the surgery so one has to plan on this in advance. The authors pioneered the use of this approach, and they usually use a single-plane implant. Personally, I have a little problem with the single-plane implant because it requires that the malignant cells be in close proximity to the plane of the implant. I would rather treat a volume implant rather than single plane. Nevertheless, the authors' results are quite good, and it is hard to argue with success.

The other point that I would make regarding such patients is that I think it is truly important to get physical therapy involved promptly. I have been places where physical therapists were not actively involved in such patients, and I have been in places where the physical therapy/rehabilitation medicine team was very actively involved. There is no question in my mind that the functional results are vastly improved when their expertise enters the picture early in the game, preferably even before RT has been given. It is common to give lip service to physical therapy and rehabilitation medicine, but it truly is a very important component to maximizing the functional outcome in such patients. I would have enjoyed this article more had the authors shown the overall survivals. This is mentioned but not shown in graphic format.

E. Glatstein, MD

Long-term Outcome of Combined Modality Therapy in Retroperitoneal and Deep-Trunk Soft-Tissue Sarcoma: Analysis of Prognostic Factors
Youssef E, Fontanesi J, Mott M, et al (Wayne State Univ, Detroit)
Int J Radiat Oncol Biol Phys 54:514-519, 2002 12–8

Background.—In patients with retroperitoneal and deep-trunk soft tissue sarcoma, an advanced stage at diagnosis leads to difficulty resecting the tumor and achieving negative margins. Also, the use of adjuvant radiotherapy is limited by the lack of tolerance of surrounding normal tissue. These factors can lead to a poor prognosis. In an effort to overcome these problems and allow high doses to be delivered, various strategies have been undertaken. The experience of 1 institution where most patients received postoperative external beam radiotherapy (EBRT) with or without brachytherapy was reported, including an analysis of prognostic factors for overall survival, disease-free survival (DFS), and local control.

Methods.—Combined surgery and radiotherapy were used for 60 patients with nonmetastatic retroperitoneal and deep-trunk soft tissue sarcoma receiving treatment at Wayne State University. Thirty-eight patients had retroperitoneal tumors and 22 were deep-trunk lesions (Table 2). For 76% of the patients, the disease was primary and for 24%, it was recurrent. Twenty-four patients had negative margins, 3 had close margins, and 33 had positive margins, of which 18 were microscopic and 15 macroscopic. Tu-

TABLE 2.—Pathologic Features

Feature	*n* (%)
Histologic type	
Malignant fibrous histiocytoma	16 (27)
Leiomyosarcoma	12 (20)
Liposarcoma	10 (17)
Fibrosarcoma	6 (9)
Other	16 (27)
Grade	
Low	15 (25)
Intermediate	10 (17)
High	35 (58)
Stage	
IA/IB	1/6 (1.5/10)
IIA/IIB	1/8 (1.5/13)
IIIA/IIIB	5/24 (8/40)
Recurrent	14 (23)
Unknown	1 (1.5)
Resection margins	
Negative	24 (40)
Close*	3 (5)
Microscopically positive	18 (30)
Grossly positive	15 (25)

*Close margin defined as presence of tumor cells within 2 mm but not at the inked margin.

(Reprinted from Youssef E, Fontanesi J, Mott M, et al: Long-term outcome of combined modality therapy in retroperitoneal and deep-trunk soft-tissue sarcoma: Analysis of prognostic factors. *Int J Radiat Oncol Biol Phys* 54:514-519, 2002. Copyright 2002, with permission from Elsevier Science.)

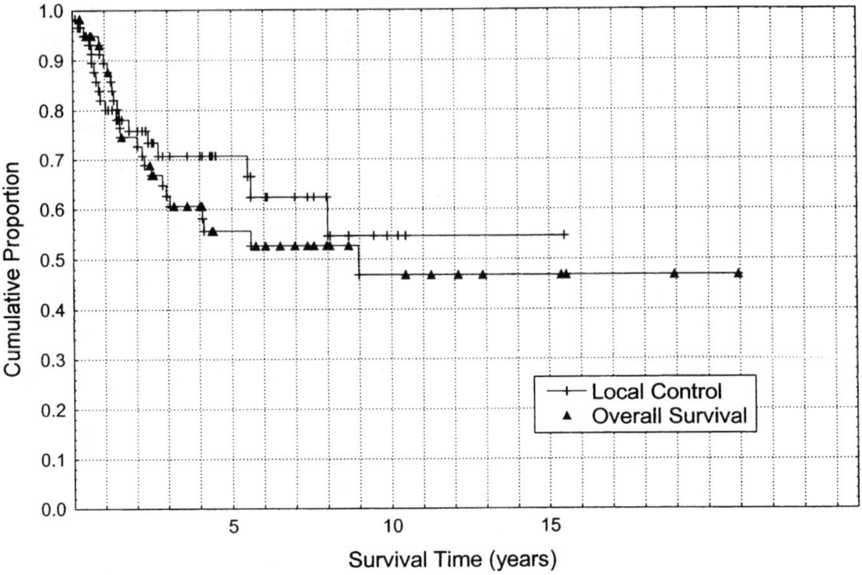

FIGURE 1.—Actuarial overall survival and local control for the entire study population. (Reprinted from Youssef E, Fontanesi J, Mott M, et al: Long-term outcome of combined modality therapy in retroperitoneal and deep-trunk soft-tissue sarcoma: Analysis of prognostic factors. *Int J Radiat Oncol Biol Phys* 54:514-519, 2002. Copyright 2002, with permission from Elsevier Science.)

mors ranged in size from 2 to 55 cm (median, 8.6 cm). Forty-four patients received a median dose of 5220 cGy EBRT and 16 had a median dose of 4200 cGy EBRT plus a median dose of 1600 cG brachytherapy. Follow-up extended for a median of 3 years, or 4.4 years in living patients.

Results.—Local recurrence was found in 6 patients, local recurrence plus distant metastases in 12, and distant metastases only in 12; 25 patients died. The DFS rate at 4 years was 53% and that at 10 years was 44%. Gender and margin status were borderline significant factors for DFS at 10 years. Local control rates were 71% at 5 years and 54% at 10 years (Fig 1). Seventy-five percent of all local relapses occurred in the first 29 months. Surgical margin status was the only significant factor in the 5-year local control rate on multivariate analysis. The distant metastasis-free survival at 5 years was 58%, while that at 10 years was 54%; distant metastases developed at a median of 15.6 months after treatment and usually involved the lung, liver, or bone. Local control was the only factor showing a significant link to distant metastasis-free survival. The survival rate at 5 years was 56% and at 10 years, it was 47%. Gender, surgical margin status, and local control were significant in determining the actuarial overall survival rate.

Conclusion.—Local control and clear margins on surgical resection proved to be significant factors in determining the survival of patients receiving treatment for soft tissue sarcoma of the retroperitoneum and deep trunk.

► This group of investigators from Wayne State looks at 60 patients with non-metastatic retroperitoneal sarcoma and also soft tissue sarcomas of the trunk. Patients had an effort at maximum surgical resection followed by local radiation therapy. Margins were negative in 24 patients and overtly positive in 33. In 15 of these 33 patients with positive margins, the positivity was macroscopic. A number of patients received brachytherapy in addition to EBRT, but the median dose of EBRT was only 52 Gy. Fifteen of these patients had low-grade tumors, making the interpretation somewhat complicated. Overall, the authors feel they have achieved local control in approximately half the patients.

The inclusion of deep trunk lesions along with retroperitoneal lesions is a confounding factor. In addition, the median period of follow-up was only approximately 3 years. This relatively short period of follow-up makes it hard to interpret what the 10-year disease-free rate really means. The authors conclude that their study demonstrates the importance of complete surgical resection, and I would agree with that.

E. Glatstein, MD

13 Neurologic

Identification of Combination Gene Sets for Glioma Classification

Kim S, Dougherty ER, Shmulevich I, et al (Texas A&M Univ, College Station; Univ of Texas, Houston; NIH, Bethesda, Md)

Mol Cancer Ther 1:1229-1236, 2002 13–1

Introduction.—A goal for the gene expression profiling of cancer is to detect signature genes that robustly distinguish various types of grades of tumors. Such signature genes would ideally contribute a molecular basis for classification and also provide insight into the molecular events underlying various cancer phenotypes. A recently developed algorithm was applied to determine single classifier genes and gene sets (combinations) for use as glioma classifiers.

Findings.—Classifier genes identified by the algorithm were demonstrated to be strong features by conservatively and collectively considering the misclassification errors of the feature sets. The best single genes were identified when this approach was applied to a test set of 2- to 3-gene combinations for identifying 4 types of glioma: (1) oligodendroglioma, (2) anaplastic oligodendroglioma, (3) anaplastic astrocytoma, and (4) glioblastoma multiforme. Some of the identified genes, including insulinlike growth factor-binding protein 2, have been shown to be linked with one of the tumor types. By using combinations of genes, the classification error rate can be significantly diminished. In many instances, neither of the individual genes of a 2-gene set performs well as a reliable classifier; the combination of the 2 genes creates a robust classifier with a small error rate.

Conclusion.—Two-gene and 3-gene combinations provide robust classifications that have the potential to translate expression microarray results into diagnostic histopathologic assays that can be used in the clinical setting.

► Unlike in the case of most hematologic malignancies, the diagnosis of glial tumors is often not supported by methods and technologies such as cytogenetics and flow cytometry. For such tumors, the use of a molecularly based classification would, therefore, potentially have a considerable impact. The report by Kim et al is an excellent starting place toward this goal. The study describes several methods of microarray RNA expression analysis and their applicability to distinguishing 4 different subtypes of glioma. In addition, subsets of the larger expression data sets are shown to have excellent predictive power to accurately classify several different glioma subtypes. This latter point is critical for future work because one of the limiting characteristics of this type of work is the small sample size. In addition, this often can present further problems in terms of that sample being representative of the truly diagnostic portion of the tumor. In part, these issues should be able to be overcome with a close collaboration of the neurosurgeon with the pathologist at the time of surgery. While the solution won't be as easy as asking for another 3 mL of bone marrow, the future is starting to look brighter in terms of the application of molecular studies to the diagnosis of brain tumors.

R. J. Arceci, MD, PhD

Metabolic Imaging of Low-Grade Gliomas With Three-Dimensional Magnetic Resonance Spectroscopy
Pirzkall A, Nelson SJ, McKnight TR, et al (Univ of California, San Francisco)
Int J Radiat Oncol Biol Phys 53:1254-1264, 2002 13–2

Introduction.—The initial treatment of choice for patients with symptomatic low-grade gliomas (LGGs) is surgery, yet complete surgical resection is not usually achievable because most of these tumors are diffusely infiltrating. The role and timing of radiotherapy in the treatment of patients with LGGs is controversial. Three-dimensional (3D) MR spectroscopy imaging (MRSI) has been reported to be useful in defining the extent of glioma infiltration. The usefulness of MRSI for metabolic imaging of LGGs was examined, along with the effect MRSI would have on the routine practice of adding 2- to 3-cm margins around MRI T2-weighted hyperintensity to produce the treatment planning clinical target volume for LGGs.

Methods.—Twenty patients with supratentorial gliomas (World Health Organization grade II) underwent both MRI and MRSI preoperatively. There were 7 astrocytomas, 6 oligoastrocytomas, and 7 oligodendroglio-

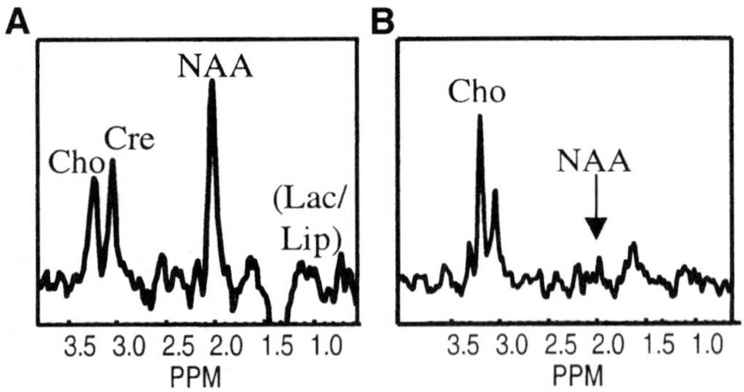

FIGURE 1.—A, Typical MR spectroscopy spectrum for normal brain. Five classes of molecules are distinct: NAA, free choline and choline-containing compounds, including phosphocholine and glycerophosphocholine (*Cho*), creatine and phosphocreatine (*Cr*), lactate (*Lac*), and lipid (*Lip*). B, MR spectroscopy spectrum for low-grade oligogastrocytoma. Cho is increased and NAA is clearly diminished. (Relatively high Cr is typical for oligoastrocytoma.) (Reprinted from Pirzkall A, Nelson SJ, McKnight TR, et al: Metabolic imaging of low-grade gliomas with three-dimensional magnetic resonance spectroscopy. *Int J Radiat Oncol Biol Phys* 53:1254-1264, 2002. Copyright 2002, with permission from Elsevier Science.)

TABLE 2.—MR Spectroscopy Imaging–Derived Choline/N-Acetyl-Aspartate Index and Creatine/*N*-Acetyl-Aspartate Index Volumes

Volume (cm^3)	Mean	Median	Range
CNI 2	32.7	29.3	10.5-72.6
CNI 3	18.7	14.4	2.6-45.9
CNI 4	9.5	6.8	0.7-31.2
CNI 6	3.1	1.5	0.1-13.3
CrNI 2	5.8	4.4	0.2-22.9

Abbreviations: CNI, Choline/*N*-acetyl-aspartate index; *CriNI,* creatine/*N*-acetyl aspartate index.
(Reprinted from Pirzkall A, Nelson SJ, McKnight TR, et al: Metabolic imaging of low-grade gliomas with three-dimensional magnetic resonance spectroscopy. *Int J Radiat Oncol Biol Phys* 53:1254-1264, 2002. Copyright 2002, with permission from Elsevier Science.)

mas. The MRI was contoured manually, with regions of interest including T2 hyperintensity and, if present, regions of contrast enhancement on T1-weighted images. The 3D-MRSI peak parameters for choline (Fig 1) and *N* acetyl aspartate, acquired voxel-by-voxel, were categorized by means of a choline/*N*-acetyl-aspartate index (CNI), which is a tool for quantitative examination of tissue metabolic levels; CNI 2 was the lowest value corresponding to tumor. The CNI data were aligned to MRI and displayed as 3D contours. The association between the anatomical and metabolic information on tumor extent was evaluated by comparing the CNI contours and other MRSI-derived metabolites to the MRI T2 volume.

Results.—The limitations in the size of the region "excited" meant that MRSI could be used to assess only a median 68% of the T2 volume (range, 38%-100%), leaving the volume T2c. The CNI 2 volume (median, 29 cm^3; range, 10-73) was contained completely within the T2c in 55% of patients (Tables 2 and 3). In the remaining cohort, the volume of CNI 2 extending beyond the T2c was small (median, 2.3 cm^3, range, 1.4-5.2).

The CNI volumes became circumferentially smaller as the value increased (Fig 3). It was not distributed uniformly about the T2c, extending up to 22 mm beyond. Two patients had small regions of contrast enhancement that corresponded to the regions of highest CNI. Other metabolites, including creatine and lactate, appeared useful for determining less and more radio-resistant areas, respectively.

TABLE 3.—Relationship of MRI T2c and MR Spectroscopy Imaging Choline/*N*-Acetyl-Aspartate Index 2 Volumes

LGG	Patients (*n*)	Mean	Median	Range
CNI 2 outside T2c (cm^3)	9	3.1	2.3	1.4-5.2
CNI 2 outside T2c (%)	9	10.9	10.0	3.0-31.2
T2c outside CNI 2 (cm^3)	20	24.9	20.0	1.6-60.0
% T2c outside CNI 2 (%)	20	44.7	43.2	14.8-74.7

Abbreviation: CNI, Choline/*N*-acetyl-aspartate index.
(Reprinted from Pirzkall A, Nelson SJ, McKnight TR, et al: Metabolic imaging of low-grade gliomas with three-dimensional magnetic resonance spectroscopy. *Int J Radiat Oncol Biol Phys* 53:1254-1264, 2002. Copyright 2002, with permission from Elsevier Science.)

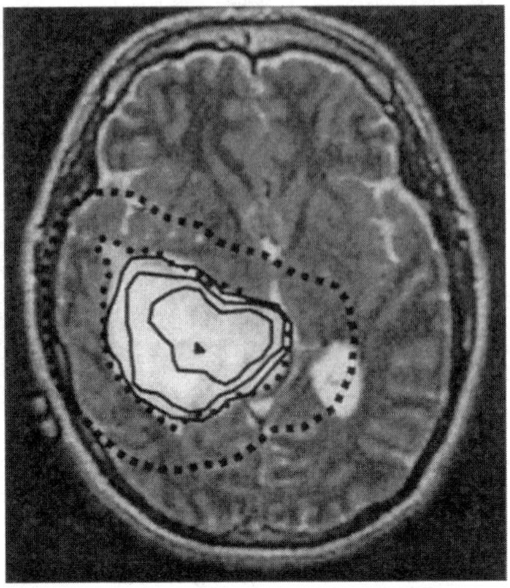

FIGURE 3.—T2-weighted fast spin echo MRI of a right temporo-occipital low-grade astrocytoma with superimposed choline/*N*-acetyl-aspartate indexes 2, 3, 4, and 6 (*solid lines, outside to inside*) and a margin of 2 cm (*outer broken line*) around T2 hyperintensity (*inner broken line*) demonstrating a typical treatment planning scenario. This particular patient would have been "overtreated" with a 2-cm uniform margin. (Reprinted from Pirzkall A, Nelson SJ, McKnight TR, et al: Metabolic imaging of low-grade gliomas with three-dimensional magnetic resonance spectroscopy. *Int J Radiat Oncol Biol Phys* 53:1254-1264, 2002. Copyright 2002, with permission from Elsevier Science.)

Conclusion.—Metabolically active tumor, as identified by MRSI, is limited primarily to the T2 hyperintensity in LGGs. It can extend outside it in a limited and nonuniform manner up to 2 cm. Thus, a CTV including T2 and areas of CNI extension beyond the T2 hyperintensity would result in a decrease in the size and a change in the shape of the standard clinical target volumes produced by adding uniform margins of 2 to 3 cm to the T2 hyperintensity.

► This team from the University of California in San Francisco has been leading the pack in the study of MRSI in the evaluation of tumors of the brain. This is a report on LGGs. The authors were able to define the tumor volume, based on metabolism, in a way that appears to be helpful. On the other hand, the issue is not how to define it, but what are the outcomes? They have to show at some point that this extra effort in definition of tumor is meaningful in terms of the outcome itself. MRSI at this point is best considered work in progress, with considerable potential, but lacking data of confirmation.

E. Glatstein, MD

In Vivo 3-T MR Spectroscopy in the Distinction of Recurrent Glioma Versus Radiation Effects: Initial Experience

Rabinov JD, Lee PL, Barker FG, et al (Harvard Med School, Boston; Stanford Med Ctr, Calif)

Radiology 225:871-879, 2002 13–3

Introduction.—After initial treatment of high-grade glioma with resection and radiation, gadolinium-enhanced areas can often be observed on conventional MRI. Yet MRI is not able to discriminate between radiation-induced changes and tumor recurrence. A blinded prospective investigation was performed to ascertain whether 3-T MR spectroscopy could provide accurate distinction of recurrent tumor from radiation effects in patients with gliomas of grade II or higher.

Methods.—Fourteen patients underwent in vivo 3-T MR spectroscopy before undergoing stereotactic biopsy. All patients had a previous diagnosis of glioma of grade II or higher and had undergone high-dose radiotherapy (over 54 Gy). Before MR spectroscopy, patients underwent conventional MR imaging at 1.5 T to identify a gadolinium-enhanced region within the irradiated volume. Diagnosis was based on histopathologic analysis of the biopsy samples.

Results.—Sixteen of 17 biopsy locations were correctly classified as predominately tumor or predominately radiation effect (Fig 2) (9 and 8 locations, respectively), based on the ratio of choline at the biopsy site to the normal creatine level using a value higher than 1.3 as the criterion for tumor. The remaining patient was classified by MR spectroscopy as having a recurrent tumor; histopathologic findings revealed a predominately radiation effect. Disease in this patient progressed to biopsy-verified recurrence within 3 months. Overall, the ratio of choline at the biopsy site to normal creatine was significantly increased ($P < .002$) in the biopsy specimens composed predominately of tumor versus those containing predominately radiation effects (9 and 8 specimens, respectively) (Fig 4). The ratio was not markedly different between the 2 histopathologic groups.

Conclusion.—In vivo 3-T MR spectroscopy has adequate spatial resolution and chemical specificity to permit distinction of recurrent tumor from radiation effects in patients with treated gliomas.

► One of the major challenges regarding patients who have high-grade gliomas is the ability to distinguish recurrent tumor from the possibility of radiation injury to the brain after treatment. These investigators from Massachusetts General Hospital and Stanford have teamed up in a small study of only 14 patients, using a 3-T MR spectroscopic study prior to stereotactic biopsy. There were 17 biopsies in the 14 patients, and in 16 of the 17, the distinction could be made on the basis of elevated choline on MR spectroscopy in areas composed predominantly of tumor.

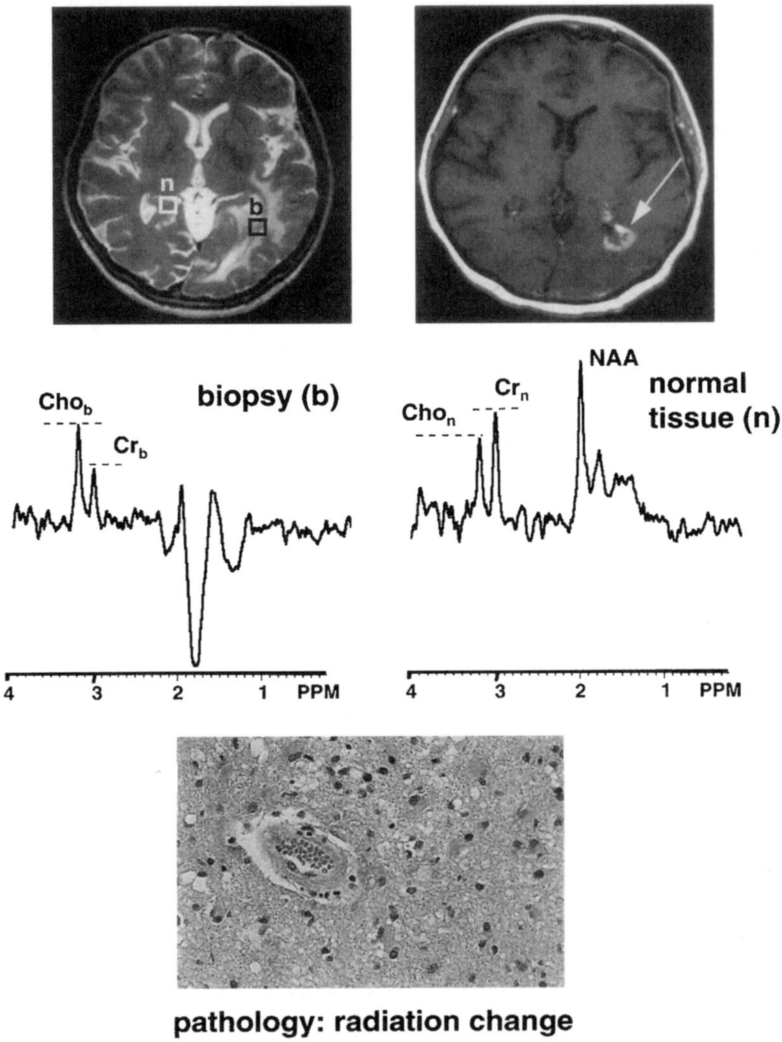

FIGURE 2.—**Upper right,** Transverse T1-weighted gadolinium-enhanced 1.5-T fast spin-echo MR image. *Arrow* indicates a focus of enhancement. **Upper left,** Transverse T2-weighted 3-T fast spin-echo MR image shows the location of the voxels corresponding to the biopsy site (*b*; middle, left spectrum) and normal tissue (*n*; middle, right spectrum). The intensity of the 2 spectra is displayed on the same (arbitrary) vertical scale. The horizontal frequency scale is in parts per million (*PPM*) relative to the magnet frequency (3 T = 126 Mhz). Choline, biopsy (Cho_b) is not elevated in relation to creatine, normal voxel (Cr_n). **Bottom,** Histopathologic specimen of the biopsy sample shows sparse cellularity with reactive glial cells and vascular fibrosis consistent with radiation effects; original magnification, ×400. (Courtesy of Rabinov JD, Lee PL, Barker FG, et al: In vivo 3-T MR spectroscopy in the distinction of recurrent glioma effects: Initial experience. *Radiology* 225:871-879, 2002. Radiological Society of North America.)

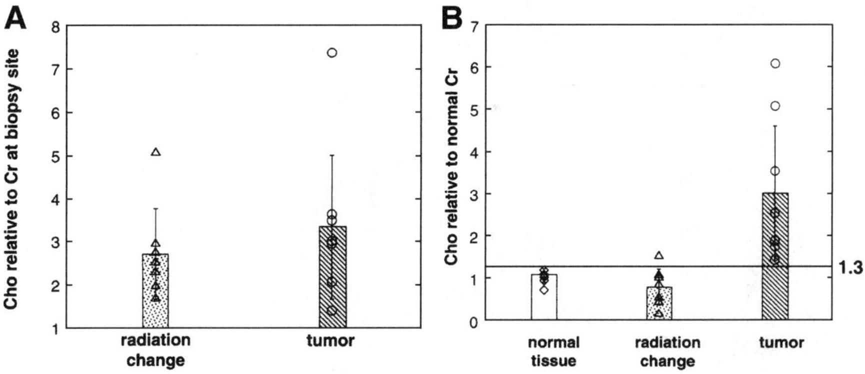

FIGURE 4.—Plots show choline/creatine (*Cho/Cr*) for all biopsy samples plotted as a function of histopathologic findings. The height of the *error bar* represents the average value. *Error bars* represent the standard deviation. **A**, Plot demonstrates that Cho/Cr from the biopsy site (Cho_b/Cr_b) is not significantly different between the 2 histopathologic groups ($P < .4$). **B**, Plot demonstrates that Cho from the biopsy site/ creatine from the normal voxel (Cho_b/Cr_n) shows a significant difference ($P < .002$) between the 2 groups. Cho/Cr from the normal voxel (Cho_n/Cr_n) is also shown. *Triangles* and *circles* indicate individual cases. (Courtesy of Rabinov JD, Lee PL, Barker FG, et al: In vivo 3-T MR spectroscopy in the distinction of recurrent glioma effects: Initial experience. *Radiology* 225:871-879, 2002. Radiological Society of North America.)

The small size of this study obviously makes it hard to make a definitive conclusion, but it certainly looks like this approach will be useful in the future. Of course, the authors seem to overlook the possibility that tumor and necrosis often coexist.

E. Glatstein, MD

External Beam Irradiation of Craniopharyngiomas: Long-term Analysis of Tumor Control and Morbidity

Varlotto JM, Flickinger JC, Kondziolka D, et al (Univ of Pittsburgh, Pa)
Int J Radiat Oncol Biol Phys 54:492-499, 2002 13–4

Background.—From 2% to 9% of all intracranial neoplasms are craniopharyngiomas, which are benign lesions derived from epithelial origin. These tumors are generally well circumscribed and encapsulated, but they are located in a critical brain area, adhering to the optic nerves or chiasm, major vessels of the circle of Willis, infundibulum, pituitary gland, and hypothalamus, with some infiltrating the infundibulum, hypothalamus, and optic nerve. In 57% to 90% of cases, the tumor can be completely removed, but recurrence is noted in 15% to 37% of cases. If an aggressive surgical approach is used, death, significant visual loss, and neurologic dysfunction can occur. An update of experience with this neoplasm was undertaken, with treatment of craniopharyngiomas using external beam radiotherapy (EBRT) and the resulting outcomes noted.

Methods.—From 1971 to 1992, 24 patients (age range, 5-69 years; median age, 29 years) with craniopharyngiomas had EBRT, with 19 treated within 3 months of subtotal resection. Two patients had had previous biop-

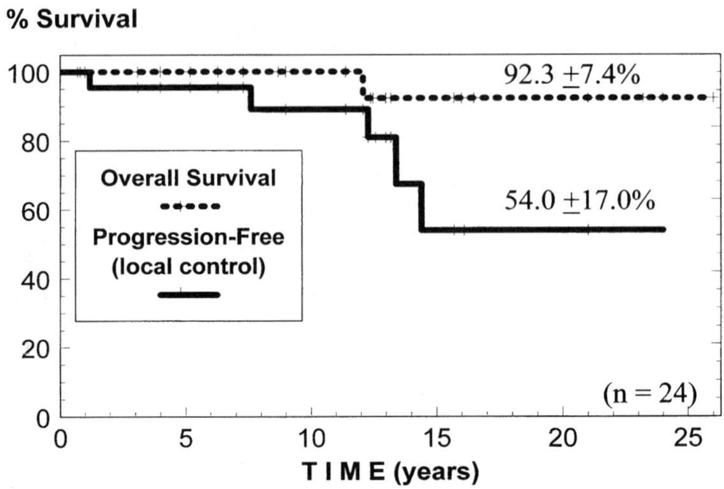

FIGURE 1.—Actuarial overall survival and progression-free survival (tumor control) after external beam radiotherapy for craniopharyngioma in 24 patients. (Reprinted from Varlotto JM, Flickinger JC, Kondziolka D, et al: External beam irradiation of craniopharyngiomas: Long-term analysis of tumor control and morbidity. *Int J Radiat Oncol Biol Phys* 54:492-499, 2002. Copyright 2002, with permission from Elsevier Science.)

sy, had gross total resection, and 2 had had no previous surgery. Patients received a total radiation dose of 36 to 70 Gy, with a median of 59.75 Gy. The normalized total dose was 28 to 83 Gy. Follow-up extended for a median of 12.1 years.

Results.—The survival rate at 10 years was 100% and at 20 years, it was 92.3% (Fig 1). Local tumor control rates were 95.4% at 5 years, 89.1% at 10 years, and 54.0% at 20 years, with local failure developing in 5 patients between 14 months and 14 years 6 months after treatment. Two patients for whom intracavitary ^{32}P was used for salvage lost visual function in 1 eye. Local failures were noted with doses less than 60 Gy (Fig 2).

Five years after completing radiotherapy, the complication-free survival rate was 80.1%; the rates for 10 and 20 years were 80.1% and 69.5%, respectively. Most complications occurred within 5 years of radiotherapy and included infarction, optic neuropathy, hemiparesis, visual field defect, mental status changes, thalamic infarct, memory loss, and left-sided visual field loss. Survival free from adverse effects was 70.1% at 10 years and 31.8% at 20 years; it was optimized with doses of 55 to 63 Gy.

A high rate of recurrence of tumor was noted with doses under 55 Gy. A high rate of complications occurred with doses of 66 to 83 Gy, although tumor control was excellent. On multivarate proportional hazards analysis, total dose showed a significant correlation with tumor control. Adverse outcome–free survival was significantly correlated with hypopituitarism on presentation.

Conclusion.—When craniopharyngiomas cannot be completely resected, EBRT presents an effective alternative treatment. The total dose of about 60

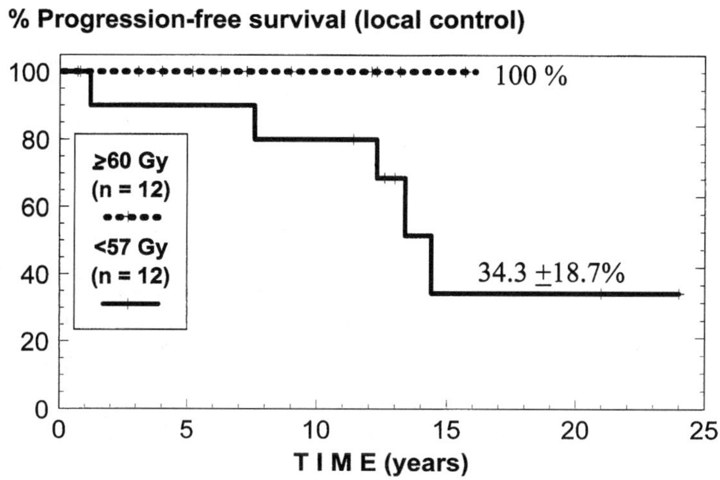

FIGURE 2.—Effect of total dose on progression-free survival (tumor control) after external beam radiotherapy for craniopharyngioma. (Reprinted from Varlotto JM, Flickinger JC, Kondziolka D, et al: External beam irradiation of craniopharyngiomas: Long-term analysis of tumor control and morbidity. *Int J Radiat Oncol Biol Phys* 54:492-499, 2002. Copyright 2002, with permission from Elsevier Science.)

Gy should be delivered in fractions of 1.6 to 1.7 Gy each to minimize long-term morbidity and prevent late treatment failures.

► Craniopharyngiomas are uncommon benign tumors within the CNS in close proximity to the suprasellar area of the brain and are thought to arise from remnants of Rathke's pouch. This series from the University of Pittsburgh is modest in size with only 24 patients receivingEBRT. The vast majority of the patients received a subtotal resection or less. The median follow-up was over 12 years, and the results show excellent survival and reasonably good local control. The 10-year figure for local control was just under 90%, but the 20-year figure was only 54%. It is not clear to me what the impact of dose was on this, as I suspect that the patients who had the lower doses were the ones treated early in the group. The authors do make the point that there were no local failures seen with doses of 60 Gy or higher. The complication rate is also acceptable.

This is a group of patients in whom radiation therapy is generally underutilized in this country. The efforts for gross total resection have considerable morbidity associated with them, and the radiation treatments are relatively easy for patients. There is an extensive review of the literature concerning treatment in this article.

E. Glatstein, MD

Surgery and Permanent ^{125}I Seed Paraspinal Brachytherapy for Malignant Tumors With Spinal Cord Compression

Rogers CL, Theodore N, Dickman CA, et al (Barrow Neurological Inst, Phoenix, Ariz; Arizona Oncology Services, Phoenix; Found for Cancer Research and Education, Phoenix, Ariz)

Int J Radiat Oncol Biol Phys 54:505-513, 2002 13–5

Introduction.—Compression of the spinal cord by metastatic epidural or locally invasive paraspinal tumors is a frequently occurring neurologic sequela of malignancy that is associated with devastating consequences. A higher rate of functional recovery has been observed when treatment is initiated before the development of severe neurologic deficits and while patients are still ambulatory. The functional outcome and predictors of response and toxicity from spinal surgery and ^{125}I brachytherapy were examined in patients with malignant tumors resulting in spinal cord compression.

Methods.—After surgical resection, 30 patients underwent 31 intraoperative paraspinal brachytherapy procedures between July 1985 and September 2001. Twenty-four patients (25 procedures) were available for follow-up. Surgical procedures focused on the location of the impinging lesion. Thirteen patients underwent corpectomy or spondylectomy and 12 underwent laminectomy. Permanent ^{125}I seeds in absorbable suture were placed with open exposure after resection was performed.

Results.—Spinal cord compression was located in the cervical, thoracic, and lumbar spine in 4 (16%), 14 (56%), and 7 (28%) patients, respectively. One patient had 2 separate procedures at different spinal sites. Twenty-two

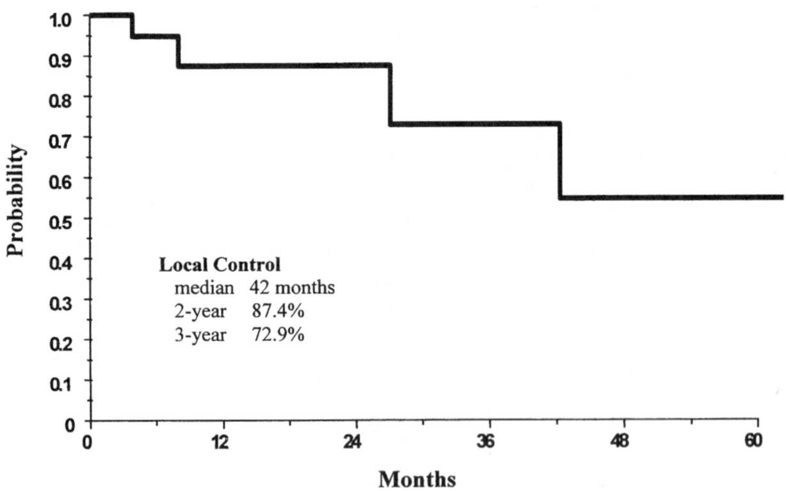

FIGURE 2.—Actuarial local control at 25 surgery and brachytherapy sites in 24 patients with spinal cord compression. (Reprinted from Rogers CL, Theodore N, Dickman CA, et al: Surgery and permanent ^{125}I seed paraspinal brachytherapy for malignant tumors with spinal cord compression. *Int J Radiat Oncol Biol Phys* 54:505-513, 2002. Copyright 2002, with permission from Elsevier Science.)

of the 25 brachytherapy sites also received external beam radiotherapy (EBRT): 5, EBRT with a planned brachytherapy boost; 4, brachytherapy and prompt EBRT after recovery; and 13, brachytherapy as salvage for local failure after prior EBRT. Three patients did not receive EBRT; 1 of these had lymphoma treated with chemotherapy, 1 had had remote previous EBRT for a childhood tumor, and 1 refused EBRT.

The mean follow-up was 19.8 months. The 2- and 3-year actuarial local control rates were 87.4% and 72.9%, respectively (Fig 2). Local failure was observed at 4 (16%) sites. The mean time for recurrent disease was 20.3 months for this subgroup. Three of these patients had failed before undergoing EBRT, with surgery and brachytherapy used for salvage. The 2- and 3-year actuarial survival rates were 24% and 16%, respectively, at a mean of 19.2 months (Fig 3).

Preoperative and postoperative ambulatory function scores were assigned as follows: I, normal ambulation; II, abnormal not requiring assistance; III, abnormal requiring assistance; and IV, unable to ambulate. One hundred percent, 91%, 67%, and 67% of patients with scores of I, II, III, and IV, respectively, were ambulatory after the procedure; 84% had either normal or improved ambulation postoperatively. There were 4 postoperative events, including 1 CSF leak, 2 wound infections treated in situ without removal of seeds or instrumentation, and 1 pulmonary embolus. There were no myelopathies or other neurologic sequelae.

Conclusion.—This is the largest published series evaluating surgery and ^{125}I brachytherapy for treatment of malignant spinal cord compression. This approach was well tolerated and resulted in durable local control and am-

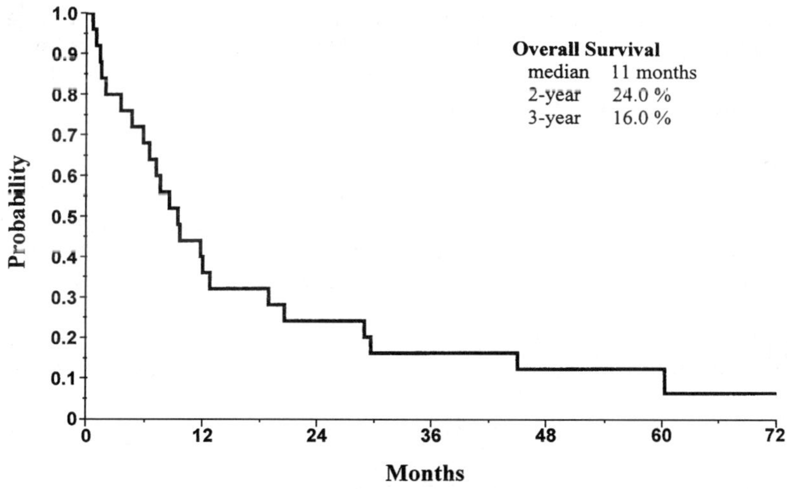

FIGURE 3.—Actuarial overall survival in 24 patients treated with surgery and brachytherapy for spinal cord compression. (Reprinted from Rogers CL, Theodore N, Dickman CA, et al: Surgery and permanent ^{125}I seed paraspinal brachytherapy for malignant tumors with spinal cord compression. *Int J Radiat Oncol Biol Phys* 54:505-513, 2002. Copyright 2002, with permission from Elsevier Science.)

bulatory function. Aggressive local therapy may be beneficial in selected patients with spinal cord compression.

► This is an interesting report that approaches patients who have spinal cord compression somewhat differently than what is usually done. In this instance, the authors have 30 patients who underwent surgical resection followed by intraoperative brachytherapy to the paraspinous region. Unfortunately, 22 of them also received external beam brachytherapy, making interpretation somewhat difficult as to what the contribution of brachytherapy truly is. Nonetheless, it is an interesting approach and one which requires close coordination between radiation oncology and neurosurgery. Treatment appears to be well tolerated and certainly worth considering in selected patients.

E. Glatstein, MD

Gene Expression-based Classification of Malignant Gliomas Correlates Better With Survival Than Histological Classification

Nutt CL, Mani DR, Betensky RA, et al (Harvard Med School, Boston; Whitehead Inst/Massachusetts Inst of Technology Ctr for Genome Research, Cambridge; Univ of Western Ontario, London, Canada; et al)
Cancer Res 63:1602-1607, 2003 13–6

Background.—The most common primary tumor of the brain is malignant glioma, which results in an estimated 13,000 deaths per year in the United States. Glial tumors are classified histologically, and the pathologic diagnosis has a greater effect than any other variable on prognostic estimation and therapeutic decisions. Among the high-grade gliomas, anaplastic oligodendrogliomas have a more favorable prognosis than histologically classic glioblastomas. Unfortunately, many malignant gliomas are diagnostically challenging because they are difficult to classify by histologic features and generate considerable interobserver variability and limited diagnostic reproducibility. The tentative pathologic diagnoses that result from histologic examination of these tumors can create a significant degree of clinical confusion. A study was undertaken to determine whether gene expression profiling, in conjunction with class prediction methods, could be used to classify high-grade gliomas in a more objective, explicit, and consistent manner than is possible with standard pathologic investigation.

Methods.—Microarray analysis was used to determine the expression of approximately 12,000 genes in a set of 50 gliomas, 28 glioblastomas, and 22 oligodendrogliomas. A 2-class prediction model was constructed on the basis of a subset of 14 glioblastomas and 7 anaplastic oligodendrogliomas with classic histology.

Results.—A 20-feature κ-nearest neighbor model correctly classified 18 of the 21 classic cases in leave-one-out cross-validation when compared with pathologic diagnoses. The model was then applied to the prediction of the classification of clinically common, histologically nonclassic samples. When tumors were classified on the basis of pathologic findings, the survival of patients with nonclassic glioblastoma and nonclassic anaplastic oligodendroglioma was not significantly different. However, a significant association was observed between class distinctions according to the old model and survival outcome. The class prediction model was found to be capable of classifying high-grade, nonclassic glial tumors objectively and reproducibly. In addition, the model provided a more accurate prediction of prognosis of malignant gliomas than could be obtained with pathologic classification.

Conclusions.—The results of this study are suggestive of the superiority of class-prediction models over standard pathologic techniques in the classification of diagnostically challenging malignant gliomas in a way that better correlates with clinical outcome.

► A major challenge in neuro-oncology is to improve treatment outcomes for patients with high-grade gliomas. Fundamental to improving therapies is the improved understanding of these malignant tumors and their classification. Currently, a substantial proportion of high-grade gliomas remain diagnostically challenging according to classic histologic methods. To better define subsets of such difficult high-grade gliomas, Nutt et al performed microarray RNA expression analysis on about 12,000 genes in a group of gliomas, glioblastomas, and anaplastic oligodendrogliomas. Using a supervised learning approach, they were able to define subsets of tumors that had a better or worse prognosis than might have been predicted with the use of only traditional pathologic methods. Importantly, the combination of pathologic and molecular analysis was critical, thus representing an excellent example of the future of brain tumor classification. Such studies are being reported for other malignant tumors as well and represent a forward-looking evolution of merging old and new technologies to improve the outcome for patients with cancer.

R. J. Arceci, MD, PhD

14 Gastrointestinal

Results of Repeat Sigmoidoscopy 3 Years After a Negative Examination

Schoen RE, for the Prostate, Lung, Colorectal, and Ovarian Cancer Screening Trial Group (Univ of Pittsburgh, Pa; et al)

JAMA 290:41-48, 2003 14–1

Background.—Several trials using tandem colonoscopy or colonoscopy by 1 practitioner followed immediately by a second colonoscopy by a second practitioner have demonstrated that adenomas, particularly small adenomas, are easily missed. The extent of adenomas and cancer in the distal colon as detected by repeat flexible sigmoidoscopy (FSG) 3 years after a negative examination was reviewed in the Prostate, Lung, Colorectal, and Ovarian Cancer Screening Trial (PLCO), a randomized, controlled, community-based investigation assessing the effectiveness of cancer screening tests on site-specific mortality rates.

Methods.—The mean patient age was 65.7 years at trial entry (1993-1995); 61.6% were men. Participants underwent screening FSG at baseline and at 3 years as part of the protocol and were referred to their personal physicians for further assessment of screen-identified abnormalities. Results from subsequent diagnostic examinations were tracked using a standardized method. Of 11,583 participants who were eligible for repeat screening FSG 3 years after an initial negative examination, 9317 (80.4%) returned for follow-up. The primary outcome measures were a polyp or mass identified in the distal colon at year 3 repeat FSG; the incidence of adenoma or cancer in the distal colon at year 3 follow-up; determination of reason for detection (increased depth of insertion or improved preparation at the 3-year examination, or detection in a previously inspected area).

Results.—A total of 1292 returning participants (13.9%) had a polyp or mass that was identified by FSG 3 years after the initial examination. In the distal colon, of 9317 participants, 292 (3.1%) had an adenoma or cancer. The incidence of advanced adenoma (n = 72) or cancer (n = 6) identified at the year 3 examination was 78 (0.8%) of 9317. Among participants with advanced distal adenomas identified at the 3-year examination, 58 of 72 (80.6%) had lesions identified in a portion of the colon that had been sufficiently examined at the initial sigmoidoscopy.

Conclusion.—Repeat FSG 3 years after a negative examination will identify advanced adenomas and distal colon cancers at a rate of 0.8%. The overall percentage with identifiable abnormalities is modest, but these data raise concerns about the impact of a prolonged screening interval after a negative FSG examination.

► The Prostate, Lung, Colorectal, and Ovarian Cancer Screening Trial is a prospective, randomized, community-based study that evaluates several screening tests on specific cancer mortality. This article reports the effectiveness of FSG examined 3 years after a prior negative examination. Approximately 1 in 7 such patients had a polyp or mass detected on repeat examination. Were these polyps missed on the initial examination, or did they develop in the interim? By the authors' evaluation, most were thought to be new neoplasms. The proper interval for undergoing an FSG remains unclear, but many recommendations currently are at the 5-year interval. Should colonoscopy be used in place of FSG? It is estimated from this and other articles that about 1% to 2% of new malignancies occur in the proximal colon and are not reached by FSG.[1,2] A colleague described the use of a FSG as similar to obtaining a screening mammogram in one breast only. Perhaps virtual colonoscopy will supplant conventional colonoscopy, but ultimately it should be recognized that endoscopy is both a screening and therapeutic modality. Optimal uses of these modalities are important on a cost-effective basis for this to be useful.

P. J. Loehrer, Sr, MD

References

1. Lieberman DA, Weiss DG, Bond JH, et al: Use of colonoscopy to screen asymptomatic adults for colorectal cancer: Veterans Affairs Cooperative Study Group 380. *N Engl J Med* 343:162-168, 2000.
2. Imperiale TF, Wagner DR, Lin CY, et al: Risk of advanced proximal neoplasms in asymptomatic adults according to the distal colorectal findings. *N Engl J Med* 343:169-174, 2000.

Neoplastic and Antineoplastic Effects of β-Carotene on Colorectal Adenoma Recurrence: Results of a Randomized Trial

Baron JA, Cole BF, Mott L, et al (Dartmouth Med School, Lebanon, NH; Univ of Southern California, Los Angeles; Univ of Minnesota, Minneapolis; et al)
J Natl Cancer Inst 95:717-722, 2003 14–2

Background.—Two large randomized lung cancer chemoprevention trials during the early 1980s investigating β-carotene unexpectedly reported that supplementation with β-carotene increased the risk of lung cancer. Most of the subjects in these studies were cigarette smokers, and the adverse effects occurred predominantly in cigarette smokers who also consumed alcohol. β-Carotene supplementation appeared not to increase the risk of cancer generally, yet it was not clear whether smoking and/or alcohol use alters the effects of β-carotene on carcinogenesis at sites outside the lung. New insight into the effects of β-carotene on carcinogenesis outside the lung was provided. The findings from a randomized double-blind trial of antioxidants, including β-carotene, as preventive agents for recurrence of large-bowel adenomas are presented.

Methods.—This study included 864 patients who had an adenoma removed and who were polyp-free. The patients were randomized to receive β-carotene (25 mg or placebo) and/or vitamins C and E in combination (1000 mg and 400 mg, respectively, or placebo) and followed with colonoscopy for recurrence of adenoma at 1 year and 4 years after the qualifying endoscopy. A total of 707 patients had 2 follow-up examinations and provided information on their smoking habits and alcohol consumption. The effects of β-carotene on adenoma recurrence were assessed with adjusted multivariate risk ratios and 95% CIs.

Results.—Among patients who did not smoke and did not consume alcohol, β-carotene was associated with a significant decrease in the risk of 1 or more recurrent adenomas. However, β-carotene supplementation conferred a modest increase in the risk of recurrence among patients who smoked (relative risk [RR] = 1.36, 95% CI = 0.70-2.62) or consumed alcohol (RR = 1.13, 95% CI = 0.89-1.43). β-carotene doubled the risk of adenoma recurrence in patients who smoked cigarettes and also consumed more than 1 alcoholic drink per day (RR = 2.07, 95% CI = 1.39-3.08).

Conclusions.—Alcohol intake and cigarette smoking appear to modify the effect of β-carotene supplementation on the risk of colorectal adenoma recurrence.

► The gist of this paper is that supplementation with β-carotene given to patients who have had an adenomatous polyp removed can either decrease or increase the risk of subsequent polyp formation. The difference in risk depends on whether subjects continue to drink alcohol or smoke cigarettes. In the latter group, β-carotene supplementation was an adverse factor. This supports the findings of other β-carotene studies with respect to lung cancer.[1,2] The importance of these findings is that a thorough social history with respect to adverse lifestyle activities (smoking, drinking) is doubly important. As we see in the paper by Calle et al (Abstract 18–6), another lifestyle habit also associated with adverse outcome is obesity.

P. J. Loehrer, Sr, MD

References

1. The effect of vitamin E and beta carotene on the incidence of lung cancer and other cancers in male smokers. The Alpha-Tocopherol, Beta Carotene Cancer Prevention Study Group. *N Engl J Med* 330:1029-1035, 1994.
2. Omenn GS, Goodman GE, Thornquist MD, et al: Effects of a combination of beta carotene and vitamin A on lung cancer and cardiovascular disease. *N Engl J Med* 334:1150-1155, 1996.

Prognostic Value of Thymidylate Synthase, Ki-67, and *p53* in Patients With Dukes' B and C Colon Cancer: A National Cancer Institute–National Surgical Adjuvant Breast and Bowel Project Collaborative Study

Allegra CJ, Paik S, Colangelo LH, et al (NIH, Bethesda, Md; Natl Surgical Adjuvant Breast and Bowel Project, Pittsburgh, Pa; Belfast City Hosp, Northern Ireland)

J Clin Oncol 21:241-250, 2003 14–3

Background.—Colorectal cancer is the third most common cancer in the United States. Approximately 60% of all patients diagnosed with colorectal carcinoma will present with locally advanced disease. For these patients, appropriate therapeutic decision making is dependent primarily on the depth of penetration of the primary tumor and malignant involvement of the regional lymph nodes. Under present guidelines, many patients will receive chemotherapy unnecessarily, yet other patients who might benefit from it are not recommended to receive chemotherapy. The value of thymidylate synthase (TS), Ki-67, and *p53* as prognostic markers in patients with stage II and III colon cancer was defined.

Methods.—A retrospective analysis was conducted of the prognostic value of TS, Ki-67, and *p53* in 706 patients with Duke's B (291 patients) or Dukes' C (415 patients) colon carcinoma who were treated with either surgery alone (275 patients) or surgery plus fluorouracil-leucovorin chemotherapy (431 patients) in National Surgical Adjuvant Breast and Bowel Project protocols C01-C03. Immunohistochemical techniques were used to analyze these 3 markers. Five years of follow-up data were used for this analysis.

Results.—This retrospective analysis found an association between the intensity of TS, Ki-67, and *p53* for recurrence-free survival and overall survival (Table 3). High TS intensity levels and positive *p53* staining were associated with a worse outcome (Fig 3). Patients with tumors that contained a high percentage of Ki-67–positive cells enjoyed an improved outcome compared with patients with tumors containing relatively few positive cells. No interaction with treatment was identified for any marker.

Conclusions.—These findings show that TS, Ki-67, and *p53* staining each had significant prognostic value in patients with Dukes' B and C colon carcinoma. However, none of these markers demonstrated sufficient power to clearly discern groups of patients who could be predicted to obtain greater or lesser benefit from the use of adjuvant chemotherapy.

► We are getting closer, but not quite there yet. This is a very elegant paper by Dr Allegra that attempts to correlate several markers to define a treatment algorithm. As expected, overexpression of TS and mutated *p53* was associated with a decreased relapse-free survival and overall survival. What is difficult to understand is that higher proliferative indices (as measured by Ki67) were associated with a better outcome. In total, these factors categorize those pa-

TABLE 3.—Five-Year Outcomes

Marker and Subset	RFS N	RFS Events	RFS Hazard Ratio	RFS P	Survival N	Survival Deaths	Survival Hazard Ratio	Survival P
p53(±)								
Dukes' B/C	379	129	1.49		379	124	1.21	
	321	77	(1.12-1.98)	.01	321	87	(.92-1.59)	.18
Dukes' B	147	35	1.50		147	33	1.26	
	141	23	(.88-2.53)	.13	141	25	(.75-2.12)	.39
Dukes' C	232	94	1.49		232	91	1.19	
	180	54	(1.06-2.09)	.02	180	62	(.86-1.64)	.30
Ki-67 (3-5/1-2)								
Dukes' B/C	361	94	.76		361	85	.62	
	342	114	(.58-1.01)	.05	342	128	(.47-.82)	.001
Dukes' B	146	32	1.25		146	29	1.05	
	145	28	(.75-2.09)	.39	145	31	(.63-1.75)	.86
Dukes' C	215	62	.62		215	56	.50	
	197	86	(.45-.87)	.005	197	97	(.36-.70)	.0001
TS Pattern (D/F)								
Dukes' B/C	451	142	1.04		451	149	1.13	
	214	63	(.77-1.41)	.79	214	61	(.84-1.53)	.42
Dukes' B	179	33	.63		179	33	.59	
	92	23	(.37-1.07)	.08	92	24	(.35-1.00)	.05
Dukes' C	272	109	1.29		272	116	1.50	
	122	40	(.89-1.36)	.18	122	37	(1.03-2.19)	.03
TS Intensity (3/0-2)								
Dukes' B/C	274	101	1.46		274	106	1.54	
	417	107	(1.11-1.92)	.01	417	106	(1.17-2.02)	.002
Dukes' B	109	23	1.12		109	25	1.27	
	174	35	(.66-1.90)	.68	174	32	(.75-2.15)	.37
Dukes' C	165	78	1.62		165	81	1.65	
	243	72	(1.17-2.24)	.004	243	74	(1.20-2.28)	.002

(Courtesy of Allegra CJ, Paik S, Colangelo LH, et al: Prognostic value of thymidylate synthase, Ki-67, and *p53* in patients with Dukes' B and C colon cancer: A National Cancer Institute–National Surgical Adjuvant Breast and Bowel Project Collaborative Study. *J Clin Oncol* 21:241-250, 2003. Reprinted with permission from the American Society of Clinical Oncology.)

FIGURE 3

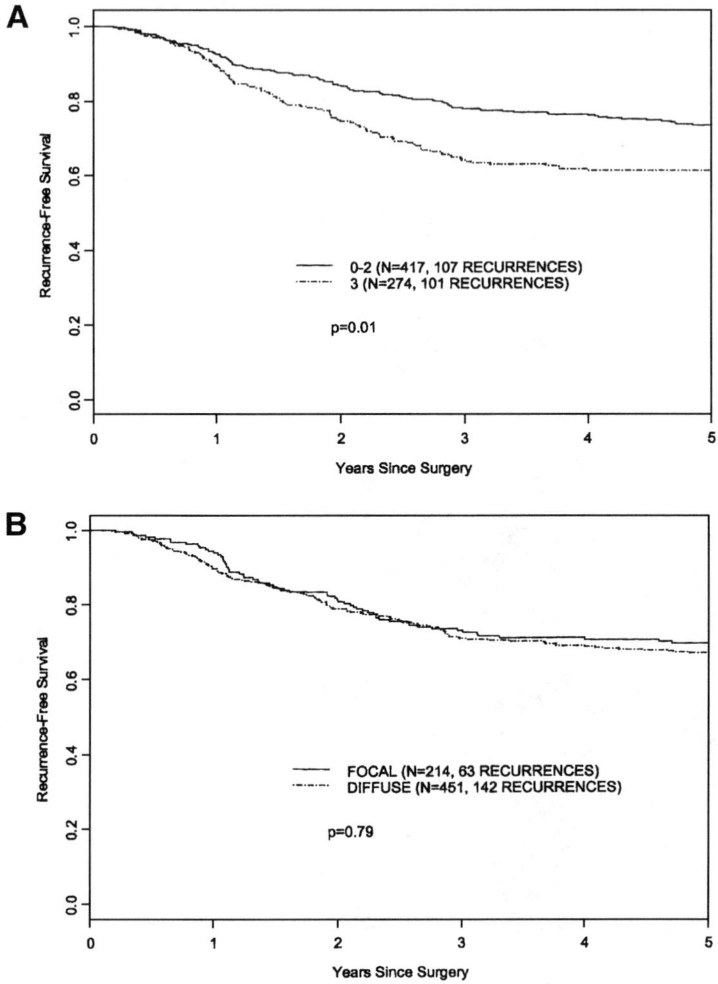

(Continued)

tients with a relatively good prognosis (80% vs 51% for relapsed-free survival). Unfortunately, this paper does not yet tease out the treatment-related outcomes as to whether those patients with poor expectations would benefit from specific therapy. This is a good start, however.

P. J. Loehrer, Sr, MD

FIGURE 3 (cont.)

C

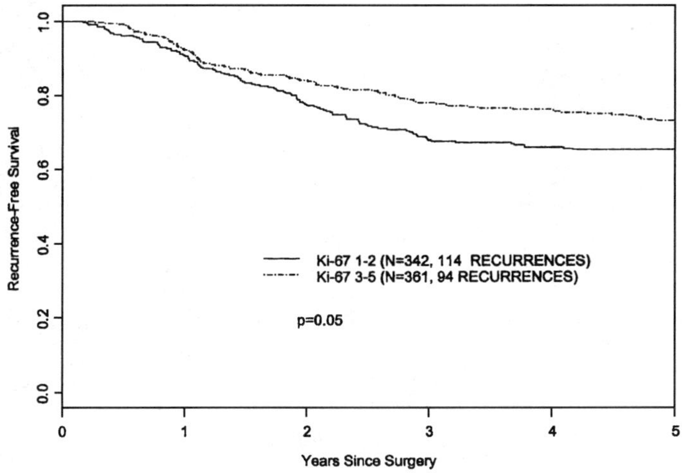

D

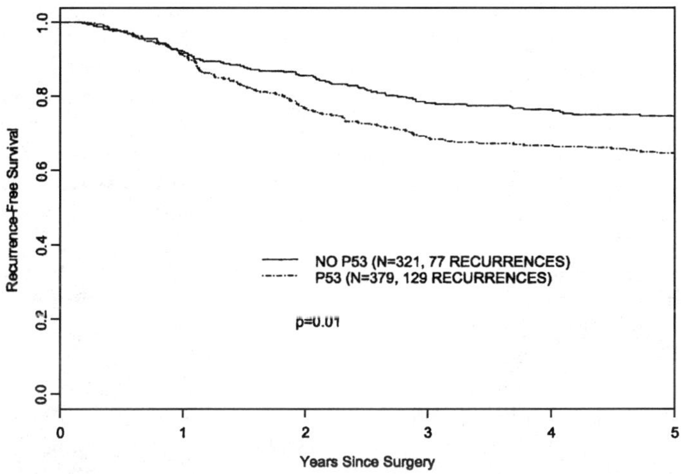

FIGURE 3.—**A,** The 5-year recurrence-free survival (*RFS*) curve for thymidylate synthase (*TS*) intensity when analyzed according to the categories listed in Table 2. **B,** The 5-year RFS curve for TS staining pattern when analyzed according to the categories listed in Table 2. Figure **C** represents the 5-year RFS curve for Ki-67 when analyzed according to the categories shown in Table 2. **D,** The 5-year RFS curve for *p53* when analyzed according to the categories listed in Table 2. (Courtesy of Allegra CJ, Paik S, Colangelo LH, et al: Prognostic value of thymidylate synthase, Ki-67, and *p53* in patients with Dukes' B and C colon cancer: A National Cancer Institute–National Surgical Adjuvant Breast and Bowel Project Collaborative Study. *J Clin Oncol* 21:241-250, 2003. Reprinted with permission from the American Society of Clinical Oncology.)

Tumor Microsatellite-Instability Status as a Predictor of Benefit From Fluorouracil-Based Adjuvant Chemotherapy for Colon Cancer

Ribic CM, Sargent DJ, Moore MJ, et al (Univ of Toronto; Mayo Found, Rochester, Minn; Queen's Univ, Kingston, Ontario, Canada; et al)

N Engl J Med 349:247-257, 2003 14–4

Background.—Colon cancers with high-frequency microsatellite instability manifest clinical and pathologic features that can be used to differentiate them from microsatellite-stable tumors. The usefulness of microsatellite-instability status as a predictor of the benefits of adjuvant chemotherapy with fluorouracil in patients with stage II and stage III colon cancer was evaluated.

Methods.—Specimens were obtained from 570 patients with colon cancer who were enrolled in randomized trials of fluorouracil-based adjuvant chemotherapy. Mononucleotide and dinucleotide markers were used to assess microsatellite instability.

Results.—Of the 570 specimens evaluated, 95 (16.7%) showed high-frequency microsatellite instability. Among 287 patients who did not receive adjuvant therapy, patients with tumors that demonstrated high-frequency microsatellite instability had a better 5-year rate of overall survival than patients with tumors that exhibited microsatellite stability or low-frequency instability (Fig 1). Among the remaining patients who received adjuvant chemotherapy, no correlation was found between high-frequency microsatellite instability and increased overall survival. Benefits of treatment were significantly different according to the microsatellite-instability status. On multivariate analysis adjusted for stage and grade, overall survival was improved by adjuvant chemotherapy in patients with microsatellite-stable tumors or tumors that demonstrated low-frequency microsatellite instability. However, there was no benefit of adjuvant chemotherapy among patients with high-frequency microsatellite instability.

Conclusions.—Fluorouracil-based adjuvant chemotherapy provided benefits to patients with stage II or stage III colon cancer with microsatellite-stable tumors or tumors exhibiting low-frequency microsatellite instability, but not patients with tumors that demonstrated high-frequency microsatellite instability.

► Patients with a higher frequency of microsatellite instability have an improved survival compared with the remainder of the colorectal cancer patients. Uncertain is the impact of adjuvant chemotherapy in patients with microsatellite instability. This is an excellent retrospective analysis of 570 tumor specimens obtained from patients entered in prospective cooperative group trials. Of note, the untreated patients with tumors displaying high-frequency microsatellite-instability (MSI) indeed do better than patients with tumors showing microsatellite-stability or low-frequency instability. Yet in those patients who received adjuvant chemotherapy, MSI did not have an impact on survival. This suggests that tumors with MSI are less responsive to chemo-

A No Adjuvant Chemotherapy

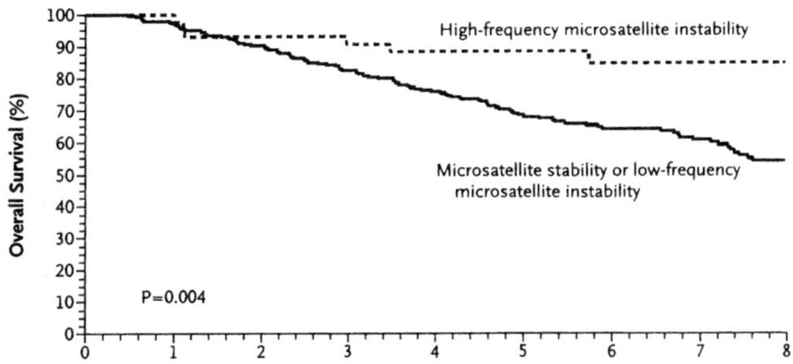

No. at Risk	0	1	2	3	4	5	6	7	8
Microsatellite stability or low-frequency microsatellite instability	245	238	220	200	176	137	105	82	53
High-frequency microsatellite instability	42	42	39	38	35	29	23	22	14

B Adjuvant Chemotherapy

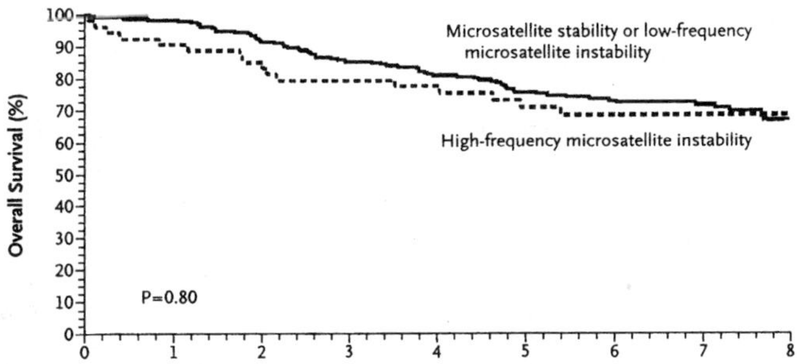

No. at Risk	0	1	2	3	4	5	6	7	8
Microsatellite stability or low-frequency microsatellite instability	230	226	209	194	181	147	123	92	59
High-frequency microsatellite instability	53	48	45	41	38	31	24	19	14

FIGURE 1.—Kaplan-Meier estimates of overall survival among patients with stage II or stage III colon cancer according to the microsatellite-instability status of the tumor. In the absence of adjuvant chemotherapy, the patients with tumors displaying high-frequency microsatellite instability had significantly longer overall survival than patients with tumors exhibiting microsatellite stability or low-frequency microsatellite instability (hazard ratio for death, 0.31 [95 percent confidence interval, 0.14 to 0.72]; $P = .004$). (**A**). When the analysis was limited to the group receiving adjuvant chemotherapy, patients with tumors exhibiting high-frequency microsatellite instability did not have a significant increase in overall survival as compared with patients with tumors exhibiting microsatellite stability or low-frequency microsatellite instability (hazard ratio for death, 1.07 [95 percent confidence interval, 0.62 to 1.86]; $P = .80$). (**B**). The analysis included data for eight years from the date of randomization. (Reprinted by permission of *The New England Journal of Medicine* from Ribic CM, Sargent DJ, Moore MJ, et al: Tumor microsatellite-instability status as a predictor of benefit from fluorouracil-based adjuvant chemotherapy for color cancer. *N Engl J Med* 349:247-257, 2003. Copyright 2003, Massachusetts Medical Society. All rights reserved.)

therapy. Whether alternative chemotherapy regimens with oxaliplatin or irinotecan would impact this population remains uncertain, but is worthy of further analysis.

P. J. Loehrer, Sr, MD

Adverse Prognostic Effect of Methylation in Colorectal Cancer Is Reversed by Microsatellite Instability

Ward RL, Cheong K, Ku S-L, et al (St Vincent's Hosp, Darlinghurst, Australia; Univ of New South Wales, Sydney, Australia)

J Clin Oncol 21:3729-3736, 2003 14–5

Background.—DNA methylation, an important biologic event in colorectal cancer, is sometimes associated with development of microsatellite instability. The prognostic significance of DNA methylation was investigated.

Methods.—A total of 625 cancer tissue samples were obtained from 605 patients, aged 29 to 99 years, undergoing curative surgery for colorectal cancer at 1 center during an 8-year period. Data from follow-up to 5 years were analyzed. Methylation-specific polymerase chain reaction (PCR) was used to determine methylation of *p16* and *hMLH1* promoters. Bisulfite-PCR was used to assess methylation at methylated-in-tumor (MINT)1, MINT2, MINT12, and MINT31 loci.

Findings.—Twelve percent of the patients had microsatellite unstable tumors. These patients had a better disease-specific survival rate than those with microsatellite stable (MSS) tumors. Three independently significant factors—tumor stage, heavy tumor methylation, and vascular space invasion—influenced the overall survival of patients with MSS tumors. Methylation at any single site did not independently predict survival in patients with MSS tumors. Favorable response to chemotherapy was not predicted by methylation or microsatellite status.

Conclusions.—In patients with colorectal cancer, DNA methylation correlates with a worse outcome. However, this adverse prognostic effect is not seen in methylated tumors showing microsatellite instability. Further research is needed to investigate the mechanisms of these events.

► Prognosticating patients with colorectal cancer via molecular markers is still in its infancy. A variety of molecular markers such as *p53, K-ras, 18q loss, c-myc,* and *HER-2* have had inconsistent results. Microsatellite instability (MSI) has been associated with an improved disease-free survival rate in patients with colorectal cancer. MSI may arise from 2 means: methylation of the *hMLH1* promoter (in sporadic colorectal cancer) and germ-line mutations of a mismatch repair gene (in hereditary nonpolyposis colorectal cancer).

This review confirms that MSI tumors are associated with a better outcome. In contrast, in patients with MSS tumors, heavy methylation was associated with a significantly worse outcome. Of interest, heavily methylated tumors in patients with MSI were not associated with worse prognostic factors. How these findings are to be incorporated into the clinical setting is not clear, but prospective evaluation of known prognostic markers may lead to more specific therapeutic options.

P. J. Loehrer, Sr, MD

Phase II, Randomized Trial Comparing Bevacizumab Plus Fluorouracil (FU)/Leucovorin (LV) With FU/LV Alone in Patients With Metastatic Colorectal Cancer

Kabbinavar F, Hurwitz HI, Fehrenbacher L, et al (Univ of California Los Angeles; Kaiser Permanente, Vallejo, Calif; Genentech, Inc, South San Francisco, Calif; et al)

J Clin Oncol 21:60-65, 2003 14–6

Background.—Inhibitors of tumor vascularization are a promising new approach to cancer treatment. Vascular endothelial growth factor (VEGF) is an important tumor angiogenic factor. Bevacizumab, a recombinant humanized monoclonal antibody to VEGF, was evaluated as a first-line treatment for metastatic colorectal cancer.

Methods.—The randomized controlled trial included 104 previously untreated patients with histologically confirmed, measurable colorectal carcinoma. There were 59 men and 45 women with liver and/or lung metastases. They were randomly assigned to receive fluorouracil/leucovorin (FU/LV), 500/500/mg/m^2 alone; FU/LV plus low-dose bevacizumab, 10 mg/kg every 2 weeks; or FU/LV plus high-dose bevacizumab, 10 mg/kg every 2 weeks. Treatment with FU/LV was given weekly through the first 6 weeks of each 8-week cycle, to a maximum of 6 cycles. Disease response and progression was evaluated.

Results.—Response rates were 17% for patients receiving FU/LV alone compared with 40% with low-dose bevacizumab and 24% with high-dose bevacizumab. The median time to disease progression was 5.2 months in the control group compared with 9.0 and 7.2 months in the low- and high-dose bevacizumab groups, respectively. The median survival was 13.8 months for LU/FV controls, 21.5 months with low-dose bevacizumab, and 16.1 months with high-dose bevacizumab. Thrombosis was the major adverse effect of bevacizumab, causing 1 death. Other adverse events included hypertension, proteinuria, and epistaxis.

Twenty-two controls were crossed over to receive single-agent treatment with bevacizumab. Partial responses occurred in 2 patients, with stable disease in another 7.

Conclusions.—This phase II randomized trial suggests that low-dose bevacizumab, combined with FU/LV chemotherapy, has significant benefits in terms of response rate and survival in patients with metastatic colorectal cancer. Ongoing phase III trials will provide further data on the role of anti-VEGF therapy with bevacizumab.

► This trial in previously untreated patients suggests that bevacizumab, a recombinant humanized monoclonal antibody to VEGF, is used to enhance the therapeutic efforts of FU/LV. A more recent trial in previously untreated patients with irinotecan, FU/LV also demonstrated improvement at the most recent American Society of Clinical Oncology meetings. The ultimate role of this drug in primary and salvage therapy needed to be defined, but these data suggest that indeed angiogenesis inhibition appears to be a valid therapeutic target in advanced colorectal cancer.

P. J. Loehrer, Sr, MD

Phase III Comparison of Two Irinotecan Dosing Regimens in Second-Line Therapy of Metastatic Colorectal Cancer

Fuchs CS, Moore MR, Harker G, et al (Dana-Farber Cancer Inst, Boston; Georgia Cancer Research Ctr, Decatur, Ga; Intermountain Hematology/Oncology Associates, PC, Salt Lake City, Utah; et al)

J Clin Oncol 21:807-814, 2003 14–7

Objective.—In phase II clinical trials, irinotecan has shown survival advantages in patients with fluorouracil-refractory colorectal cancer. One research group recommended a weekly regimen of irinotecan at a dose of 125 mg/m², whereas another recommended treatment once every 3 weeks at a dose of 350 g/m². A phase III trial was performed to compare these 2 irinotecan schedules for efficacy, safety, and quality of life.

Methods.—The multicenter open-label trial included 291 patients with recurrent or progressive metastatic colorectal cancer after fluorouracil-based chemotherapy. In a 1:2 ratio, patients were randomly assigned to the weekly or once every 3 weeks irinotecan schedules. In the latter group, the irinotecan dose was reduced to 300 mg/m² in patients who were aged 70 years or older, had an Eastern Cooperative Oncology group performance status of 2, or had previously undergone pelvic irradiation. Efficacy, safety, and quality of life outcomes were compared.

Results.—At a median follow-up of 15.8 months, efficacy outcomes were similar between groups. One-year survival was 46% with the weekly irinotecan regimen and 41% with the once every 3 weeks regimen. The median survival was 9.6 and 9.9 months and median time to progression was 4.0 and 3.0 months, respectively. The rate of grade 3/4 diarrhea was 36% on the once-weekly regimen compared with 19% on the once every 3 weeks regimen, whereas the rate of grade 3/4 neutropenia was 29% compared with 34%, respectively. Treatment-related death was somewhat more likely in the weekly group, at 5.3% versus 1.6%.

Conclusions.—In patients with fluorouracil-refractory metastatic colorectal cancer, the weekly and once every 3 weeks irinotecan regimens result in comparable survival and quality of life outcomes. The latter regimen results in a lower rate of severe diarrhea and a nonsignificantly lower risk of treatment-related death.

► This is a well-conceived industry-sponsored trial that sought to determine the optimal dose and schedule for irinotecan in patients with advanced colorectal cancer. The study was powered to detect a 15% improvement of survival at 1 year, which was not seen. The incidence of severe (grade 3/4) diarrhea, however, was nearly doubled (36% vs 19%) in the weekly group compared with the every 3 weeks group. A similar trend was noted in treatment-related mortality rate. For those patients who are candidates for single agent CPT-11, this may be at least one means to improve morbidity rate.

P. J. Loehrer, Sr, MD

Superiority of Oxaliplatin and Fluorouracil-Leucovorin Compared With Either Therapy Alone in Patients With Progressive Colorectal Cancer After Irinotecan and Fluorouracil-Leucovorin: Interim Results of a Phase III Trial

Rothenberg ML, Oza AM, Bigelow RH, et al (Vanderbilt-Ingram Cancer Ctr, Nashville, Tenn; Princess Margaret Hosp, Toronto; Sanofi-Synthelabo Research, Malvern, Canada)

J Clin Oncol 21:2059-2069, 2003 14–8

Introduction.—In the United States, the most common form of front-line chemotherapy for metastatic colorectal cancer is the combination of irinotecan, fluorouracil, and leucovorin (IFL). There is currently no effective therapeutic option for patients with progressive metastases after failure of IFL. Oxaliplatin, alone and in combination with fluorouracil and leucovorin, was evaluated for use in patients with progressive colorectal cancer.

Methods.—The randomized trial included 463 patients from 120 North American centers who had progression of metastatic colorectal cancer after initial IFL treatment. One group received bolus and infusional fluorouracil and leucovorin (LV5FU2), another received single-agent therapy with oxaliplatin, and a third received oxaliplatin in combination with fluorouracil/leucovorin (FOLFOX4). Interim analysis of this initial patient cohort included the outcomes of response rate, time to tumor progression (TTP), and effects on tumor-related symptoms.

Results.—On the basis of independent radiologic assessments, the objective response rate was 9.9% with FOLFOX4 compared with 0% with LV5FU2 and 1.3% with oxaliplatin alone. All responses were partial. FOLFOX4 had a median TTP of 4.6 months compared with 2.7 months for patients receiving LV5FU2 and 1.6% with oxaliplatin only. Thirty-three percent of the FOLFOX4 group had relief of tumor-related symptoms compared with 12% with LV5FU2. Clinical toxicity was more frequent with FOLFOX4 than with LV5FU2, but these predictable adverse effects did not increase the rate of treatment discontinuation or 60-day mortality rate.

Conclusions.—For patients with metastatic colorectal cancer that progresses after initial IFL treatment, the FOLFOX4 combination regimen is a promising form of second-line therapy. FOLFOX4 is superior to LV5FU2 in all efficacy end points measured, including response rate, time to progression, and symptom reduction. Oxaliplatin alone is no more effective than LV5FU2.

► It would not seem logical that one would use 5-fluorouracil (5-FU) as part of salvage therapy in patients who had already progressed on 5-fluorouracil. Preclinical data from 7 research institutes many years ago demonstrated synergy of cisplatin plus 5-fluorouracil. As a result, this simple phase III trial in patients who have progressive colorectal cancer has rather important clinical relevance. Rothenberg et al confirm a potential synergy with these 2 drugs with respect to response rates and time to progression. These differences are modest; however, I believe they are clinically relevant.

P. J. Loehrer, Sr, MD

Impact of T and N Substage on Survival and Disease Relapse in Adjuvant Rectal Cancer: A Pooled Analysis

Gunderson LL, Sargent DJ, Tepper JE, et al (Mayo Clinic, Scottsdale, Ariz; Mayo Clinic, Rochester, Minn; Univ of North Carolina, Chapel Hill; et al)

Int J Radiat Oncol Biol Phys 54:386-396, 2002 14–9

Background.—The staging classifications for cancers of the large bowel depend on the depth of primary tumor invasion, both within and beyond the bowel wall, as well as on the presence or absence of nodal or distant metastases. Differences in the staging systems or incorrect interpretations of these systems may create difficulties when comparing treatment results. The National Institutes of Health Consensus conference noted that a modification of the Astler-Coller rectal cancer staging system (MAC) is commonly used in the United States, but the conference made a plea for more standard use of the Tumor, Node, Metastasis (TNM) system. The rates of survival and disease control by TNM and MAC stage in 3 randomized North American rectal adjuvant studies were investigated.

Methods.—Data were obtained for 2551 eligible patients from the NCCTG 79-47-51, the NCCTG 86-47-51, and the INT 114 trials. All of the patients received postoperative radiation, and 96% were randomly assigned to concomitant and maintenance chemotherapy. Five-year follow-up was available for 94% of patients, and 7-year follow-up was available for 84%. The distribution of overall survival (OS) and disease-free survival (DFS) was estimated with Kaplan-Meier analysis. The log-rank test was used to determine *P* values, and time to local and distant relapse was estimated with cumulative incidence methodology. Analyses were adjusted for treatment effect using Cox proportional hazards modeling.

Results.—OS and DFS depended on both TN stage and NT stage (Figs 1 and 2). T stage influenced OS, even among N2 patients (Tables 4A and 4B). As a result of these findings, 3 risk groups of patients were defined: intermediate (T3N0, T1-2N1), moderately high (T4N0, T1-2N2, T2N1), and high (T3N2, T4N1, T4N2).

For group 1 (intermediate), the 5-year OS was 74% and 81% and DFS was 66% and 74% (Table 5A). For group 2 (moderately high), the 5-year OS ranged from 61% to 69%, and for group 3 (high), the 5-year OS ranged from 33% to 48% (Table 5B). The cumulative incidence rates of local relapse and distant metastases showed similar differences by TN and NT stage.

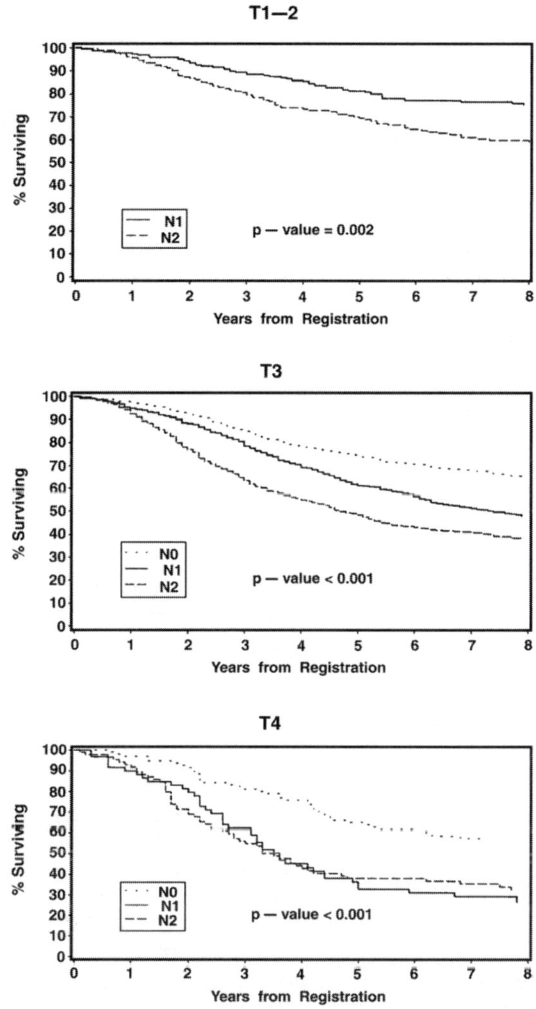

FIGURE 1.—Impact of TN stage on overall survival in the rectal cancer pooled analysis. *P* values reflect pairwise comparisons between the adjacent TN stages of patients (the impact of N substage within the 3 separate T stages; T1-2N1 vs T1-2N2; R3N0 vs T3N1, T3N2; T4N0 vs T4N1, T4N2). (Reprinted from Gunderson LL, Sargent DJ, Tepper JE, et al: Impact of T and N substage on survival and disease relapse in adjuvant rectal cancer: A pooled analysis. *Int J Radiat Oncol Biol Phys* 54:386-396, 2002. Copyright 2002, with permission from Elsevier Science.)

Conclusion.—For patients with rectal cancer with a single high-risk factor of either extension beyond the rectal wall (T3N0) or nodal involvement (T1-2N1), OS and DFS and disease control have improved when compared with those with both high-risk factors. The different survival rates and rates of relapse for intermediate-risk versus moderately high or high-risk patients

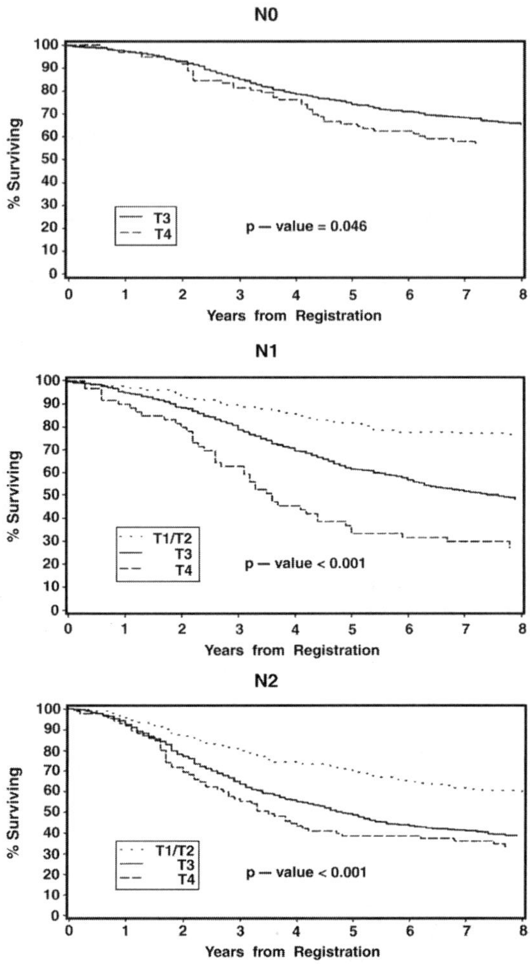

FIGURE 2.—Impact of NT stage on overall survival in the rectal cancer pooled analysis. *P* values reflect pairwise comparisons between the adjacent NT stages of patients (the impact of T substage within the 3 separate N stages). (Reprinted from Gunderson LL, Sargent DJ, Tepper JE, et al: Impact of T and N substage on survival and disease relapse in adjuvant rectal cancer: A pooled analysis. *Int J Radiat Oncol Biol Phys* 54:386-396, 2002. Copyright 2002, with permission from Elsevier Science.)

may warrant different treatment strategies for these groups. It may be preferable in the future to perform separate studies for each of these risk groups.

► This article represents pooled data from 3 different randomized studies of postresection radiation therapy, usually with concurrent chemotherapy in patients with rectal cancer. Both primary stage and nodal status were relevant

TABLE 4A.—Pooled Rectal Analysis: Impact of T stage and TN Stage on Survival

	Overall Survival*			Disease-free Survival*		
Classification	No.	5-yr (%)	*P* Value	No.	5-yr (%)	*P* Value
(T stage)						
T1-T2	412	76		412	69	
T3	1896	61	<0.001	1880	52	<0.001
T4	241	47		241	39	
(TN stage)						
T1-2N1	225	81	0.002	225	74	<0.001
N2	180	69		180	62	
T3N0	668	74		664	65	
N1	544	61	<0.001	536	51	<0.001
N2	663	48		659	38	
T4N0	95	65		95	54	
N1	59	33	<0.001	59	30	<0.001
N2	84	38		84	30	

*Unadjusted Kaplan-Meier estimates.

(Reprinted from Gunderson LL, Sargent DJ, Tepper JE, et al: Impact of T and N substage on survival and disease relapse in adjuvant rectal cancer: A pooled analysis. *Int J Radiat Oncol Biol Phys* 54:386-396, 2002. Copyright 2002, with permission from Elsevier Science.)

prognostically. The greater the number of negative factors, the worse the prognosis turned out to be. This all seems reasonable and predictable. The authors argue that these factors may have to be taken into account for future prospective studies.

TABLE 4B.—Impact of T Stage and TN Stage on Disease Relapse

		Local Recurrence†		Distant Metastases†	
Classification	No.	5-yr (%)	*P* Value	5-yr (%)	*P* Value
(T stage)					
T1-2	412	7		20	
T3	1880	11	<0.001	32	<0.001
T4	241	18		40	
(TN stage)					
T1-2N1	225	6	0.06	15	<0.001
N2	180	8		26	
T3N0	664	8		19	
N1	536	11	<0.001	34	<0.001
N2	659	15		45	
T4N0	95	15		28	
N1	59	22	0.48	39	0.004
N2	84	19		50	

†Cumulative incidence rates.

(Reprinted from Gunderson LL, Sargent DJ, Tepper JE, et al: Impact of T and N substage on survival and disease relapse in adjuvant rectal cancer: A pooled analysis. *Int J Radiat Oncol Biol Phys* 54:386-396, 2002. Copyright 2002, with permission from Elsevier Science.)

TABLE 5A.—Pooled Rectal Analysis: Impact of N Stage and NT Stage on Survival

	Survival - 5 yr (%)*					
Stage	No	OS	*P* Value	No.	DFS	*P* Value
(N stage)						
N0	763	73		759	64	
N1	828	65	<0.001	820	56	<0.001
N2	929	52		925	42	
(NT stage)						
N0T3	668	74	0.046	664	66	0.05
T4	95	65		95	54	
N1T1-2	225	81		225	74	
T3	544	61	<0.001	536	50	<0.001
T4	59	33		59	30	
N2T1-2	180	69		180	62	
T3	663	48	<0.001	659	39	<0.001
T4	84	38		84	30	

*Unadjusted Kaplan-Meier estimates.
Abbreviations: OS, Overall survival; *DFS*, disease-free survival.
(Reprinted from Gunderson LL, Sargent DJ, Tepper JE, et al: Impact of T and N substage on survival and disease relapse in adjuvant rectal cancer: A pooled analysis. *Int J Radiat Oncol Biol Phys* 54:386-396, 2002. Copyright 2002, with permission from Elsevier Science.)

There are subgroups within any and all staging categories. This is inherent because staging groups patients together largely on the basis of the anatomy of their disease. This "lumping" process inevitably creates interest in "splitting" subgroups out. This whole area really depends on whether one is more interested in the similarities among patients or their differences. That is what "makes for horse races."

E. Glatstein, MD

TABLE 5B.—Impact of N and NT Stage on Disease Relapse

	Disease Relapse - 5 yr (%)*				
Stage	No.	Local	*P* Value	Distant	*P* Value
(N stage)					
N0	759	9		20	
N1	820	10	<0.001	29	<0.001
N2	925	14		42	
(NT stage)					
N0T3	664	8	0.04	19	0.04
T4	95	15		28	
N1T1-2	225	6		15	
T3	536	11	0.002	34	<0.001
T4	59	22		39	
N2T1-2	180	8		26	
T3	659	15	0.14	45	<0.001
T4	84	19		50	

*Cumulative incidence rates.
(Reprinted from Gunderson LL, Sargent DJ, Tepper JE, et al: Impact of T and N substage on survival and disease relapse in adjuvant rectal cancer: A pooled analysis. *Int J Radiat Oncol Biol Phys* 54:386-396, 2002. Copyright 2002, with permission from Elsevier Science.)

Macroscopic Evaluation of Rectal Cancer Resection Specimen: Clinical Significance of the Pathologist in Quality Control

Nagtagaal ID, for the Cooperative Clinical Investigators of the Dutch Colorectal Cancer Group (Leiden Univ, The Netherlands; et al)

J Clin Oncol 20:1729-1734, 2002 14–10

Introduction.—In the quality assessment of surgical procedures, indirect parameters (complications, recurrence, survival rates) are of limited value for the individual surgeon. Direct assessment of the result of surgery is potentially more useful. Standardization of treatment for rectal cancer was able to be accomplished in the Dutch trial of radiotherapy plus total mesorectal excision (TME). The quality of the mesorectal excision of patients treated in this trial was assessed by examining the resection specimen on arrival in the pathology department. Criteria by which pathologists can judge the quality or completeness of the resection specimen were assessed.

Methods.—The pathology reports of all patients seen between January 1996 through December 1999 from this large randomized multicenter trial were reviewed. To guarantee a standard surgical technique within the trial, instructor surgeons supervised the first 5 TME procedures performed by any participating surgeon. All participating pathologists were instructed in workshops and videos in how to obtain a standardized pathology workup. A 3-tiered classification was applied to evaluate completeness of the TME. The prognostic value of this classification system was examined by log-rank analysis of Kaplan-Meier survival curves with the data of all patients who did not undergo any adjuvant treatment.

Results.—Of 180 patients for whom data were available concerning the quality of the mesorectum reports, 102 (56.6%) specimens were classified as complete, 35 (19.4%) as nearly complete, and 43 (23.9%) as incomplete mesorectum. Forty-one patients had a positive resection margin (tumor cells within 1 mm of the inked resection margin). In 44%, the specimens were incomplete, compared with 11% in patients with margins more than 1 cm ($P <$ .001). In 44% of the tumor, node, metastases stage III patients in whom margin involvement was ascertained by the primary tumor, the mesorectum was incomplete. This was significantly higher compared with patients with a negative margin (24%; $P <$ .05). The groups with complete and nearly complete mesorectum were combined for analyses because there were no differences in their prognoses. The overall recurrence rates were worse in the incomplete group at 2-year follow-up compared with the combined group (35.6% vs 21.5%; $P =$ .01) (Fig 2). Survival rates were similar (76% vs 85%; $P =$ .10). In patients with a positive resection margin, the quality assessment of surgery on prognosis conferred no added benefit ($P =$ .97). In patients with negative resection margins, the overall rate of recurrence was higher in the group with incomplete mesorectum (28.6% vs 14.9%; $P =$ .03), with both local recurrence (11.4% vs 5.5%; $P =$ .09) and distant recurrence (19.2% vs 11.4%; $P =$ .11) contributing to this effect. Survival was 90.5% in patients with complete mesorectum compared with 76.9% in those with an incomplete mesorectum ($P <$ .05).

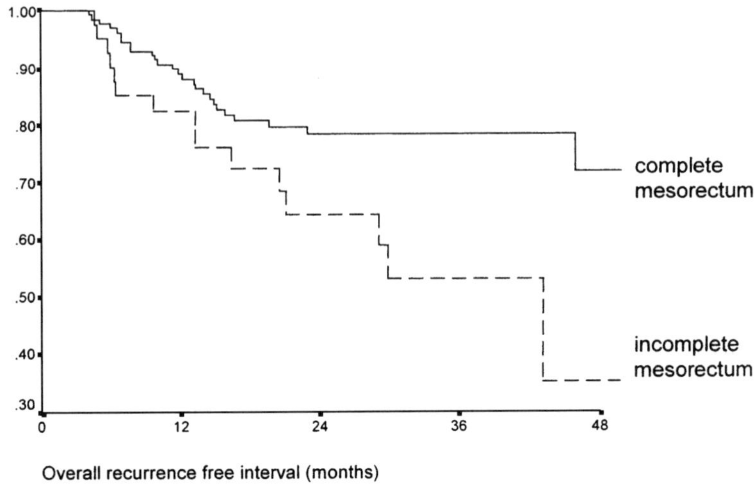

FIGURE 2.—Relation of completeness of mesorectal excision with overall recurrence rates. Patients with a complete mesorectum show significantly lower overall recurrence rates than patients with an incomplete mesorectum ($P = .010$). Log-rank testing was used. (Courtesy of Nagtagaal ID, for the Cooperative Clinical Investigators of the Dutch Colorectal Cancer Group: Macroscopic evaluation of rectal cancer resection specimen: Clinical significance of the pathologist in quality control. *J Clin Oncol* 20:1729-1734, 2002. Reprinted with permission from the American Society of Clinical Oncology.)

Conclusion.—Pathologists are able to judge the quality of TME in patients with rectal cancer. With the aid of this direct interdisciplinary evaluation instrument, a new role in quality control has been created for the pathologist.

► Although clinical trials of adjuvant therapy have detailed entry criteria and follow-up procedures to ensure standardization, little attention has been paid to the potential impact of lack of surgical quality control on protocol outcomes. Variation in the surgical procedure has the potential to result in inaccurate staging and may have a direct impact on survival. A major problem with surgical quality control has been the difficulty in assessing the quality of the surgical procedure by reviewing the operative note. In this innovative study from Nagtagaal et al and the Dutch Colorectal Cancer Group, the ability of the pathologist to assess the completeness of total mesorectal excision was evaluated. A significant relationship between the assessment of the completeness of the resection and the outcomes of local recurrence and survival (in patients with negative margins) was observed. Of note, pathologists were trained by videos, newsletters, and workshops—all low-cost, portable techniques. This suggests that a targeted pathology exam can survive as a surrogate for intraoperative observation as a quality control measure, at least in the case of total mesorectal excision. Surgical quality control is useful not only to ensure that optimal results are obtained from trials of adjuvant therapy, but also allows individual surgeons to audit their own practices.

M. Morrow, MD

Long-term Control of T2-T3 Rectal Adenocarcinoma With Radiotherapy Alone

Gerard J-P, Chapet O, Ramaioli A, et al (Centre Hospitlier Lyon Sud, France; Centre Antoine-Lacassagne, Nice, France)

Int J Radiat Oncol Biol Phys 54:142-149, 2002 14–11

Background.—Abdominoperineal resection is the usual treatment for low-lying T2-T3 rectal adenocarcinomas in most institutions. Combined approaches with the addition of radiotherapy (RT) have been used to improve local control and possibly increase sphincter preservation. However, radical surgery is not performed in some patients with T2-T3 low-lying rectal adenocarcinomas, either because the patient is considered inoperable due to age, performance status, or comorbidity, or the patient refuses abdominoperineal resection as the only option. In some cases, selected operable patients choose to undergo RT alone with salvage surgery in case of RT failure.

It is well-recognized that preoperative external beam RT (EBRT) in sufficient doses can shrink the tumor and, in some cases, sterilize it in the operative specimen. The dose to the rectal tumor can be further increased by the use of endocavitary irradiation either by contact X-ray therapy or by interstitial ^{192}Ir brachytherapy. This study assessed the long-term results in patients with T2-T3 rectal adenocarcinomas treated with curative intent by RT alone, using a combination of contact RT, EBRT, and ^{192}Ir brachytherapy.

Methods.—Sixty-three patients (mean age, 72 years) were enrolled in this pilot study from 1986 to 1998. All of these patients had T2-T3, N0-N1, M adenocarcinoma of the middle or lower rectum involving less than two thirds of the circumference and underwent RT beam with contact X-rays (80 Gy in 3 fractions for 21 days) followed by EBRT for 17 days (39 Gy in 13 fractions) with a concomitant boost (4 Gy in 4 fractions). After 4 to 6 weeks, an iridium implant delivered a completion dose of 20 Gy to the tumor. None of the patients received chemotherapy.

Results.—T2 tumors were present in 41 patients, and 22 patients had T3 tumors. The mean distance of the tumor from the anal verge was 3.6 cm. All of the patients completed the treatment according to the protocol, with the exception of 7 patients who did not undergo brachytherapy. The rate of primary local control was 63% with a mean follow up of 54 months. After pelvic surgery, the ultimate pelvic control was 73%.

The 5-year overall survival rate was 64.4%. Among the 42 patients younger than 80 years of age, the 5-year survival rate was 78%, and 10 patients were alive and well at 10 or more years of follow-up. There was no severe grade 3 or 4 toxicity. Most patients developed acute proctitis but did not require treatment interruption. Late rectal bleeding occurred in 24 patients, but only 1 patient needed blood transfusion. Good anorectal function was maintained in 92% of patients alive at this writing. The T stage was found to be a strong prognostic factor; the 5-year overall survival rate for patients younger than 80 years with T2 tumors was 84%; those with T3 tumors had a 5-year survival rate of 53%.

Conclusion.—These initial findings show that long-term local control and survival can be achieved by RT alone in patients with US-staged T2-T3 rectal adenocarcinoma. High-dose irradiation to a small volume can provide a high therapeutic ratio for these tumors.

► These French investigators present their experience using RT alone for T2 and T3 rectal adenocarcinoma. They have used a combination of contact RT treatment, EBRT, and brachytherapy utilizing iridium. These patients were considered unsuitable for surgery because of comorbid disease or because they were adamant not to undergo surgery.

The authors report 63 patients with adenocarcinoma of the middle or lower rectum involving less than two thirds of the circumference. They have a median period of follow-up of 54 months with primary local control of 63%. Salvage surgery was able to retrieve another 10%. Their overall survival rate was 64% at 5 years and for those patients who were less than 80 years of age, the survival rate at 5 years was really quite good at 78%. The treatment appeared to be well tolerated in most patients, although there was some late rectal bleeding, but only 1 patient required transfusion.

I do not think these results are likely to replace surgical resection, but they do suggest that if a patient is adamant or simply a poor candidate for surgery, radiation treatment can be a valuable alternative with a curative potential.

E. Glatstein, MD

The Continuing Increase in the Incidence of Hepatocellular Carcinoma in the United States: An Update

El-Serag HB, Davila JA, Petersen NJ, et al (Houston Veterans Affairs Med Ctr; Baylor College of Medicine, Houston; Natl Cancer Inst, Bethesda, Md; et al)

Ann Intern Med 139:817-823, 2003 14–12

Background.—A previous study has reported an increase in the incidence and mortality rates of hepatocellular carcinoma in the United States. However, there are several possible alternative explanations for this observed increase in hepatocellular carcinoma, including changes in the demographic structure of the underlying populations, resulting in an increasing number of persons at high risk for hepatocellular carcinoma, better detection of the disease as a result of improved diagnostic testing, or an increase in high-risk sex or racial or ethnic groups of the population residing in one or a few high-risk geographic regions. Temporal trends in the incidence of hepatocellular carcinoma were examined.

Methods.—Data for this study were obtained from population-based registries of the Surveillance, Epidemiology, and End Results program. The study population included persons given a diagnosis of hepatocellular carcinoma between 1975 and 1998. A linear Poisson multivariate regression model, with adjustment for differences in age, sex, race or ethnicity, and geographic region, was calculated among patients with hepatocellular carcinoma in the underlying population.

Results.—There was an increase in the overall age-adjusted incidence rates of hepatocellular carcinoma from 1.4 per 100,000 from 1975 to 1977 to 3.0 per 100,000 from 1996 to 1998. A 25% increase occurred during the last 3 years compared with the preceding 3 years. Age groups older than 40 years were most affected by this increase, with the greatest increase in incidence occurring in the 45- to 49-year-old age group. Men had the greatest increase (31%) in the last time period (1996 to 1998) compared with 1993 to 1995. The Poisson regression model confirmed the findings of a nearly 2-fold increase in the incidence rate ratio for hepatocellular carcinoma between 1975 and 1977 and 1996 and 1998.

Conclusions.—There has been a rapid increase in the incidence of hepatocellular carcinoma in the United States, with the fastest increase in rates occurring in white men aged 45 to 54 years. The findings of this study are consistent with a true increase in incidence. It is likely that the incidence of hepatocellular carcinoma will continue to increase in the near future because persons infected with the hepatitis C virus ultimately have cirrhosis develop unless there is improvement in the secondary prevention of hepatocellular carcinoma.

► Hepatocellular carcinoma is one of the most common cancers worldwide. It is associated with chronic liver disorders (eg, hepatitis B, alcoholic and nonalcoholic cirrhosis). Hepatitis C virus (HCV) leads to chronic hepatitis in approximately 80% of exposed individuals, despite antibodies to the virus. This study highlights a disturbing picture of the rapid rise of a very malignant disease. The findings are consistent with HCV infections acquired 30 to 40 years ago. As treatment options for advanced malignancies are limited, increased secondary measures to prevent HCV exposure and infection are clearly needed.

P. J. Loehrer, Sr, MD

Results of Postoperative Radiotherapy for Resectable Hilar Cholangiocarcinoma

Gerhards MF, van Gulik TM, González DG, et al (Univ of Amsterdam)
World J Surg 27:173-179, 2003 14–13

Background.—Surgical resection is the only chance for a cure in patients with carcinoma of the extrahepatic bile duct. Most of these cholangiocarcinomas are hilar cholangiocarcinomas, which are relatively small and slow growing and difficult to treat. A previous series reported that resection with postoperative radiotherapy showed a significantly improved survival compared with resection alone in patients with hilar cholangiocarcinomas. The long-term survival and complications associated with radiotherapy, particularly intraluminal brachytherapy, after resection of hilar cholangiocarcinoma were assessed.

Methods.—One hundred twelve patients underwent resection of a hilar cholangiocarcinoma from 1983 to 1998. This study included findings in 91

TABLE 5.—Number of Patients Still Alive, Median Survival, and 5-Year Survival After Resection of Hilar Cholangiocarcinoma

	No Irradiation (n = 20) Number (%)	External Beam Irradiation With Brachytherapy (n = 41) Number (%)	External Beam Irradiation Alone (n = 30) Number (%)	Total (n = 91) Number (%)	*P*
Alive	0 (0)	6 (15)	15 (50)	21 (23)	<0.01
Median survival (months)	8 (5-11)*	21 (13-29)*	30 (6-54)*	21 (17-25)*	<0.01‡
5-years survival†	2/18 (11)	6/36 (17)	4/17 (24)	12/71 (17)	0.62

Note: The 91 patients were subdivided according to the use and type of adjuvant radiation therapy.
*95% confidence interval.
†Patients operated on more than 5 years previously.
‡Log-rank test.
(Courtesy of Gerhards MF, van Gulik TM, González DG, et al: Results of postoperative radiotherapy for resectable hilar cholangiocarcinoma. *World J Surg* 27:173-179, 2003. Copyright Springer-Verlag.)

patients who survived the postoperative period (mortality rate, 19%). Twenty patients had no adjuvant radiotherapy. In the remaining patients, radiotherapy was given either externally (30 patients) or as a combination of external and intraluminal brachytherapy (41 patients) via the Roux-en-Y loop used for the biliary-enteric anastomoses. The patients were subdivided into 3 groups as follows: no irradiation, external radiation in combination with intraluminal brachytherapy, and external radiation only. The groups did not differ significantly in gender, age, or tumor type.

Results.—Overall, late complications occurred in 88% of patients, with a significantly higher rate of complications among patients receiving external beam irradiation and brachytherapy. Abdominal pain was the most frequent complication (56% of patients), followed by cholangitis (49%), which occurred significantly more often in patients who had received brachytherapy. Retrograde bile leakage occurred after closure of the temporary jejunostomy in 24% of patients treated with brachytherapy. The overall median survival was longer after treatment with adjuvant radiotherapy (24 months) than after resection without additional radiation (8 months). However, there was no significant benefit obtained from the use of intraluminal brachytherapy (Table 5).

Conclusion.—In patients with resectable hilar cholangiocarcinoma, adjuvant radiotherapy after resection significantly improved survival. It is recommended that adjuvant radiotherapy be delivered by external beam irradiation rather than intraluminal brachytherapy.

▶ These investigators from The Netherlands report on a series of patients who underwent a resection for cholangiocarcinoma of the hepatic hilum region. The series covers a 15-year period during which 112 patients underwent such a resection. Ninety-one of them survived the postoperative period and 20 received no additional therapy, but 30 received external beam radiotherapy alone and another 41 had both external plus intraluminal brachytherapy.

The authors conclude that radiation therapy, particularly external, significantly improved survival. The data are not that overwhelming, and it is reasonably clear that the brachytherapy approach had a lot of morbidity with it which may have contributed to a relatively poor survival in those patients who received brachytherapy. One wonders what could be achieved using fiberoptics in the biliary tree and using photodynamic therapy. One would almost certainly have to use one of the newer radiosensitizers which are not yet approved by the FDA in order to get a longer wavelength of activation.

I am sure it can be done, although what the benefits would be is unclear. This is still a problem for which surgery is the major thrust of treatment, although not terribly effective long-term. These tumors are particularly difficult to deal with and they have a propensity to seed the peritoneal cavity.

E. Glatstein, MD

Radiofrequency Ablation of Liver Tumors: Influence of Technique and Tumor Size

Kuvshinoff BW, Ota DM (Univ of Missouri, Columbia)
Surgery 132:605-612, 2002 14–14

Introduction.—Most patients with hepatocellular carcinoma (HCC) or metastatic colorectal cancer to the liver are not candidates for surgical resection, which is unfortunate since hepatic resection is a potentially curative treatment for these patients. Radiofrequency ablation (RFA) of liver tumors has become more widespread, based on ease of use, safety, reasonable cost, and applicability to minimally invasive techniques. An initial experience with RFA in 45 patients with hepatic malignancies was described.

Methods.—All patients with primary or secondary hepatic malignancies seen between March 1999 and April 2001 who were not candidates for resection underwent US-guided RFA under general anesthesia. The end points were recurrence within or adjacent to the ablation zone or new hepatic or

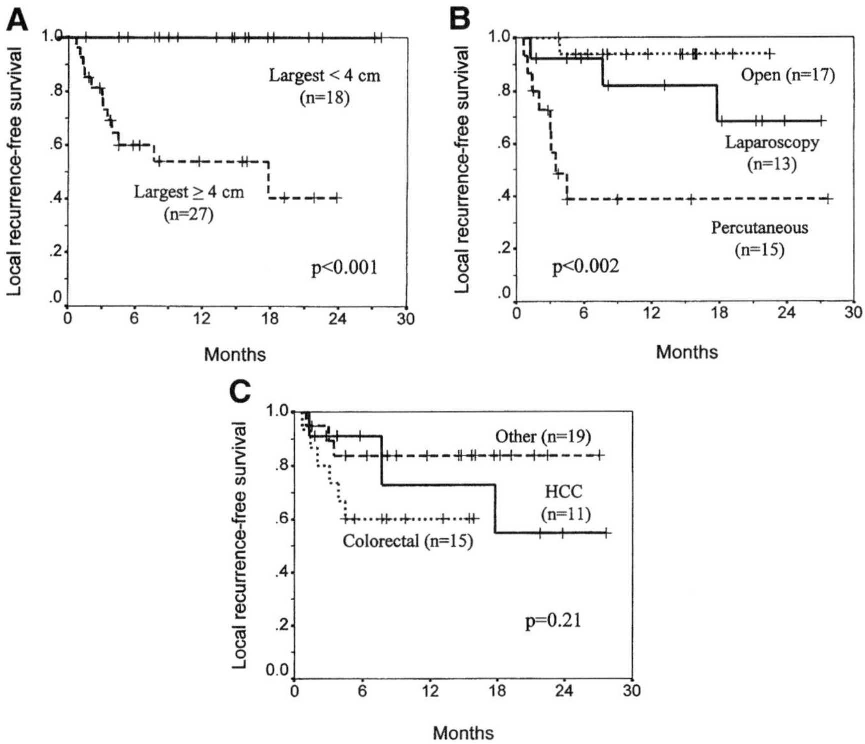

FIGURE 1.—Local (ablation site) recurrence-free survival from the time of initial radiofrequency ablation on the basis of (**A**) largest ablated tumor size (<4 cm vs ≥4 cm), (**B**) type of radiofrequency ablation procedure performed (percutaneous, laparoscopic, or laparotomy), and (**C**) type of disease treated (hepatocellular carcinoma, colorectal cancer, or other metastatic tumors). (Reprinted by permission of the publisher from Kuvshinoff BW, Ota DM: Radiofrequency ablation of liver tumors: Influence of technique and tumor size. *Surgery* 132:605-612, 2002. Copyright 2002 by Elsevier.)

extrahepatic lesions. Product limit survival estimates for both ablation site recurrence-free survival and disease-free survival were determined and compared for tumor size (<4 cm and ≥4 cm), operative approach (percutaneous, laparoscopy, or open surgery), and tumor type (HCC, colorectal cancer, or other metastatic disease).

Results.—Eleven patients with HCC and 34 with secondary hepatic malignancies had 84 lesions that underwent RFA. The median follow-up was 12 months. The largest ablated tumor size of 4 cm or greater ($P < .001$) and the percutaneous approach ($P < .02$) were correlated with worse ablation site recurrence-free survival (Fig 1) but not overall disease-free survival ($P = .06$). The 15 patients with colorectal cancer had worse disease-free survival than other tumor types ($P < .01$).

Conclusion.—RFA of hepatic malignancies can be performed with the use of a percutaneous, laparoscopic, or open approach. Local control seems to be superior for tumors of less than 4 cm and when an open surgical approach is used. The difficulty in accomplishing prolonged disease-free survival, particularly in colorectal cancer, shows the need to examine multimodal approaches that include local ablative techniques. Future RFA investigations should consider tumor size, surgical technique, and tumor type in trial design.

▶ RFA has enjoyed considerable use in recent years, especially for the treatment of lesions of the liver, which usually are not resectable. Radiofrequency thermal ablation is a form of hyperthermia, but unlike the hyperthermia of 15 to 20 years ago, it uses a greater temperature elevation in order to induce coagulation necrosis. It is generated by radiofrequency techniques and clearly is able to control lesions for a long period of time, particularly if they are small (less than 4 cm) and particularly if the techniques for using the RFA are either open surgical or laparoscopic.

It is hard to know where this kind of treatment will really end up in the long haul because the sorts of patients who are being treated generally represent metastatic disease. The rest of their tumor(s) is usually not amenable to this type of treatment.

E. Glatstein, MD

High Prognostic Value of *p16*^{INK4} Alterations in Gastrointestinal Stromal Tumors

Schneider-Stock R, Boltze C, Lasota J, et al (Otto-von-Guericke Univ, Magdeburg, Germany; Armed Forces Inst of Pathology, Washington, DC)
J Clin Oncol 21:1688-1697, 2003 14–15

Background.—Gastrointestinal stromal tumors (GISTs) are a distinctive but histologically heterogeneous group of neoplasms and are the most common mesenchymal tumors of the gastrointestinal tract. The malignant potential of these tumors is often uncertain. Immunohistochemically, GISTs are defined as KIT (CD117, stem cell factor receptor)-positive tumors. A cyc-

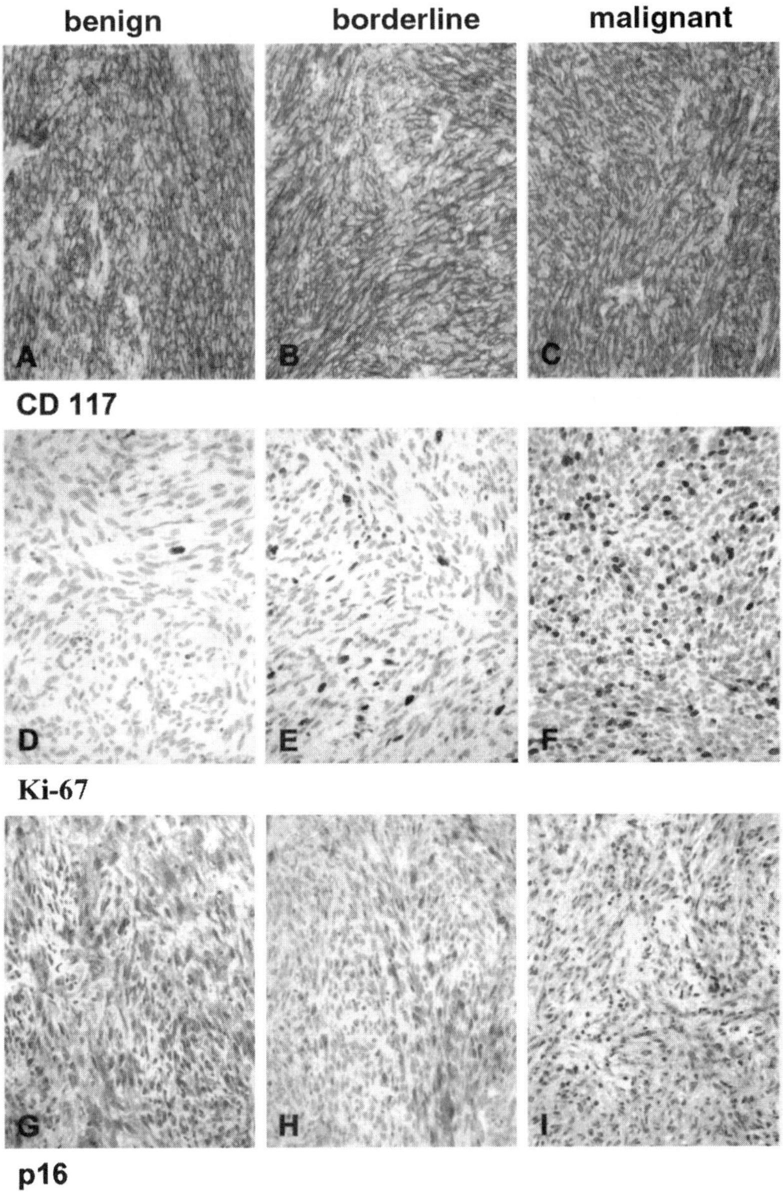

FIGURE 1.—CD117 staining (**A-C**); Ki-67 (Mib1) (**D-F**); and *p16*^{INK4} (**G-I**) in benign (tumor 9), borderline (tumor 16), and malignant gastrointestinal stromal tumors (GISTs; tumor 36). CD117 was equally expressed. The brownish stained nuclei (**D-F**) show the highest proliferation rate (Ki-67) in the malignant GIST (**F**); *p16*^{INK4} expression was higher in the nuclei and cytoplasm of the benign GIST (**G**). (Courtesy of Schneider-Stock R, Boltze C, Lasota J, et al: High prognostic value of *p16*^{INK4} alterations in gastrointestinal stromal tumors. *J Clin Oncol* 21:1688-1697, 2003. Reprinted with permission from the American Society of Clinical Oncology.)

lin-dependent kinase 4 inhibitor ($p16^{INK4}$) gene located at 9p21 has been shown to be inactivated in a variety of tumors by homozygous deletions, point mutations, or de novo methylation of its promoter region. The prognostic relevance of $p16^{INK4}$ alterations in GISTs was determined by investigation of a larger group of GISTs and correlation of the genetic findings with clinicopathologic factors and patient survival.

Methods.—A total of 43 GISTs in 39 patients were evaluated for methylation status of the promoter by methylation-specific polymerase chain reaction (PCR), the presence of mutations by PCR-SSCP-sequencing, the loss of heterozygosity at the $p16^{INK4}$ locus, and the immunohistochemical expression of $p16^{INK4}$ protein (Fig 1).

Results.—Alterations of $p16^{INK4}$ were identified in 25 of 43 GISTs (58.1%), with no differences in the type and frequency of alterations among benign, borderline, or malignant GISTs. $p16^{INK4}$ alterations were correlated with a loss of $p16^{INK4}$ protein expression. Patients with tumors with $p16^{INK4}$ alterations had a poorer prognosis compared with patients with tumors that had no $p16^{INK4}$ alterations. In terms of clinical outcome, a high predictive value for $p16^{INK4}$ alterations was found only in patients with benign and borderline GISTs. Univariate Cox proportional hazard regression analysis showed a strong correlation between $p16^{INK4}$ alterations, tumor size, mitotic index, and overall survival rate. However, multivariate analysis showed that only $p16^{INK4}$ alterations were an independent prognostic factor.

Conclusions.—The evaluation of $p16^{INK4}$ alteration status in patients with gastrointestinal stromal tumors is a helpful prognostic tool, particularly in patients with benign and borderline tumors.

▶ There is more to know about GISTs than the presence of *c-kit* mutations. Patients in this series with $p16^{INK4}$ alterations have strikingly different outcomes. This provides critical prognostic information and serves as further focus of research in this modern model of treatable malignancies.

P. J. Loehrer, Sr, MD

Factors Associated With Progression of Carcinoid Heart Disease

Møller JE, Connolly HM, Rubin J, et al (Mayo Clinic, Rochester, Minn)

N Engl J Med 348:1005-1015, 2003 14–16

Introduction.—Carcinoid tumors release serotonin and other vasoactive substances into the circulation that can cause right-sided valvular heart disease. Knowledge concerning the mechanisms involved in the progression of the cardiac lesions may lead to the development of treatments that attenuate the process. Factors associated with the progression of valvular dysfunctions in patients with metastatic carcinoid disease were reviewed retrospectively.

Methods.—Seventy-one patients with carcinoid syndrome who underwent serial echocardiographic evaluations performed more than 1 year apart, and 32 patients referred directly for surgical intervention after an initial echocardiographic examination were evaluated. A score for carcinoid heart disease was assigned based on an assessment of valvular anatomy and function and the function of the right ventricle. An increase of more than 25% in the score between studies was regarded as suggestive of disease progression. Tumor progression was based on abdominal CT scans and changes in the level of urinary 5-hydroxyindoleacetic acid (5-HIAA), a metabolite of serotonin.

Results.—Among patients who underwent serial echocardiographic evaluations, 25 (35%) had an increase of more than 25% in the cardiac score. Compared with patients whose score changed by 25% or less, these patients had higher urinary peak 5-HIAA levels (median, 265 mg per 24 hours [interquartile range, 209-593] vs 189 mg per 24 hours [interquartile range, 75-286]; $P = .004$) and were more likely to have biochemical progression (10/25 patients vs 9/46; $P = .05$) and to have received chemotherapy (13/25 vs 10/46; $P = .009$). Logistic regression analysis revealed that a higher peak urinary 5-HIAA level and previous chemotherapy were predictive of an increase in the cardiac score that exceeded 25% (odds ratio for each increase in 5-HIAA of 25 mg per 24 hours, 1.08 [95% confidence interval, 1.03-1.13]; $P = .009$). The odds ratio linked with chemotherapy was 3.65 (95% confidence interval, 1.74-7.48; $P = .001$).

Conclusion.—Serotonin is associated with progression of carcinoid heart disease. The risk of progressive heart disease is higher among patients who undergo versus those who do not undergo chemotherapy.

▶ Carcinoid tumors are rare, with about 20% to 30% presenting with advanced disease. The carcinoid syndrome is well known (diarrhea, cutaneous vasomotor flushing, bronchospasm), but less well described are the cardiac abnormalities associated with chronic exposure to serotonin and other vasoactive substances. This is an excellent article and review on the topic.

P. J. Loehrer, Sr, MD

Administration of Optimal Biological Dose and Schedule of Interferon α Combined With Gemcitabine Induces Apoptosis in Tumor-Associated Endothelial Cells and Reduces Growth of Human Pancreatic Carcinoma Implanted Orthotopically in Nude Mice

Solorzano CC, Hwang R, Baker CH, et al (Univ of Texas, Houston)

Clin Cancer Res 9:1858-1867, 2003 14–17

Background.—More than 80% of patients have locally advanced or metastatic disease by the time their pancreatic cancer is diagnosed. Only 3% to 4% of all patients with adenocarcinoma of the pancreas are still alive 5 years after diagnosis. Whether long-term interferon α (INF-α) treatment at optimal biologic doses inhibits angiogenesis of human pancreatic carcinoma in the pancreas of nude mice was determined.

Methods.—Seven days after implantation of human pancreatic cancer line L3.6pl cells into the pancreas of nude mice, groups of animals received subcutaneous injection with IFN-α alone, 50,000 units biweekly or 10,000 units daily; intraperitoneal injection with gemcitabine alone, 125 mg/kg biweekly; or injection with IFN-α daily plus gemcitabine biweekly for 35 days.

Findings.—Biweekly IFN-α treatments were not effective. However, daily IFN-α injections alone reduced tumor volume by 53%. Biweekly gemcitabine injections alone decreased tumor volume by 70%, and combined IFN-α and gemcitabine by 87%. In an immunohistochemical analyses, treatment with IFN-α alone or with IFN-α plus gemcitabine inhibited the expression of the proangiogenic molecules' basic fibroblast growth factor and matrix metalloproteinase 9 times more than did gemcitabine treatment alone. These treatments also reduced the staining of proliferating cell nuclear antigen in the tumor, inducing apoptosis in tumor-related mouse endothelial cells, resulting in reduced microvessel density.

Conclusions.—In this murine model, IFN-α treatment at an optimal biologic dose and schedule combined with gemcitabine induced apoptosis in tumor-related endothelial cells. It also decreased the growth of human pancreatic cancer cells in the pancreas, resulting in significantly increased length of survival.

► The investigators carried out experiments in nude mice assessing a dose-response relationship between low-dose INF-α and gemcitabine in the treatment of pancreatic cancer. This laboratory has for years assessed the role of low-dose INF in the treatment of cancer as an antiangiogenic therapy. Since pancreatic cancer represents a disease for which no effective therapy truly exists, the ability to modify this treatment and enhance its activity has been a long-standing interest. In this study the investigators identified that low doses of INF-α alone had activity that appears to be mediated in part by the antiangiogenic effects of this therapy. Not only was it seen for single-agent therapy, but also for combination with gemcitabine where it increased the survival of mice in combination with gemcitabine. This study suggests that antiangiogenic strategies for the treatment of pancreatic cancer should be considered and that rational combinations could be defined based on the activity of INF-α on basic fibroblast growth factor–expressing tumors.

M. S. Gordon, MD

Comparison of Gemcitabine Versus the Matrix Metalloproteinase Inhibitor BAY 12-9566 in Patients With Advanced or Metastatic Adenocarcinoma of the Pancreas: A Phase III Trial of the National Cancer Institute of Canada Clinical Trials Group

Moore MJ, Hamm J, Dancey J, et al (Univ Health Network, Toronto; Natl Cancer Inst of Canada Clinical Trials Group, Kingston, Ont, Canada; Centre Hospitalier de L'Universite Montreal Pavillon Saint-Luc, Montreal; et al;)

J Clin Oncol 21:3296-3302, 2003 14–18

Background.—Pancreatic adenocarcinoma carries a 5-year survival rate of less than 5%, the worst in the Surveillance, Epidemiology and End Results database. Improvements in systemic treatments are clearly needed. The selective matrix metalloproteinase inhibitor BAY 12-9566 was compared with the nucleoside analog gemcitabine in patients with advanced pancreatic cancer.

Methods.—Two hundred seventy-seven patients with advanced pancreatic adenocarcinoma previously untreated with chemotherapy were enrolled in the trial. By random assignment, 138 received BAY 12-9566, 800 mg orally bid continuously, and 139 received gemcitabine, 1000 mg/m^2, given intravenously on days 1, 8, 15, 22, 29, 36, and 43 for the first 8 weeks, then on days 1, 8, and 15 of subsequent 28-day cycles.

Findings.—The median survival in the BAY 12-9566 and gemcitabine groups were 3.7 and 6.6 months, respectively. The median progression-free survival rates were 1.7 and 3.5 months, respectively. In both groups, the rates of serious toxicity were low. Quality of life was found to be better with gemcitabine than with BAY 12-9566.

Conclusions.—In this study of patients with advanced pancreatic adenocarcinoma and no previous chemotherapy, gemcitabine was significantly more effective than BAY 12-9566. This matrix metalloproteinase inhibitor does not appear to be a useful treatment in advanced pancreatic cancer.

► Several years ago, Burris et al demonstrated an improvement in clinical benefit and survival with gemcitabine over 5-fluorouracil in advanced pancreatic cancer.[1] Many skeptics felt that this represented serendipity rather than real findings. As a result, comparison trials were initiated looking at other agents compared with gemcitabine. The rationale of looking at matrix metalloproteinase inhibitors in various malignancies has been strong. Unfortunately, it did not pan out in this trial. This trial was unable to document activity or survival advantage for patients treated with the matrix metalloproteinase and thus gives indirect further support for gemcitabine as a standard of care for patients with advanced disease. Once again, this emphasizes the importance of prospective randomized trials.

P. J. Loehrer, Sr, MD

Reference

1. Burris HA III, Moore MJ, Andersen J, et al: Improvements in survival and clinical benefit with gemcitabine as first-line therapy for patients with advanced pancreas cancer: a randomized trial. *J Clin Oncol* 15:2403-2413, 1997.

Randomized Phase II Comparison of Dose-Intense Gemcitabine: Thirty-Minute Infusion and Fixed Dose Rate Infusion in Patients With Pancreatic Adenocarcinoma

Tempero M, Plunkett W, van Haperen VR, et al (Univ of Calif, San Francisco; Univ of Texas, Houston; Sarah Cannon Cancer Ctr, Nashville, Tenn; et al)

J Clin Oncol 21:3402-3408, 2003 14–19

Background.—Gemcitabine, a potent cytotoxic agent, has demonstrated a broad spectrum of activity in pancreatic, bladder, lung, ovarian, and breast

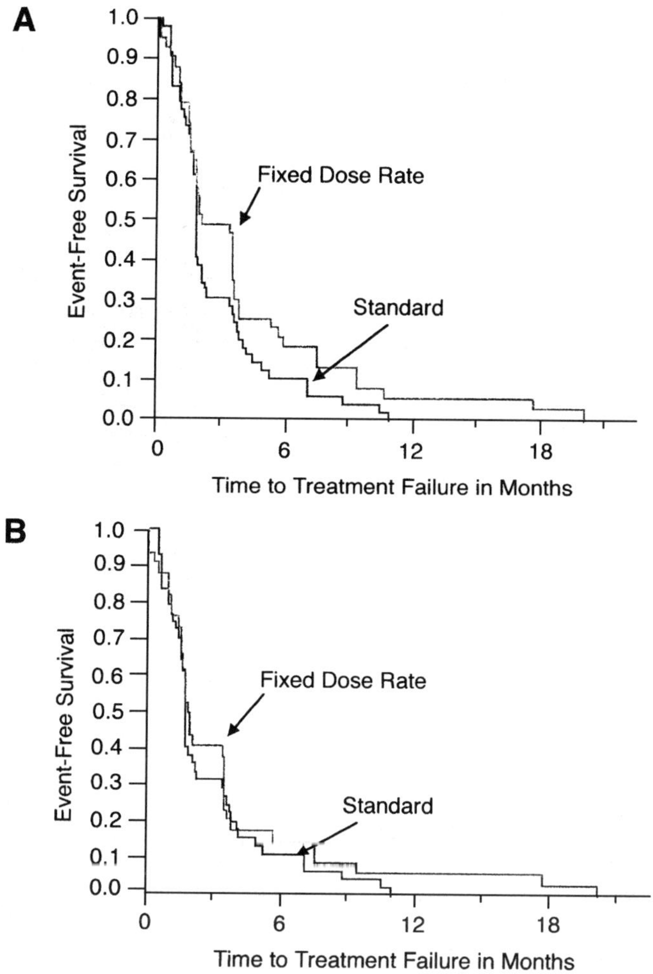

FIGURE 1.—Time to treatment failure for all patients (**A**) and for patients with metastases (**B**) on the standard arm (2200 mg/m^2 over a 30-minute period) and on the FDR arm (1500 mg/m^2 over a 150-minute period). (Courtesy of Tempero M, Plunkett W, van Haperen VR, et al: Randomized phase II comparison of dose-intense gemcitabine: Thirty-minute infusion and fixed dose rate infusion in patients with pancreatic adenocarcinoma. *J Clin Oncol* 21:3402-3408, 2003. Reprinted with permission from the American Society of Clinical Oncology.)

cancer. The effects of dose-intense gemcitabine in a standard 30-minute infusion or at the fixed dose rate (FDR) infusion, 10 mg/m^2 per minute, in patients with pancreatic adenocarcinoma were investigated in a randomized phase II study.

Methods.—Ninety-two patients were enrolled in the prospective trial. All had locally advanced or metastatic pancreatic adenocarcinoma. Treatment consisted of 2200 mg/m^2 gemcitabine given over a 30-minute period (in the standard arm) or 1500 mg/m^2 gemcitabine given over a 150-minute period (in the FDR arm) on days 1, 8, and 15 of 4-week cycles.

Findings.—Ninety-one percent of the patients had metastatic disease. Time to treatment failure was similar in the 2 treatment arms (Fig 1). However, the median survival for 8 months in the FDR arm compared with 5 months in the standard arm. The median survival for patients with metastases in these 2 treatment groups was 7.3 months and 4.9 months, respectively. Survival at 1 year was 9% for those in the standard arm and 28.8% for those in the FDR arm. At 2 years, survival was 2.2% and 18.3%, respectively. More hematologic toxicity occurred in the FDR infusion group. Pharmacokinetic analyses showed a 2-fold increase in intracellular gemcitabine triphosphate levels in patients receiving FDR infusion.

Conclusions.—Time to treatment failure, time to progression, and objective response were comparable in the 2 treatment arms of this trial, but the FDR administration method was associated with a modest overall improvement in survival and unusually high survival rates at 1, 2, and 3 years. Thus, continued evaluation of the FDR infusion strategy for gemcitabine, alone or combined with other agents, is warranted.

▶ This randomized phase II trial was presented at ASCO in 1999 and has received great interest in the years since. Fixed-dose administration of gemcitabine makes pharmacologic sense, but its therapeutic impact in patients with pancreatic cancer remains uncertain. This trial would suggest that there may be a favorable advantage. However, this advantage seems to be largely found in patients with locally advanced disease with respect to time to treatment failure. As appropriate, this concept is now being tested in a prospective randomized trial through the Eastern Cooperative Oncology Group comparing it with standard administration of gemcitabine and with oxaliplatin plus gemcitabine.

P. J. Loehrer, Sr, MD

Multiple Approach to the Exploration of Genotype-Phenotype Correlations in Familial Adenomatous Polyposis

Bertario L, Russo A, Sala P, et al (Natl Cancer Inst, Milan, Italy; Local Health Authority of Milan, Italy; Natl Cancer Inst, Genoa, Italy)

J Clin Oncol 21:1698-1707, 2003 14–20

Background.—Familial adenomatous polyposis (FAP) is a syndrome that predisposes affected persons to colorectal cancer. It is caused by an adenomatous polyposis coli (*APC*) gene mutation, its severity related to the position of the mutation on the gene. Several other clinical conditions have been associated with FAP. Associations among major clinical manifestations were identified in a large series of patients with FAP and mutation sites correlated with specific disease manifestations.

Methods and Findings.—Nine hundred fifty-three patients with FAP from 187 families were studied for *APC* mutations. Analysis indicated *APC* germline mutations between codons 156 and 2011 of the *APC* gene. Mutations varied across the region between codons 543 and 1309, but these mutations correlated strongly with congenital hypertrophy of retinal pigment epithelium. Mutations between codons 1310 and 2011 correlated with a 6-fold increase in risk of desmoid tumors compared with the low-risk reference region. Early colorectal cancer development was associated with codon 1309 mutations. Mutations between codons 976 and 1067 correlated with a 3- to 4-fold increase in the risk of duodenal adenomas. Mutations between codons 976 and 1067 carried the highest cumulative frequency of extracolonic manifestations, followed by mutations between 1310 and 2011.

Conclusions.—By analyzing the associations between APC mutation site and phenotype, FAP patient subgroups at increased risk for major extracolonic disease can be identified. Such data are useful for surveillance and prevention.

► FAP is an autosomal dominant disorder associated with an excessive number of colonic adenomas. When the colon is left intact in such patients, virtually 100% will ultimately develop colorectal cancer. FAP is associated with a number of other physical findings, including desmoid tumors, osteomas, congenital hypertrophy of retinal pigment epithelium, upper gastrointestinal polyps, and other malignancies. What seems logical is that phenotypic variants are associated with specific genotypic abnormalities. This may be quite helpful in the targeted screening of FAP patients.

P. J. Loehrer, Sr, MD

Multiple Colorectal Adenomas, Classic Adenomatous Polyposis, and Germ-Line Mutations in *MYH*

Sieber OM, Lipton L, Crabtree M, et al (Cancer Research UK, London; St Mark's Hosp, Harrow, England; Guy's Hosp, London; et al)

N Engl J Med 348:791-799, 2003 14–21

Background.—Recessive inheritance of multiple colorectal adenomas has been associated with germ-line mutations in the base-excision-repair gene *MYH*. Tumors from affected patients have been shown to have excess somatic transversions of a guanine-cytosine pair to a thymine-adenine pair in the *APC* gene. A large series of patients were screened for germ-line *MYH* mutations.

Methods.—One hundred fifty-two patients with multiple colorectal adenomas (ranging from 3 to 100) and 107 *APC* mutation–negative probands with classic familial adenomatous polyposis (defined as more than 100 adenomas) were included in the study (Table 3). Changes in the related genes *MTH1* and *OGG1* were analyzed. In addition, adenomas were examined for somatic *APC* mutations.

Findings.—Biallelic germline *MYH* variants were documented in 6 patients with multiple adenomas and in 8 with polyposis (Table 4). Missense and protein-truncating mutations were identified. The spectra of mutations were comparable between the 2 groups. In the biallelic mutation carriers, all somatic *APC* mutations in tumors studies were G:C→T:A transversions. Approximately one third of the patients with more than 15 adenomas in the

TABLE 3.—Characteristics of Patients With Classic Adenomatous Polyposis in Relation to Germ-Line *MYH* Mutation Status

Characteristic	Germ-Line *MYH*-Mutation Status		
	Negative (N=95)	Single Mutation (N=4)	Biallelic Mutation (N=8)
Age at presentation			
Age known—no. of patients (%)	55 (58)	4 (100)	8 (100)
Median—yr	30	31	48
Range—yr	7-72	30-54	30-70
No. of polyps—no. of patients (%)			
100-1000	68 (72)	4 (100)	8 (100)
>1000	27 (28)	0	0
Family history of colorectal cancer —no. of patients (%)			
Yes	29 (31)	0	4 (50)
None reported	66 (69)	4 (100)	4 (50)

(Reprinted by permission of *The New England Journal of Medicine* from Sieber OM, Lipton L, Crabtree M, et al: Multiple colorectal adenomas, classic adenomatous polyposis, and germ-line mutations in *MYH*. *N Engl J Med* 348:791-799, 2003.)

multiple adenoma group had biallelic *MYH* mutations. Among patients with polyposis, none of those with biallelic *MYH* mutations had severe disease, but 3 had extracolonic tumors. None of the *MTH1* or *OGG1* mutations identified were clearly pathogenic.

Conclusions.—These data indicate that germ-line *MYH* mutations predispose persons to a recessive phenotype, multiple adenomas, or polyposis coli. Genetic MYH testing is indicated in patients with 15 or more colorectal adenomas, especially when no germ-line *APC* mutation has been found and family history is consistent with recessive inheritance. The clinical care of persons with biallelic *MYH* mutations is comparable to that of patients with classic or attenuated familial adenomatous polyposis.

► As previously noted in Abstract 14–20, familial adenomatous polyposis is associated with hundreds to thousands of adenomatous polyps that ultimately lead to colon cancer. This study by Sieber et al carefully characterizes another syndrome that phenotypically is similar to familial adenomatous polyposis in that patients may present with hundreds of polyps, but with a recessive inheritance. This syndrome is a result of a germ-line mutation in the base-excision-repair gene *MYH*. By these authors' estimate, *MYH* mutations are found in 5% of patients who have moderate numbers of adenomas (3 to 100).

P. J. Loehrer, Sr, MD

TABLE 4.—Patients With Classic Adenomatous Polyposis and Germ-Line *MYH* Mutations

Patient No.	First *MYH* Mutation	Second *MYH* Mutation	Sex	Age at Diagnosis	No. of Polyps	Colorectal Cancer	Family History of Classic Adenomatous Polyposis	Extracolonic Features
				yr				
13	Y165C	Y165C	Male	41	100-1000	None reported	Yes	Congenital hypertrophy of the retinal pigment epithelium
14	Y165C	G382D	Female	50	100-1000	None reported	Yes	None reported
15	G382D	G382D	Male	30	100-1000	None reported	None reported	Duodenal adenomas
16	252delG	137insIW	Male	38	100-1000	Yes	None reported	Duodenal adenomas
17	Y165C	Y165C	Female	45	100-1000	Yes	Yes	None reported
18	Y165C	V232F	Male	70	100-1000	None reported	None reported	None reported
19	Y165C	G382D	Male	51	210	Yes	None reported	None reported
20	Y165C	G382D	Female	69	115	Yes	Yes	None reported
21	G382D	None detected	Male	32	100-1000	None reported	Yes	None reported
22	1209V	None detected	Female	54	100-1000	None reported	None reported	Osteoma
23	Y165C	None detected	Male	30	100-1000	None reported	None reported	None reported
24	Y165C	None detected	Male	30	750	None reported	Yes	None reported

(Reprinted by permission of *The New England Journal of Medicine* from Sieber OM, Lipton L, Crabtree M, et al: Multiple colorectal adenomas, classic adenomatous polyposis, and germ-line mutations in *MYH*. *N Engl J Med* 348:791-799, 2003.)

15 Cancer Biology

Micro-magnetic Resonance Lymphangiography in Mice Using a Novel Dendrimer-Based Magnetic Resonance Imaging Contrast Agent

Kobayashi H, Kawamoto S, Star RA, et al (NIH, Bethesda, Md; Johns Hopkins Univ, Baltimore, Md)

Cancer Res 63:271-276, 2003 15–1

Introduction.—Important advances in cancer biology and immunology have been attained with the use of mouse models. Few methods are currently available to image the deep lymphatic system. A new micromagnetic resonance lymphangiography (micro-MRL) method in mice was created that uses dendrimer-based MRI contrast agents. Due to its long survival in the circulatory system with minimal leakage from vessels, PAMAM-G8 was compared with gadolinium-diethylenetriaminepentaacetic acid (Gd-DTPA)-dimeglumine (control) in mouse inflammation/infection, proliferative lesion/lymphoma, and lymphangitis models.

Findings.—Micro-MRL imaging clearly visualized most of the mouse lymphatic system, including both lymphatics and lymph nodes. This approach was able to identify and distinguish dilation of lymphatic vessels in a lymphangitis model, proliferative or neoplastic lymph node swelling in a lymphoproliferative model, and inflammatory lymph node swellings in an infectious/inflammation model (Fig 4). It was possible to visualize changes in the lymphoid system of transgenic mice overexpressing interleukin-15. Abnormal enlarged lymph nodes identified via micro-MRL were selectively removed and examined to determine their cell type, receptor expression, and clonality in individual mice.

Conclusion.—Enhanced resolution of this noninvasive micro MRL can identify and classify lymphatic and lymph node abnormalities in mice, which should provide wide applicability to the evaluation of immunology and cancer in both experimental animals and clinical medicine.

▶ Ordinarily I do not include preclinical research as materials to include in the YEAR BOOK, but the pictures that are seen in this article dealing with "micro-magnetic resonance lymphangiography" in mice are so spectacular in terms of the detail that I think it is of interest. The authors have exploited new contrast imaging agents for MRI, and they are able to visualize in remarkable detail most of the mouse lymphatic system, both lymphatic channels as well as the nodes.

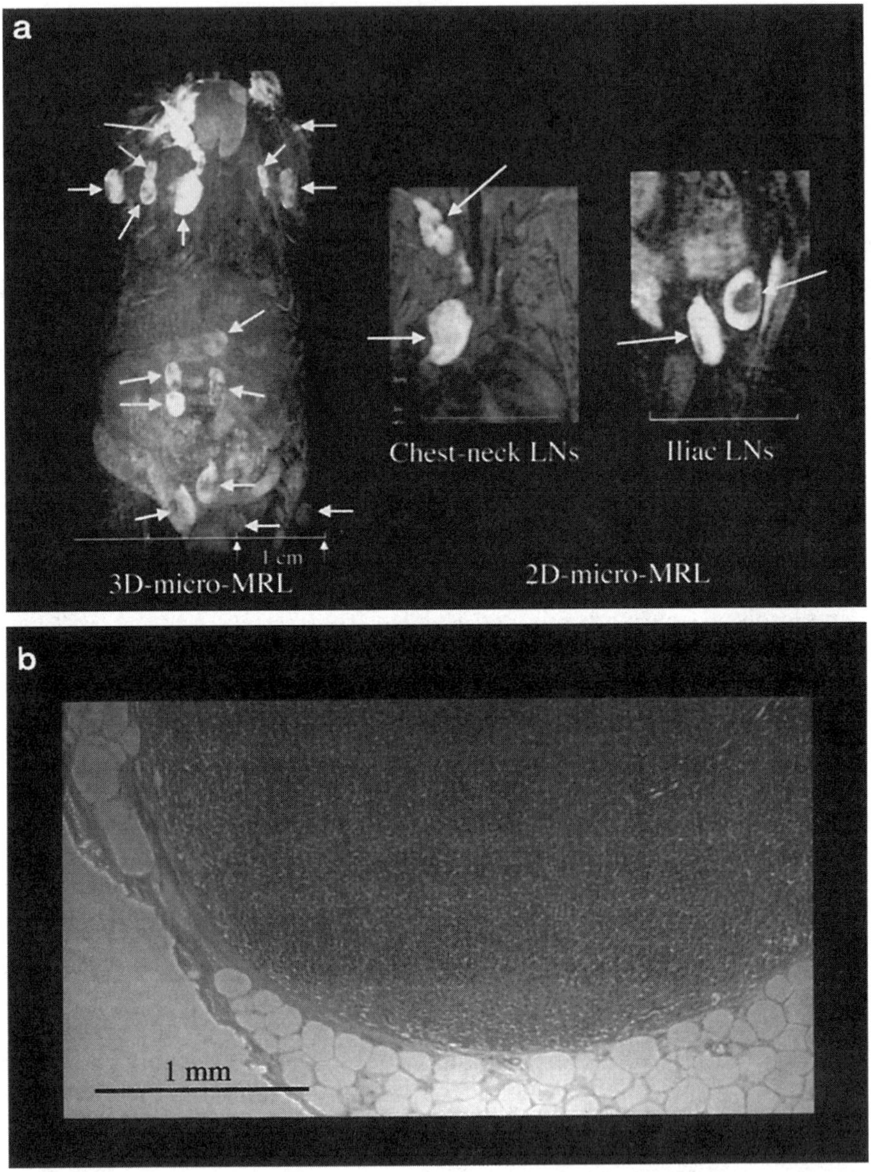

FIGURE 4.—Whole body 3-dimensional micro-MR and neck and pelvis 2-dimensional micro-MR lymphangiograms (MRL) of interleukin-15 transgenic-induced lymphoadenopathy with CD8+ T cells (**A**) injected with 0.005 mmol gadolinium/kg of PAMAM-G8-(1BAM-Gd)$_{1024}$. In addition, a microscopic picture (×20) of an enlarged lymph node (**B**) obtained from an interleukin-15 transgenic mouse is shown. The germinal center structure was no longer seen in these lymph nodes and was replaced by a homogeneous dense infiltration of lymphoid cells. All animals were given injections of contrast agents intracutaneously into fingers. All of the images were obtained at 45 minutes post injection. (Courtesy of Kobayashi H, Kawamoto S, Star RA, et al: Micro-magnetic resonance lymphangiography in mice using a novel dendrimer-based magnetic resonance imaging contrast agent. *Cancer Res* 63:271-276, 2003.)

One of the serious problems with diagnostic CT is the utilization of nodal size as the only criteria for what is normal or abnormal. The cutoffs that are employed are obviously arbitrary. The lymphangiograms of the past had nodal architecture as a major feature of the interpretation. It was my experience to see many nodes which had abnormal architecture but normal size. These nodes were usually confirmed histologically at the time of a staging laparotomy.

Therein lies part of the dilemma. If we had CT first and then developed the classic lymphangiogram that is not done any more, we would be oohing and aahing about the detail that one can see with lymphangiography. This detail is usually insufficient for carcinomas, because they frequently involve nodes in the peripheral sinuses and do not necessarily cause expansion of nodal size until the node is extensively replaced. However, it is exceedingly helpful in lymphoma, including Hodgkin's disease.

It is clear that the lymphangiogram as a standard procedure is dead. This kind of technology may cause resuscitation in the interest of nodal architecture that could be very useful for patients in the future.

E. Glatstein, MD

The Radiosensitivity of the Human Oocyte

Wallace WHB, Thomson AB, Kelsey TW (Univ of Edinburgh, Scotland; Univ of St Andrews, Scotland)

Hum Reprod 18:117-121, 2003 15–2

Background.—Cancer treatments involving abdominal, pelvic, or total body irradiation may damage the ovary permanently and cause primordial follicles to be lost, resulting in impaired fertility and premature menopause. The pool of primordial follicles is fixed in any female, with depletion leading to premature exhaustion of the pool and menopause well before the normal age of 51 years. The size of the follicle pool can be estimated with the use of a mathematical model of decline and the age of menopause calculated for patients who have had radiotherapy if the extent of radiation-induced damage to the follicle pool is determined. Then patients can receive counseling regarding their reproductive life span and pinpoint the window of opportunity for fertility. The best model available for natural follicle decline in healthy women was used to estimate the radiosensitivity of the human oocyte, leading to the calculation of age of menopause.

Methods.—Six patients aged 12.5 to 16.0 years who received total body irradiation at ages 4.9 to 15.1 years were diagnosed with ovarian failure. The estimated radiation dose needed to destroy 50% of the oocytes was less than 4 Gy. A model proposed by Faddy and Gosden was applied to yield the oocyte population for any given age in healthy untreated women between birth and age 51 years (Fig 1).

Two cohorts of women with ovarian failure resulting from radiotherapy treatment for childhood cancer were evaluated; 1 consisted of 8 postpubertal women aged 15.4 to 21.5 years who had been treated for leukemia without ovarian shielding and the other comprised 19 women treated for an in-

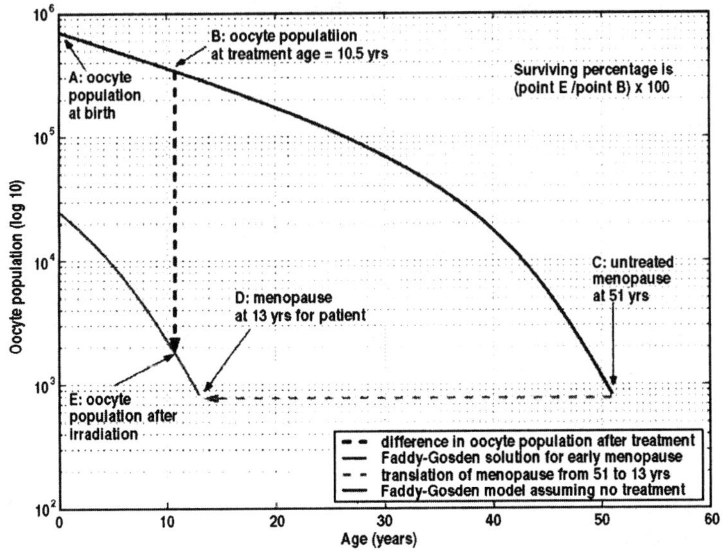

FIGURE 1.—The Faddy-Gosden model. The solution of the Faddy-Gosden equation enables the size of the oocyte pool to be determined for any given age from birth to menopause, at an estimated age of 51 years. The calculation of an estimated surviving fraction for case 5 in Table 1 is shown: ovarian failure occurred at age 13 years in case 5. By applying the Faddy-Gosden model, we can determine the size of the surviving fraction following radiotherapy at age 10.5 years to be 0.56%. (Courtesy of Wallace WHB, Thomson AB, Kelsey TW: The radiosensitivity of the human oocyte. *Hum Reprod* 18:117-121, 2003. Copyright European Society for Human Reproduction and Embryology, by permission of Oxford University Press.)

tra-abdominal tumor using whole abdominal radiotherapy, surgery, and chemotherapy. Ovarian failure developed in six women in the first cohort (median age, 13.2 years) and in 18 in the second cohort (median age, 12.7 years).

Results.—Following the model, age at irradiation and age at diagnosis of ovarian failure were used to determine the percentage of oocytes surviving. Included in the calculation was the solution to the differential equation of Faddy and Gosden. The number of follicles left after irradiation was given as $sol(51 - s + r)$, where r equals age at treatment, s equals age at diagnosis of ovarian failure, and 51 years is the average age of menopause. The surviving fraction of oocytes, given as a percentage, is 100 times this number divided by $sol(r)$.

For the first cohort, the mean surviving fraction was 0.66%. Previously, the surviving fraction for each patient in the second cohort was determined and plotted logarithmically against the dose of radiation received (Fig 2) to determine the point at which 50% of the oocytes remain (LD_{50}), which was less than 4 Gy. More recent findings suggested that the decay of primordial follicles does not follow a simple logarithmic decline but rather is an instantaneous rate of temporal change based on the remaining population pool. By using a revised mathematical model, the LD_{50} of the human oocyte was determined to be just under 2 Gy.

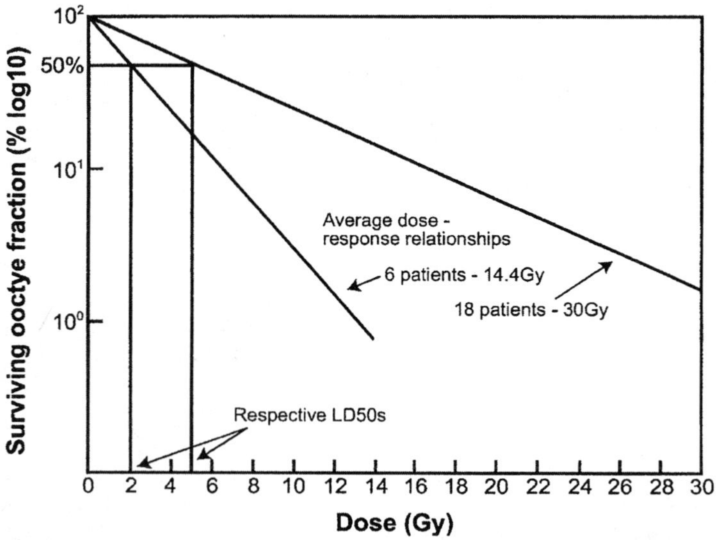

FIGURE 2.—Dose-response relationships for the human oocyte. The mean surviving fraction of oocytes for each patient has been calculated and plotted against the dose of radiation received: (1) for the 6 patients who received 14.4 Gy, and (2) for the 18 patients who received 30 Gy. These lines represent the estimated (fractionated) dose-response relationship for the human oocyte. The LD_{50} is given by the dose required to leave a surviving fraction of 50%. Our revised LD_{50} of less than 2 Gy is taken from the relationship obtained by data from the cohort of 6 patients. (Courtesy of Wallace WHB, Thomson AB, Kelsey TW: The radiosensitivity of the human oocyte. *Hum Reprod* 18:117-121, 2003. Copyright European Society for Human Reproduction and Embryology, by permission of Oxford University Press.)

Conclusion.—The surviving fraction of oocytes after irradiation was calculated and the LD_{50} of the human oocyte determined by using new data and a revised mathematical model of natural oocyte decline. Calculating the dose of radiation each ovary receives and using this more accurate estimate of the human oocyte's radiosensitivity should allow counseling that is more scientifically defensible for young women at risk for premature menopause after cancer treatment.

▶ This represents a mathematical effort to assess the dose of radiation that is required to knock out a human oocyte. These investigators from Scotland have done a fairly thorough and thoughtful analysis and come up with a dose of approximately 2 Gy as an estimate of the LD_{50} for human oocytes.

There is just one problem with this article. It is an estimate based on 2 groups of patients, 1 of which received total body irradiation as part of leukemia management; and, although they do not say anything about other treatment, I assume that the patients received fairly extensive chemotherapy as well as a bone marrow transplant. The second group of patients consisted of 19 patients treated for abdominal neoplasm with whole body abdominal radiation therapy. These included 12 patients with Wilms tumor, 3 patients with ovarian dysgerminoma, 1 with adrenal carcinoma, 1 with a sacrococcygeal teratoma, 1 with a bladder rhabdomyosarcoma, and 1 with an abdominal neuroblastoma. Eight of these 19 patients received no chemotherapy, but the other

11 received agents that are classified as not being "gonadotoxic," although exactly what that means is not clear.

Then there is the basic problem of how to define ovarian failure, which in this study is defined as failure to undergo or complete pubertal development or the onset of a premature menopause before the age of 40. This is supposedly seen in association with elevated follicle-stimulating hormone and luteinizing hormone levels and low estrodiol.

The point is that these are complicated patients who had received a lot of treatment, and it is hard to believe that the chemotherapeutic agents have absolutely no affect on ovarian function. It is clear to me that radiation to the ovaries has a risk of causing menopause and destroying human oocytes. On the other hand, in this group of patients, I think it is little naïve to assume that the disease has no impact, that chemotherapy has no impact, and that the entire compromise of ovarian function is a reflection of radiation alone.

E. Glatstein, MD

Epigenetic Inactivation of Laminin-5-Encoding Genes in Lung Cancers

Sathyanarayana UG, Toyooka S, Padar A, et al (Univ of Texas, Dallas; Aichi Cancer Ctr, Nagoya, Japan; Centre Hospitalier Regional Universitaire, Grenoble, France)

Clin Cancer Res 9:2665-2672, 2003 15–3

Background.—Invasion and destruction of the basement membrane are the earliest morphological characteristics of invasive carcinomas. Laminins are the major component of the basement membrane, playing an important role in anchorage dependence. This study investigated the loss of expression of 3 laminin-5 (LN5)-encoding genes in lung cancer cell lines and defined the mechanism of inactivation of the genes in lung cancer cell lines and tumors.

Methods.—Forty-nine lung cancer cell lines were examined by reverse transcription–polymerase chain reaction to determine expression of LN5-encoding genes. Expression-negative cell lines were treated with a demethylating agent, and restoration of expression was assessed by reverse transcription–polymerase chain reaction. The methylation patterns of CpG sites unique to the promoter regions of LN5-encoding genes were dissected out by bisulfite genomic sequencing of expression-negative cell lines. In addition, methylation patterns were investigated in 36 primary non–small cell lung cancers (NSCLCs), 26 small cell lung cancers (SCLCs), and 24 carcinoid tumors.

Findings.—Losses of expression in NSCLC and SCLC cell lines were frequent. Loss of expression of 1 or more genes was documented in 90% of SCLC cell lines and in 65% of NSCLC cell lines. In all cases, demethylating agent treatment of expression-negative cell lines restored expression. Methylation of LN5-encoding genes was more common in SCLC cell lines than in NSCLC cell lines. One or more genes were methylated in 95% of SCLC and in 60% of NSCLC cell lines. Statistically significant concordances were found between loss of expression and methylation in 40 lung cancer cell lines for the 3 genes. Methylation was more frequent in SCLC than in NSCLC or carcinoid tumors. At least 1 gene was methylated in 92% of the SCLC tumors, 47% of the NSCLC tumors, and 33% of the carcinoids.

Conclusion.—Epigenetic inactivation of LN5-encoding genes is frequent in lung cancers. The current findings may have important clinical implications.

► LN5 is a component of the extracellular matrix which is secreted by the overlying epithelial cells and plays a major role in anchorage independence and cell attachment. Epithelial cells must attach to the extracellular matrix to survive. Their transmembrane receptors are known as integrins. LN5 is specific to the epithelium and is pivotal to the binding of integrins. Because LN5 is a component of the basement membrane, which is a major barrier to the invasion of cancer, it is postulated that the loss of LN5, with a consequent failure of cell anchoring, may lead to an invasive and metastatic phenotype.

Since 1 method for downregulating or inactivating many genes, as discussed above, is via aberrant methylation of the CpG islands in their promoter regions, in this study, Sathyanarayana and coworkers looked at whether LN5 expression is inactivated in lung tumors. They demonstrate that not only are LN5 genes frequently inactivated in lung cancer cell lines and human tumors, particularly SCLC, the mechanism for this inactivation is hypermethylation of the LN5 encoding genes.

J. H. Schiller, MD

Rapid Akt Activation by Nicotine and a Tobacco Carcinogen Modulates the Phenotype of Normal Human Airway Epithelial Cells

West KA, Brognard J, Clark AS, et al (Natl Cancer Inst, Bethesda, Md; Lovelace Respiratory Research Inst, Albuquerque, NM)

J Clin Invest 111:81-90, 2003 15–4

Background.—The serine/threonine kinase Akt (protein kinase B) controls important cellular processes such as glucose metabolism, cell cycle progression, and apoptosis. Active Akt can contribute to tumorigenesis in vivo in lymphoid, breast, ovarian, prostate, and brain tissue. Akt is often activated in tumor cells through activation of growth factor receptors or Ras or through inactivation of phosphatase-and-tensin-homologue-deleted-on-chromosome-10 (PTEN), a phosphatase whose tumor suppressor function is dependent on dephosphorylation of 3'-phosphoinositide products of the upstream kinase PI3K. The described studies demonstrated an early biochemical effect of tobacco components in normal human lung epithelial cells—the activation of the PI3K/Akt pathway.

Methods.—Nonimmortalized normal human bronchial epithelial cells (NHBEs) and small airway epithelial cells (SAECs) were treated with 100 μM nicotine or 1 μM NNK, a potent, tobacco-specific carcinogen.

Results.—Activation of the Akt pathway by nicotine or NNK occurred within minutes at concentrations achievable by smokers and was dependent on α3-/α4-containing or α7-containing nicotine acetylcholine receptors, respectively. Activated Akt increased phosphorylation of downstream substrates such as GSK-3, p70^{S6K}, 4EBP-1, and FKHR. Nicotine or NNK treatment attenuated apoptosis caused by etoposide, UV irradiation, or hydrogen peroxide and partially induced a transformed phenotype evidenced by a loss of contact inhibition and loss of dependence on exogenous growth factors or adherence to ECM. In the in vivo study, active Akt was detected in airway epithelial cells and lung tumors from NNK-treated A/J mice and in human lung cancer specimens obtained from smokers.

Conclusions.—These studies demonstrated activation of the serine/threonine kinase Akt in nonimmortalized human airway epithelial cells in vitro by 2 components of cigarette smoke. The findings presented in these studies are consistent with the hypothesis that tumorigenesis is promoted by carcinogens through both biochemical and genetic mechanisms. The presence of active Akt in human lung cancers is an indication that Akt may be a legitimate target for therapeutic approaches in patients with established non–small-cell lung carcinoma.

► Although the carcinogenic effects of cigarette smoke have been described, the effects of nicotine on signaling pathways in normal cells has not. Activation of the serine/threonine kinase Akt results in inhibition of apoptosis, resulting in unregulated cell survival and tumor growth. In this article, West and colleagues report the activation of Akt by nicotine or the tobacco carcinogen NNK in both immortalized human bronchial epithelial cells in vitro, in preclinical murine models, and in human lung cancer, often occurring within minutes of concentrations achieved by smokers. The mechanism appears to be via nicotinic acetylcholine receptors, which are expressed in human airway epithelial cells, although subunit expression is different, depending on whether the cells were derived from proximal or distal airways. Thus, nicotinic activation of the Akt pathway may play a role in lung tumor carcinogenesis and may be an important target that may have therapeutic implications.

J. H. Schiller, MD

Comparison of Antiangiogenic Activities Using Paclitaxel (Taxol) and Docetaxel (Taxotere)

Grant DS, Williams TL, Zahaczewsky M, et al (Thomas Jefferson Univ, Philadelphia)

Int J Cancer 104:121-129, 2003 15–5

Background.—The taxanes, paclitaxel and docetaxel, are novel antimitotic agents whose exact mechanism of action is not completely understood. The effect of these drugs on angiogenesis has not been investigated. The effect of the taxanes on in vitro and in vivo angiogenic processes was examined.

Methods.—The effect of increasing dosages of paclitaxel and docetaxel on cultured human umbilical vein endothelial cell (HUVEC) and tumor cell proliferation, apoptosis, migration, tube formation, and aortic ring sprouting was investigated. The effect of the taxanes on tumor growth in nude mice was also assayed.

Results.—Both taxanes were effective at targeting endothelial cell activities, but docetaxel was 10 to 100 times more effective than paclitaxel at inhibiting proliferation, differentiation, and cell death in vitro and in vivo.

Conclusions.—Both taxanes are effective at targeting endothelial cells, but docetaxel is 10 to 100 times more potent than paclitaxel. Docetaxel may be a better therapeutic choice because it can be administered in lower doses, which may decrease toxicity.

Inhibition of Endothelial Cell Function In Vitro and Angiogenesis In Vivo by Docetaxel (Taxotere): Association With Impaired Repositioning of the Microtubule Organizing Center

Hotchkiss KA, Ashton AW, Mahmood R, et al (Albert Einstein College of Medicine, Bronx, NY)

Mol Cancer Ther 1.1191-1200, 200 15–6

Background.—Docetaxel (Taxotere) is a microtubule-binding drug with antitumor properties. The effects of the taxanes, Taxotere and Taxol, on endothelial cell functions were investigated.

Methods.—The 2 assays of endothelial cell function were in vitro chemokinetic migration with and without angiogenesis factors and in vivo 3-dimensional Matrigel tubule formation with rat fat pad endothelial cells or human umbilical vein endothelial cells.

Results.—Taxotere was active in all assays at concentrations that were not cytotoxic and did not inhibit endothelial cell proliferation. Human umbilical vein endothelial cells migration was more sensitive to Taxotere than Taxol. Taxotere was a 1000 times more potent inhibitor of cell migration. Taxotere also had antiangiogenic activity in vivo in the Matrigel plug assay.

Conclusions.—Taxotere is a potent inhibitor of endothelial cell migration and angiogenesis both in vitro and in vivo. Its antiangiogenic activity may contribute to its antitumor activity.

► With current therapy, 75% of patients with advanced ovarian carcinoma will achieve a clinically complete response. Unfortunately, 75% of these complete responders will eventually relapse. Over the last 2 decades, multiple approaches have been evaluated as consolidation or maintenance therapy in an attempt to reduce or delay these relapses. None of these has been successful. Based on observations that the taxanes, when dosed long term, have antiangiogenic effects (Abstracts 15–5 and 15–6) and on observations of delayed responses until the tenth, eleventh, or twelfth cycle of therapy in the initial phase II trials of paclitaxel, the Southwest Oncology Group initiated a trial of prolonged paclitaxel therapy as maintenance therapy in clinically complete responders. This trial was joined subsequently by the Gynecologic Oncology Group.

Patients were randomized to either 3 additional cycles of paclitaxel given monthly or 12 additional cycles given monthly. A prospectively defined interim analysis of the first 225 patients revealed highly significant improvement in the progression-free survival of those receiving 12 additional cycles of paclitaxel and led to the closure of the study. Because of demand by those patients assigned to 3 cycles for 9 more cycles of paclitaxel, meaningful survival information is unlikely.

This is the first study of maintenance therapy that has employed a therapy for which a solid rationale existed. The results are unequivocally positive. The study did not include a quality of life component, so no comment regarding "clinical benefit" can be made. In addition, one positive does not change the standard of care. Nevertheless, the study does provide convincing evidence of improved progression-free survival with maintenance paclitaxel. Improvement in progression-free survival in patients with ovarian carcinoma has led to even larger improvement in overall survival in most other trials of advanced disease (GOG 111, OV 10, etc).

How then should the physician use the results of this study? The results should be discussed with each patient, and the patient should be given the option of electing to take maintenance paclitaxel. If maintenance paclitaxel is to be used, it should be given in the manner that has been shown to work: 12 cycles given monthly at a starting dose of 175 mg/m^2 with dose reduction if toxicity necessitates. A confirmatory trial is planned by the GOG in the immediate future.

J. T. Thigpen, MD

16 Supportive Care

Influenza Vaccination in Elderly Patients With Advanced Colorectal Cancer
Earle C (Harvard Med School, Boston)
J Clin Oncol 21:1161-1166, 2003 16–1

Background.—Yearly influenza vaccination is recommended for people aged 65 years and older, especially those with underlying immunosuppressive disorders. There is debate over the use of influenza vaccine in patients with cancer, reflecting concerns about the resulting antibody response or possible immunosuppression. The outcomes of influenza vaccination in older adults with advanced colorectal cancer were analyzed.

Methods.—The National Cancer Institute's Survival, Epidemiology, and End Results registry was used to identify Medicare patients treated for stage IV colorectal cancer between 1993 and 1998. All patients had survived at least 4 months with colorectal cancer and were alive during the fall months, making them potentially eligible for influenza vaccination. Medicare data were used to determine whether the patients received influenza vaccination and to assess their subsequent outcomes. A total of 1225 patients met the study criteria, receiving chemotherapy over a total of 1577 person-years of observation.

Results.—The rate of influenza vaccination was 39.7% overall, increasing from 26% to 43% in the years studied. More than two thirds of vaccinated patients received the vaccine from their primary care physician. Factors associated with influenza vaccination included white race, higher socioeconomic status, and increased comorbidity. During treatment, vaccinated patients were less likely to be diagnosed as having influenza or pneumonia. Vaccination was also associated with a lower rate of chemotherapy interruptions and an increased chance of survival to the start of fall the next year (hazard ratio, 0.88). Vaccinated patients also had a slight reduction in health care resource utilization.

Conclusions.—For elderly patients with advanced colorectal cancer, the benefits of influenza vaccination appear comparable to those of cancer-free older adults. Vaccination rates are relatively low in this population, particularly for minority and lower income patients. Oncologists should advocate yearly influenza vaccinations for patients being treated for advanced cancer.

▶ This year will mark one of the most severe influenza seasons in this country. Oncologists become the primary care providers for many patients diagnosed with cancer. As physician caretakers, responsibility for other typically nononcologic medical needs falls to us. This study is a reminder.

P. J. Loehrer, Sr, MD

Minidose Warfarin Prophylaxis for Catheter-Associated Thrombosis in Cancer Patients: Can It Be Safely Associated With Fluorouracil-Based Chemotherapy?

Masci G, Magagnoli M, Zucali PA, et al (Istituto Clinico Humanitas, Rozzano, Milan, Italy)

J Clin Oncol 21:736-739, 2003 16–2

Purpose.—In patients undergoing central venous catheter (CVC) insertion, low-dose oral warfarin can reduce the rate of thromboembolic complications at a low risk of bleeding. Warfarin has a known adverse interaction with fluorouracil (FU). However, the frequency of this complication and its occurrence in response to minidose warfarin are unclear. The effects of minidose warfarin on international normalized ratio (INR) alterations and bleeding events were studied in patients receiving continuous-infusion FU chemotherapy.

Methods.—The 2-year retrospective study included 95 consecutive patients receiving FU-based chemotherapy for cancer, including liver metastases in 43%. A Groshong CVC was in place in 83% of patients and a Port-a-Cath in 17%. All received minidose warfarin prophylaxis, 1 mg/d orally starting the day after catheter placement. The rate of INR alterations—defined as an increase to more than 1.5—was assessed along with potential predictive factors.

Results.—Thirty-three percent of patients had INR elevations, including INR levels greater than 3.0 in 19%. Bleeding occurred in 8% of patients, with all but 1 showing INR elevations. The rate of INR elevations differed for patients receiving differing FU regimens: 57% with FU, folinic acid, and oxaliplatin; 27.5% with FU and folinic acid; and 26% with FU, folinic acid, and irinotecan.

Conclusions.—Patients receiving FU-based cancer chemotherapy and minidose warfarin prophylaxis have a high rate of INR elevations. These abnormalities are particularly frequent among patients receiving the FU, folinic acid, and oxaliplatin chemotherapy regimen. Patients receiving warfarin and FU need close monitoring of the prothrombin time.

▶ The administration of minidose (1 mg) warfarin for prevention of an indwelling catheter has become common. This study highlights the problems with drug interaction, which can lead to a markedly elevated INR when administered with fluoropyrimidine-based chemotherapy. One needs to continue to be mindful in such patient populations.

P. J. Loehrer, Sr, MD

High Incidence of Angina Pectoris in Patients Treated With 5-Fluorouracil: A Planned Surveillance Study With 102 Patients

Wacker A, Lersch C, Scherpinski U, et al (Ludwig-Maximilians-Universität München, Deutschland, Germany)

Oncology 65:108-112, 2003 16–3

Background.—5-Fluorouracil (5-FU) is a widely used form of cancer chemotherapy that has unexplained cardiotoxic effects. Previous reports have described cardiac events including angina pectoris, arrhythmia with sudden death, and myocardial infarction in patients receiving 5-FU. The incidence of angina pectoris was assessed in a series of patients receiving 5-FU chemotherapy.

Methods.—The surveillance study included 102 consecutive, unselected patients receiving 5-FU: 70 men and 32 women, median age 62 years. Twelve had a history of coronary artery disease. Before the start of chemotherapy, all patients underwent 12-lead ECG monitoring, echocardiography, and radionuclide ventriculography. Holter monitoring was performed during 5-FU infusion; all studies were repeated at 3 months' follow-up. The incidence and duration of ischemic symptoms were assessed along with other outcomes.

Findings.—Nineteen patients had reversible angina pectoris within 24 hours after starting 5-FU treatment. The symptoms persisted for up to 12 hours after the end of 5-FU infusion and were accompanied by ECG changes in most cases. Six of these 19 patients underwent coronary angiography, which found no evidence of coronary artery disease. However, 2 patients had reduced ventricular ejection fraction less than 50%, which did not improve during follow-up.

Holter monitoring showed a significantly increased rate of bradycardia and ventricular extrasystoles during treatment compared with follow-up studies 3 months later. At follow-up, the QTc time showed significantly prolongation compared with baseline.

Conclusions.—Patients receiving 5-FU chemotherapy show a high incidence of angina pectoris. The mechanism of cardiotoxicity remains unproven, but reversible vasospasm is the most likely explanation. Patients receiving 5-FU need close monitoring continuing past the drug's half-life because symptoms and ECG changes may persist up to 12 hours after discontinuation.

► Although this is a study about an old drug, it is worth mentioning a clinical syndrome that is often missed.

P. J. Loehrer, Sr, MD

Risk Factors for Traumatic and Bloody Lumbar Puncture in Children With Acute Lymphoblastic Leukemia

Howard SC, Gajjar AJ, Cheng C, et al (St Jude Children's Research Hosp, Memphis, Tenn; Univ of Tennessee, Memphis)
JAMA 288:2001-2007, 2002 16–4

Background.—Lumbar puncture (LP) is generally safe, but there is a risk of trauma. Blood can be introduced into the cerebrospinal fluid (CSF) when LPs are difficult to perform or when repeated attempts are necessary. Traumatic or bloody LP reduces the diagnostic value of the procedure and may worsen the outcome of patients with acute lymphoblastic leukemia. However, little is known of the risk factors for traumatic and bloody LP. An attempt was made to determine the risk factors for traumatic and bloody LP.

Methods.—This retrospective cohort study enrolled 956 consecutive patients with newly diagnosed childhood acute lymphoblastic leukemia who were treated at a pediatric cancer center between February 1984 and July 1998. Each of the patients underwent a diagnostic LP followed by a median of 4 LPs to instill intrathecal chemotherapy. Traumatic LP was defined as an LP in which CSF contained at least 10 red blood cells per microliter and bloody LP as CSF containing at least 500 red blood cells per microliter.

Results.—A total of 5609 LPs were evaluated, of which 1643 (29%) were traumatic and 582 (10%) were bloody. Estimated odds ratios for traumatic LP were 1.5 for black versus white race, 2.3 for age younger than 1 year versus 1 year or older, 1.4 for early versus recent treatment era, 1.5 for platelet count of $100 \times 10^3/\mu L$ or more compared with less than $100 \times 10^3/\mu L$, 10.8 for short (1 day) versus longer (more than 15 days) interval since the previous LP, and 1.4 for the least versus the most experienced practitioners. Similar results were obtained on analysis for bloody LP.

Conclusions.—Among the unmodifiable risk factors for traumatic and bloody LP were black race, age less than 1 year, a traumatic or bloody previous LP performed within the past 2 weeks, and a previous LP when the platelet count was $50 \times 10^3/\mu L$ or less. Among the modifiable risk factors were procedural factors reflected in treatment era, platelet count of $100 \times 10^3/\mu L$ or less, an interval of 15 days or less between LPs, and a less experienced practitioner.

► The presence of leukemic blasts in the CSF of patients with acute lymphoblastic leukemia (ALL) increases the risk of relapse and requires additional therapy directed at eradicating that disease and preventing central nervous system relapse. The introduction of leukemic blasts into the CSF from a traumatic LP at the time of diagnosis has also been associated with an increased risk of CNS relapse. Factors that could contribute to traumatic LPs are therefore important. The study by Howard et al retrospectively examined 956 consecutive patients with newly diagnosed ALL who had LPs done. A traumatic LP was defined as one in which 10 or more red blood cells per microliter were present and a bloody LP as one in which 500 or more red blood cells per microliter were present. Of the 5609 LPs examined, nearly 30% were considered traumatic and 10% were bloody. An examination of the potential contributing factors to a traumatic or bloody tap included the patient being black, an age younger than 1 year, a previous traumatic or bloody LP, and a previous LP done when the platelet count was 50,000 or less per microliter. Potential modifiable factors contributing to traumatic or bloody LPs included the platelet count, a short interval between LPs, and the experience of the person performing the LP. While information regarding effectiveness of sedation or types of needles used was lacking, this study raises several important potential interventions that could be pursued to lower the risk of traumatic and bloody LPs in patients with ALL. The results also raise the interesting question as to who should be allowed to do LPs on such patients.

R. J. Arceci, MD, PhD

Analysis of Patients With Epithelial Ovarian Cancer or Fallopian Tube Carcinoma Retreated With Cisplatin After the Development of a Carboplatin Allergy

Dizon DS, Sabbatini PJ, Aghajanian C, et al (Mem Sloan-Kettering Cancer Ctr, New York)

Gynecol Oncol 84:378-382, 2002 16–5

Background.—Among patients with ovarian cancer treated with carboplatin, 5% to 34% will have an allergic reaction. Such a reaction is usually manifest after a median of 8 rounds of carboplatin therapy. Outcomes are reported in 7 patients who were treated for recurrent ovarian cancer with cisplatin after having an allergic reaction to carboplatin.

Case Report.—Woman, 67, with no significant past medical history was diagnosed with stage IIC papillary serous peritoneal carcinoma, FIGO grade 3, in 1996. She underwent a total abdominal hysterectomy, bilateral salpingo-oophorectomy, and full surgical staging and was optimally debulked. She then received 6 cycles of cisplatin and paclitaxel on an every-3-week cycle, which was well tolerated. She was diagnosed with recurrent disease 7 months later, at which time she was treated with carboplatin and paclitaxel for 5 cycles with partial response, followed by progression of disease. She was then treated with doxorubicin and etoposide sequentially, with progression. The patient was re-treated with 80 mg of carboplatin after a platinum-free interval of 14 months and had shortness of breath, facial flushing, sinus tachycardia, and hypertension. The reaction subsided after treatment with diphenhydramine and dexamethasone, and the patient was released. After 24 months her progressive disease was treated with cisplatin, which resulted in a fatal anaphylactic reaction. After this fatal reaction, the experience of patients at the authors' institution who were treated with cisplatin after manifesting a carboplatin allergy was reviewed.

Methods.—Records of patients treated from 1993 to 2000 were reviewed, and 6 patients were identified. Electronic medical records for these patients were reviewed for relevant treatment and outcome data.

Results.—Of these 6 patients, 5 were successfully treated without further allergic reactions. One patient with platinum-refractory disease had an allergic reaction to carboplatin and then to cisplatin.

Conclusions.—Few patients at this study's institution were treated with cisplatin after manifesting a carboplatin allergy. One patient died from a serious hypersensitivity reaction after retreatment. It would appear from this limited experience that cross allergy can exist, although the true incidence of this phenomenon is unknown. Thus, routine retreatment of carboplatin-allergic patients with cisplatin in the relapsed setting cannot be recommended without careful consideration of potential risks and benefits.

Successful Administration of Carboplatin in Patients With Clinically Documented Carboplatin Hypersensitivity

Rose PG, Fusco N, Smrekar M, et al (Case Western Reserve Univ, Cleveland, Ohio; Univ Hosps of Cleveland, Ohio; MetroHealth Med Ctr, Cleveland, Ohio)

Gynecol Oncol 89:429-433, 2003 16–6

Background.—Current standard first-line chemotherapy regimen for ovarian cancer in the United States is the combination of carboplatin and paclitaxel. Most patients are clinically responsive to this regimen but have recurrent disease develop at an average of 10 to 20 months after initial treatment, depending on the extent of residual disease after initial surgery. The time to recurrence is often used to guide the selection of second-line therapy. Patients who have recurrence more than 6 months after initial platinum therapy are considered potentially platinum sensitive. The tolerance and effectiveness of carboplatin rechallenge was evaluated by a prolonged desensitizing carboplatin infusion regimen in patients with clinically documented moderate to severe carboplatin hypersensitivity.

Methods.—Computerized pharmacy records were used to identify patients admitted for carboplatin infusion, and a retrospective analysis of these patients was performed.

Results.—A total of 33 patients were identified, including 27 with recurrent ovarian, 4 with peritoneal, 1 with tubal, and 1 with cervical cancer. The patients were treated with a prolonged desensitizing carboplatin infusion. The patients had received a median of 10 courses of carboplatin (range, 3-33) before manifesting the moderate to severe hypersensitivity reaction. A total of 215 courses were administered, with patients receiving a median of 5 treatments and a range of 1 to 52 treatments. A total of 29 patients (88%) were successfully rechallenged. Four patients had a recurrent moderate to severe carboplatin hypersensitivity reaction, which precluded further administration of carboplatin. Recurrent moderate to severe carboplatin hypersensitivity recurred in 3 additional patients (9%) after 2, 3, and 6 subsequent courses despite initial tolerance of the infusion schedule. Objective responses to therapy were observed in 22 (79%) of 28 evaluable patients.

Conclusions.—A prolonged desensitizing carboplatin infusion regimen is tolerated by most patients who have had moderate to severe carboplatin hypersensitivity.

Carboplatin Hypersensitivity Reactions: Re-treatment With Cisplatin Desensitisation

Jones R, Ryan M, Friedlander M (Prince of Wales Hosp, Randwick, NSW, Australia; Royal Hosp for Women, Randwick, NSW, Australia)

Gynecol Oncol 89:112-115, 2003 16–7

Background.—Hypersensitivity reactions to carboplatin therapy have been reported to occur in 5% to 34% of women with ovarian cancer treated with carboplatin. These reactions usually manifest after the patient has had at least 6 cycles of carboplatin and nearly always occur when the patient is re-treated with carboplatin as a second-line or third-line treatment. In addition, these reactions are usually seen in the second cycle of carboplatin administered in the relapse setting. Typically these patients have previously received carboplatin with no allergic reactions and may then develop a hypersensitivity reaction ranging from minor to life threatening. The feasibility of re-treating patients who have had a hypersensitivity reaction to carboplatin with cisplatin after desensitization was evaluated.

Methods.—Five patients with recurrent ovarian cancer who had a documented hypersensitivity reaction to carboplatin and a good clinical indication for continuing treatment with platinum were re-treated after cisplatin desensitization. All the patients were rechallenged with cisplatin after a lengthy desensitization protocol, and the initial 4 patients subsequently received cycles with a shortened protocol in an effort to shorten and simplify the procedure.

Results.—All the patients tolerated their first cycle of cisplatin on rechallenge with the full desensitization protocol, and none had adverse reactions. However, 2 patients who received further treatment with a shortened cycle had further adverse hypersensitivity reactions. Two patients received 1 additional cycle with a shortened protocol and did not have problems with hypersensitivity; however, treatment was stopped because of evidence of disease progression. The fifth patient underwent 2 additional cycles with the full desensitization protocol without adverse reactions, but treatment was halted because of evidence of disease progression.

Conclusions.—The indication of these findings is that a full cisplatin desensitization protocol is an effective method for retreatment of patients with previously documented hypersensitivity reaction to carboplatin. Efforts to shorten the procedures were associated with additional allergic reactions, which indicates that it may be necessary to follow the full protocol with each treatment.

▶ These 3 articles concern an increasingly common problem seen more often in the second-line therapy of ovarian carcinoma by retreatment of platinum-sensitive patients with a carboplatin-based regimen: the problem of hypersensitivity reactions to carboplatin. Some of these reactions are clearly life threatening and pose significant problems as to whether the most active agents in ovarian carcinoma, the platinum compounds, must be dropped from the patient's treatment regimen. The article by Dizon et al (Abstract 16–5) documents that cross allergy can exist between carboplatin and cisplatin. The other 2 articles (Abstracts 16–6 and 16–7) present desensitization regimens for carboplatin and cisplatin that have been successfully used to enable further treatment with a platinum compound.

J. T. Thigpen, MD

Sensitivity of a Blood Culture Drawn Through a Single Lumen of a Multilumen, Long-term, Indwelling, Central Venous Catheter in Pediatric Oncology Patients

Robinson JL (Univ of Alberta, Edmonton, Canada)

J Pediatr Hematol Oncol 24:72-74, 2002 16–8

Background.—Bacteremia is common among pediatric oncology patients; blood cultures drawn from these patients because of fever will be positive in approximately 10% of cases. These blood cultures are often drawn from long-term, indwelling, central venous catheters because this prevents the need for venipuncture; however, these cultures may have a higher sensitivity than do peripheral blood cultures. In many centers, it has become common practice to draw simultaneous blood cultures from all lumens when long-term, indwelling, central venous catheters have multiple lumens. This practice increases the incidence of contaminated blood cultures, yet it may also increase the detection rate of true bacteremias. The sensitivity of a blood culture drawn from only 1 lumen of a multilumen, long-term, indwelling, central venous catheter was assessed in pediatric oncology patients.

Methods.—Records of a microbiology laboratory were used to conduct a retrospective review of all positive blood cultures obtained from pediatric oncology patients admitted to 1 center from January 1994 through March 1999. Episodes of positive findings on blood culture were included only if cultures were sent simultaneously from multiple lumens of a long-term, indwelling, central line and if the culture was thought to represent a true bacteremia.

Results.—Discordant findings occurred in 13 (32%) of 41 episodes of blood cultures drawn simultaneously from different lumens. The estimated sensitivity of a culture obtained from a single lumen was 84%, which is lower than the minimum acceptable standard of 95%.

Conclusions.—It is recommended that blood cultures should be drawn from all lumens in patients with central venous catheters with multiple lumens because the sensitivity of a blood culture from a single lumen in a pediatric patient with a long-term, indwelling, venous catheter appears to be lower than the minimum acceptable sensitivity of 95%. Drawing blood cultures from multiple lumens increases the risk of obtaining a contaminated blood culture and can introduce infections, but the failure to recognize bacteremia or a delay in making the diagnosis increases the risk of septic shock and secondary seeding and may increase the need for removal of the line or prolongation of hospital stay.

► The issue of where to draw blood cultures from patients with central venous catheters that have single or multiple lumens is addressed in this study. Importantly, the results demonstrate a 32% discordance in cultures drawn simultaneously from different lumens. The sensitivity of a culture from a single lumen was 84%. While the volume of blood drawn is also known to affect the sensitivity of blood cultures, the results of this study would argue for sampling all lumens of multilumen catheters to increase the sensitivity of detecting bacteremia.

R. J. Arceci, MD, PhD

Relationship Between Changes in Hemoglobin Level and Quality of Life During Chemotherapy in Anemic Cancer Patients Receiving Epoetin Alfa Therapy

Crawford J, Cella D, Cleeland CS, et al (Duke Univ, Durham, NC; Evanston Northwestern Healthcare, Ill; Univ of Texas, Houston; et al)

Cancer 95:888-895, 2002 16–9

Background.—Quality of life (QOL) is an important factor in the treatment of patients with cancer, even when survival is the primary objective of therapy. The relations among hemoglobin, functional status, and patient-reported QOL have not been well studied. The relations among baseline hemoglobin levels and QOL, the change in hemoglobin levels during epoetin alfa therapy and change in QOL, and incremental change in hemoglobin levels during epoetin alfa therapy and incremental change in QOL were evaluated.

Methods.—Data for this study were obtained from 2 open-label, community-based trials of epoetin alfa therapy that used 4382 anemic cancer patients undergoing chemotherapy. The data were used to evaluate the relation between hemoglobin changes and QOL changes. QOL was measured with the Linear Analog Scale Assessment (LASA) and the more detailed, disease-specific Functional Assessment of Cancer Therapy-Anemia (FACT-An).

Results.—On cross-sectional analyses, a nonlinear relation and significant positive correlation were seen between high hemoglobin levels and high LASA and FACT-An scores. Patients with hemoglobin increases of 2 g/dL or more reported statistically significant improvements in 5 FACT-An items selected specifically to reflect functional capacity.

Conclusions.—There is a direct relation between increases in hemoglobin during epoetin alfa therapy and corresponding improvement in QOL in cancer patients receiving chemotherapy across the clinically relevant hemoglobin range of 8 to 14 g/dL. The indication is that the maximal incremental gain in QOL occurs with hemoglobin at a level of 11 to 13 g/dL.

Multivariate Regression Analyses of Data From a Randomized, Double-blind, Placebo-controlled Study Confirm Quality of Life Benefit of Epoetin Alfa in Patients Receiving Non-platinum Chemotherapy

Fallowfield L, for the Epoetin Alfa Study Group (Univ of Sussex, Brighton, England; et al)

Br J Cancer 87:1341-1353, 2002 16–10

Background.—Fatigue is now the most common and often the most bothersome side effect of patients with cancer receiving chemotherapy. Surveys of patients with cancer in both Europe and the United States have reported prevalence rates between 58% and 90%. The efficacy of epoetin alfa was evaluated for the treatment of cancer-related anemia.

Methods.—A total of 375 anemic patients with cancer receiving non–platinum-based chemotherapy were included in this multinational, double-blind, placebo-controlled trial. Cancer-specific measures of quality of life, including the general scale (FACT-G Total) and fatigue subscale (FACT-An Fatigue subscale) of the Functional Assessment of Cancer Therapy-Anemia and the Cancer Linear Analogue Scales, were used to measure energy, ability to perform daily activities, and overall quality of life. These assessment tools were also used to evaluate the relation between hemoglobin levels and quality of life. Univariate and multivariate analyses and linear regression analyses were performed.

Results.—Findings of the univariate analysis have been presented in a previous report and were confirmed on multivariate analysis, which adjusted for the effects of disease progression and several other potentially confounding variables. Specifically, a significant advantage for epoetin alfa over placebo was demonstrated in the multivariate analysis on all 5 assessment scales used. For cancer-specific measures, significant correlations were observed between baseline hemoglobin and quality of life and between change in hemoglobin levels and change in quality of life.

Conclusions.—It was demonstrated by these findings that the quality of life in patients with cancer can be significantly improved by administration of epoetin alfa.

Epoetin Alfa Treatment Results in Clinically Significant Improvements in Quality of Life in Anemic Cancer Patients When Referenced to the General Population

Cella D, Zagari MJ, Vandoros C, et al (Northwestern Univ, Evanston, Ill; Ortho Biotech UKI, Bucks, UK; Janssen-Cilag Pharmaceutical SACI, Pefki, Athens, Greece; et al)

J Clin Oncol 21:366-373, 2003 16–11

Background.—Anemia is a common occurrence among patients with cancer and is often a cause of cancer-related fatigue, which adversely affects the patient's quality of life. Randomized clinical trials have shown that epoetin alfa is effective in raising hemoglobin levels, reducing fatigue, decreasing transfusion requirements, and improving overall quality of life in patients with cancer-related anemia and fatigue. However, these conditions continue to be undertreated, possibly because scales and measures of quality of life are relatively unfamiliar to most clinicians and because there is a lack of population-based references, which make it difficult to interpret the results of clinical trials. Population-based data were developed that will provide a better perspective on the quality of life changes observed in clinical trials of epoetin alfa in patients with cancer-related fatigue.

Methods.—The Functional Assessment of Cancer Therapy-Anemia (FACT-An) quality of life instrument was administered to a nationally representative sample of 1400 people by using an Internet survey panel in the United States. Findings from this survey were then compared with quality of life data from a randomized, double-blind clinical trial that evaluated epoetin alfa versus placebo in 375 cancer patients with anemia.

Results.—The FACT-An displayed good psychometric properties when administered to the survey population and was able to discriminate between survey respondents with a history of specified illnesses, including anemia and cancer, and respondents without a history of specified illnesses. The comparison of the population norm and clinical trial data demonstrated that treatment with epoetin alfa provided statistically significant and clinically relevant improvements in quality of life.

Conclusions.—The interpretation of clinical trial results in which the FACT-An is used can now be aided by reliable population norm data. In this study, treatment with epoetin alfa was shown to be effective in overcoming much of the quality of life deficit that is seen in cancer patients with anemia compared with the norm population sample.

Pretreatment Haemoglobin Levels Significantly Predict the Tumour Response to Primary Chemotherapy in Human Breast Cancer

Bottini A, Berruti A, Brizzi MP, et al (Azienda Ospedaliera Istituti Ospitalieri, Cremona, Italy; Azienda Ospedaliera San Luigi, Orbassano, Italy)

Br J Cancer 89:977-982, 2003 16–12

Background.—Several studies have shown that tumor hypoxia plays an important role in the outcome of cancer patients. The oxygenation status of tumors primarily depends on the availability of oxygen from the blood and the diffusional flux from the microvessel to the oxygen-consuming cell. Hemoglobin concentration has been shown to be an important predictive factor for the outcome of radiotherapy or chemoradiotherapy in the treatment of a variety of cancers. Whether tumor response to primary chemotherapy in breast cancer is affected by baseline hemoglobin status was evaluated.

Methods.—A total of 157 patients with T2 to T4, N0-1 M0 breast cancer were treated with chemotherapy comprising either the cyclophosphamide, methotrexate, 5-fluorouracil regimen plus tamoxifen (the first 76 patients) or the single-agent epirubicin (the remaining 81 patients) before definitive surgery. Of these patients, 144 were available for inclusion in the final study analysis. Ki67, p53, bcl-2, c-erbB2, steroid hormone receptor, and microvessel density were evaluated immunohistochemically in tumor specimens obtained before chemotherapy and at surgery.

Results.—Tumor shrinkage of more than 50% occurred in 72.1% of patients. Those who responded to treatment had higher baseline hemoglobin levels and red blood cell counts compared with nonresponders. The distribution of disease response according to increasing cutoffs of baseline hemoglobin status showed that from 12.5 mg/L and higher, patients with hemoglobin levels above the cutoff obtained a greater response rate than patients with lower hemoglobin values. The difference was statistically significant at 12.5 g/dL (76.1% vs 59.5%) and 13.0 g/dL (81% vs 57.6%) cutoffs, respectively. the predictive role of hemoglobin levels persisted on multivariate analysis after adjustment for clinical and biologic characteristics and treatment regimen. Patients whose baseline hemoglobin levels were 13 g/dL or lower had a lower treatment-induced reduction in Ki67 expression and higher Ki67 expression at postoperative evaluation than other patients.

Conclusions.—It would appear from these findings that low levels of hemoglobin may adversely affect the response rate of chemotherapy in breast cancer patients, with the inhibition of antiproliferative activity as a potential mechanism for this effect.

► A growing body of literature documents the importance of hemoglobin levels in patients who are receiving treatment with chemotherapy or radiotherapy or both. The first 3 of these articles (Abstracts 16–9 to 16–11) report on the association of quality of life and hemoglobin levels and suggest that maintaining hemoglobin levels above 13 g/dL is important in optimizing quality of life for these patients. The fourth article by Bottini et al (Abstract 16–12) provides suggestive evidence that the efficacy of the chemotherapy or radiotherapy is improved in those patients with hemoglobin levels that exceed 13 g/dL during therapy. These articles further bolster the importance of maintaining hemoglobin levels in cancer patients undergoing definitive chemotherapy or radiotherapy.

J. T. Thigpen, MD

17 Late Effects of Treatment

Psychosocial Considerations: Cognitive and Psychosocial Functioning of Pediatric Hematopoietic Stem Cell Transplant Patients: A Prospective Longitudinal Study

Kupst MJ, Penati B, Debban B, et al (Med College of Wisconsin, Milwaukee)

Bone Marrow Transplant 30:609-617, 2002 17–1

Introduction.—Understanding regarding the posttreatment cognitive and behavioral functioning of children and adolescents undergoing hematopoietic stem cell transplantation (HSCT) is emerging. Until recently, research in this area has been limited to clinical descriptions, individual case studies, or a single-occasion evaluation of a small number of children and adolescents. Potential correlates of cognitive outcome (age at HSCT), dose of total body irradiation, sex, and treatment regimen have been assessed in several trials, with age and pre-HSCT functioning being the strongest correlates. A prospective, longitudinal investigation of cognitive and psychosocial functioning in patients undergoing pediatric HSCT was performed on 3 occasions: pre-HSCT, 1 year after HSCT, and 2 years after HSCT.

Methods.—A total of 153 children and adolescents were assessed before HSCT and at 1 year after. Two-year data were available in 74 children. Longitudinal analyses of Wechsler IQ data was performed in 100 children (longitudinal exact test), and repeated measures analysis was performed in 52 children.

Results.—Cognitive evaluations revealed stability of IQ scores over time. The strongest predictor of IQ was pre-HSCT cognitive functioning. Psychosocial evaluates showed a low prevalence of behavior and social problems and stability in functioning over time. The pre-HSCT functioning was strongly predictive of later functioning.

Conclusion.—This may be the largest number of children and adolescents prospectively evaluated from before HSCT to 2 years after HSCT. It may provide the most comprehensive analysis to date regarding variables associated with cognitive and psychosocial functioning in a longitudinal sample. Patient IQ remained stable and there was a low prevalence of behavior and social problems and stability over time in this series; pre-HSCT scores were strongly predictive of later functioning in all measures.

► The psychological and neurocognitive functioning of children treated for cancer and for those undergoing bone marrow transplantation are important and well studied. The study by Kupst et al reports on these characteristics in children undergoing stem cell transplantation both before and up to 2 years after transplantation. The results are consistent with most previous studies, although the current study includes a larger number of patients and extends observations out to 2 years. There was a low prevalence of behavioral and social problems with stability in functioning over the period studied. In addition, the pretransplant functioning was found to be the most important predictor of posttransplant functioning. While these results are important and encouraging, there remains a need for more detailed analysis of the younger subgroup of patients as well as analysis of more extended periods of follow-up.

R. J. Arceci, MD, PhD

Pulmonary Complications in Survivors of Childhood and Adolescent Cancer: A Report From the Childhood Cancer Survivor Study

Mertens AC, Yasui Y, Liu Y, et al (Univ of Minnesota, Minneapolis; Fred Hutchinson Cancer Research Ctr, Seattle; Univ of Texas, Houston; et al)

Cancer 95:2431-2441, 2002 17–2

Introduction.—The Childhood Cancer Survivor Study is a multi-institutional trial involving persons who survived for 5 or more years after treatment for carcinoma, leukemia, tumors, or similar illnesses diagnosed during childhood or illness. The results of the long-term effects of malignant disease and its associated therapy on the pulmonary conditions and complications were examined in a large cohort of 5-year survivors of childhood cancer.

Methods.—Data were used from questionnaires from 12,390 childhood cancer survivors and 3546 randomly selected siblings. The incidence of first occurrence of 15 selected pulmonary conditions were assessed in 3 periods: during therapy, from therapy completion to 5 years after diagnosis, and 5 or more years after diagnosis. The relative risks (RR) with 95% confidence intervals (CI) were calculated by multivariate analyses to assess reported pulmonary conditions by exposure to these treatment variables: radiation therapy to the chest; bleomycin, cyclophosphamide, busulfan, lomustine (CCNU); and carmustine (BCNU).

Results.—Compared with siblings, survivors had a statistically significant increased RR during all 3 periods for lung fibrosis, recurrent pneumonia, chronic cough, pleurisy, use of supplemental oxygen, abnormal chest wall, exercise-induced shortness of breath, bronchitis, recurrent sinus infection, and tonsillitis. During the period of more than 5 years after diagnosis, statistically significant correlations were observed for lung fibrosis and chest radiation (RR, 4.3; $P = .001$); supplemental oxygen use and chest radiation (RR, 1.8; $P < .001$), BCNU (RR, 1.4; $P = .05$), bleomycin (RR, 1.7; $P =$

.001), busulfan (RR, 3.2; *P* = .002), CCNU (RR, 2.1; *P* < .001), and cyclophosphamide (RR, 1.5; *P* = .01); recurrent pneumonia and chest radiation (RR, 2.2; *P* = .001) and cyclophosphamide (RR, 1.6; *P* = .04); chronic cough and chest radiation (RR, 2.0; *P* < .001), bleomycin (RR, 1.9; *P* < .001), and cyclophosphamide (RR, 1.3; *P* = .004); and pleurisy and chest radiation (RR, 1.4; *P* = .02) and busulfan (RR, 5.1; *P* = .02). Chest radiation was linked with a 3.5% cumulative rate of lung fibrosis at 20 years after diagnosis.

Conclusion.—Treatment-associated factors that continue to manifest more than 5 years after diagnosis and treatment are important determinants of risk. Continued follow-up is necessary in survivors of childhood cancer to assess the impact of pulmonary conditions on quality of life.

► The adverse effects of radiation and chemotherapy on pulmonary structure and function have been known for many years. More recently, reports have data that children with cancer may have a nearly 10-fold increase from death from pulmonary complications compared with control groups. The report by Mertens et al uses data from the Childhood Cancer Survivor Study to examine the short- and long-term pulmonary complications experienced by survivors of childhood cancer. Importantly, although the greatest number of complications occur during treatment, a substantial number of late complications, such as pulmonary fibrosis, recurrent pneumonias, exercise-induced shortness of breath, and oxygen use, occur more than 5 years after diagnosis. As expected, exposure to many of the known culprits, such as radiation, busulfan, bleomycin, and other lung-toxic chemotherapies, were reported to be associated with a higher incidence of complications. Even though such a survey is compromised because of the self-reporting nature of the data, these striking findings are important and underline the need to find alternative, effective therapies. In addition, until that day comes, increased education of survivors and intervention to prevent other "lung-toxic behaviors" such as smoking tobacco or marijuana, as well as work choices, should become a priority.

R. J. Arceci, MD, PhD

Risk of Disease Recurrence and Second Neoplasms in Survivors of Childhood Cancer Treated With Growth Hormone: A Report From the Childhood Cancer Survivor Study

Sklar CA, Mertens AC, Mitby P, et al (Mem Sloan-Kettering Cancer Ctr, New York; Univ of Minnesota, Minneapolis; Fred Hutchinson Cancer Research Ctr, Seattle)

J Clin Endocrinol Metab 87:3136-3141, 2002 17–3

Introduction.—Growth hormone (GH) deficiency is frequently observed in survivors of childhood cancer, particularly those who undergo radiation of the brain. The effect of GH therapy on disease recurrence has been examined in these patients, yet few data are available concerning the risk of disease recurrence in survivors of other types of tumors who undergo GH therapy. The risk of second neoplasms (SNs) linked with GH use has also not been systematically examined. These relations were examined in 361 GH-treated survivors (including 172 brain tumor survivors) from among 13,539 survivors enrolled in the Childhood Cancer Survivor Study, a cohort of 5-year survivors of childhood cancer.

Methods.—A time-dependent Cox model was used to compare the risk of recurrent disease, risk of SN, and risk of death between survivors who did and did not undergo GH treatment.

Results.—The relative risk for disease recurrence was 0.83 (95% confidence interval, 0.37-1.86; P = .65) for survivors who received GH. The relative risk for recurrent disease was not increased for any of the major cancer diagnoses. GH–treated patients had 15 SNs; all were solid tumors and none were secondary leukemias. The overall relative risk was 3.21 (95% confidence interval, 1.88-5.46; $P < .0001$). This was primarily the result of a small excess number of SNs in GH-treated survivors of acute leukemia. The risk of death was not linked with GH use (P = .43).

Conclusion.—Treatment with GH does not seem to increase the risk of disease recurrence or death in survivors of childhood cancer. The risk of an SN, especially in survivors of acute leukemia, is of concern; these data need to be interpreted with caution because the numbers are small.

► The risk of using GH replacement in survivors of childhood cancer remains a controversial area in pediatric oncology. A study by Leung et al[1] last year examined the impact of GH replacement in children with acute lymphoblastic leukemia and found no significant adverse outcomes as a result of its use. The study by Sklar et al examines 361 GH-treated survivors of childhood cancer, including 172 with brain tumors. Their results show no increased risk of recurrence in any of the major cancer diagnoses. Taken together, these 2 studies show that there does not appear to be an increase in cancer recurrence or secondary neoplasm in cancer survivors who are taking GH. However, clinicians should be cautious in discussions with patients and families in that the numbers of patients studied prospectively remain relatively small.

R. J. Arceci, MD, PhD

Reference

1. Leung W, Rose SR, Zhou Y, et al: Outcomes of growth hormone replacement therapy in survivors of childhood acute lymphoblastic leukemia. *J Clin Oncol* 20:2959-2964, 2002.

Second Malignancies in Children With Neuroblastoma After Combined Treatment With ¹³¹I-Metaiodobenzylguanidine

Garaventa A, Gambini C, Villavecchia G, et al (G Gaslini Children's Hosp, Genova, Italy; Galliera Hosp, Genova, Italy; Univ of Catania, Italy; et al)

Cancer 97:1332-1338, 2003 17–4

Background.—The long-term survival rate of children with inoperable or disseminated neuroblastoma diagnosed after age 1 year is unsatisfactory because the disease cannot be eradicated with currently available treatment. Iodine 131 metaiodobenzylguanidine (^{131}I-MIBG) is selectively taken up by cells that originate in the neural crest, which facilitates the targeted radiotherapy of tumors such as neuroblastoma and pheochromocytoma. Radiotherapy may provide additional benefits in the treatment of neuroblastoma, with moderate side effects such as hematologic and thyroid toxicity. However, other complications may develop with longer follow-up. The experience with second cancers occurring in children treated with ^{131}I-MIBG and chemotherapy was described.

Methods.—This retrospective review included the clinical records of 119 consecutive patients with neuroblastoma treated with ^{131}I-MIBG at a single institution from 1984 to 2001. These records were reviewed for the occurrence of a second malignant neoplasm.

Results.—Second malignant neoplasm developed in 5 of 119 patients, including 2 patients with myeloid leukemia and 1 patient each who developed angiomatous fibrous histiocytoma, malignant schwannoma, and rhabdomyosarcoma, respectively. The schwannoma and rhabdomyosarcoma developed within the residual neuroblastic mass in patients who had undergone first-line therapy.

Conclusions.—The risk of development of a second malignant neoplasm must be considered if ^{131}I-MIBG is more widely used in the treatment of neuroblastoma. An international registry of patients treated with ^{131}I-MIBG may more clearly elucidate the frequency and features of second malignancies after combined treatment with ^{131}I-MIBG and chemotherapy.

▶ One of the most challenging problems that faces survivors of childhood cancer is the risk of secondary malignancies. There is also increasing evidence that the intensification of therapy, particularly with alkylating agents and topoisomerase inhibitors, can result in the development of secondary leukemias and sometimes solid tumors. The study by Garaventa et al raises the issue of second malignancy development in children with neuroblastoma treated with ^{131}I-MIBG, which selectively targets neuroblastoma cells. One of the issues with this agent is that scatter radiation may harm bystander cells. In some cases, these could be normal solid organ tissues but also hematopoietic precursors. Current estimates suggest that secondary malignancies in patients with neuroblastoma occur with a cumulative risk of approximately 2% to 3% up to 20 years after initial diagnosis. In the group of patients reported by Garaventa et al, the authors estimate a 20% cumulative risk for patients with neuroblastoma treated with ^{131}I-MIBG. Of further interest is that the secondary malignancies included 2 cases of leukemia as well as cases of histiocytoma, schwannoma, and rhabdomyosarcoma. Such data raise the important issue of what criteria should be used to proceed with introduction of a new agent into patients with newly diagnosed disease versus stopping further testing of an agent except in the relapsed setting. The decision to bring such an agent into up-front therapy for patients with the poorest prognosis may be reasonable, but extending its use to better prognostic patients should be done with extreme caution and close monitoring for secondary malignancies.

R. J. Arceci, MD, PhD

Phase III Study of Interferon Alfa-NL as Adjuvant Treatment for Resectable Renal Cell Carcinoma: An Eastern Cooperative Oncology Group/Intergroup Trial

Messing EM, Manola J, Wilding G, et al (Univ of Rochester, NY; Dana-Farber Cancer Inst, Boston; Univ of Wisconsin, Madison; et al)

J Clin Oncol 21:1214-1222, 2003 17–5

Introduction.—Locally advanced renal cell carcinoma is challenging to manage. Even with the widespread use of abdominal imaging to evaluate nonspecific symptoms, stage T3+ or N+ disease is detected in 21% to 25% of patients on initial evaluation. The role of adjuvant interferon alfa was examined after complete resection of locally extensive renal cell carcinoma.

Methods.—Between May 1987 and April 1992, 283 eligible patients with pT3-4a or node-positive disease were randomly assigned after radical nephrectomy and lymphadenectomy to either observation or treatment with interferon alfa-NL administered daily for 5 days every 3 weeks up to 12 cycles. Patients were stratified on the basis of pathologic stage. Treatment was continued until confirmed recurrence, excessive toxicity, or patient/physician preference deemed removal appropriate.

Results.—At a median follow-up of 10.4 years, the median survival was 7.4 years for patients in the observation arm and 5.1 years for the treatment arm (P = .09). The median recurrence-free survival was 3.0 years and 2.2 years in the observation and interferon arms, respectively (P = .33). Multivariate analysis revealed that performance status (P = .003), nodal status (N2 vs N0; P < .0001), and tumor stage (P = .0002) were significant prognostic factors. Random assignment to interferon treatment (P = .009) and shorter time to recurrence (P < .0001) were independent predictors of shorter survival after recurrence. There were no lethal toxicities. Among patients assigned to treatment with interferon, 11.4% experienced severe toxicities (grade 4), including neutropenia, myalgia, fatigue, depression, and other neurologic toxicities.

Conclusion.—Random assignment to treatment with adjuvant lymphoblastoid interferon alfa-NL in the dosage used versus observation did not provide a benefit for patients with locally or regionally extensive, completely resected renal cell carcinomas.

► This article represents one of the largest randomized trials of adjuvant therapy in patients with resected renal cell cancer. Unfortunately, this patient population is without adequate adjuvant therapy for any patient population (high or low risk). The use of interferons in renal cell cancer is well established, and the rationale for the study was sound. Standard doses of interferon were used and, as a result, patients experienced interferon-related toxicities, with approximately 10% suffering from grade 4 toxicities. The results of the study failed to demonstrate any benefit for the interferon arm compared with observation. Patients in the interferon arm actually tended to have a shorter relapse-free survival and shorter median survival, although these did not reach statistical significance. One of the confounders of the trial may be the relative lower percentage of high-risk patients (nodal involvement) compared with higher T stage (T3) patients. Overall, this study reaffirms the lack of activity for interferon in the adjuvant setting of renal cell cancer and establishes observation as the standard for this patient population. In a similarly designed trial, a small study of high-dose interleukin-2 compared to observation suggested a trend to improvement but showed no statistical benefit over observation.[1]

M. S. Gordon, MD

Reference

1. Clark JI, Atkins MB, Urba WJ, et al: Adjuvant high-dose bolus interleukin-2 for patients with high-risk renal cell carcinoma: A cytokine working group randomized trial. *J Clin Oncol* 21:3133-3140, 2003.

Pregnancy Outcome of Female Survivors of Childhood Cancer: A Report From the Childhood Cancer Survivor Study

Green DM, Whitton JA, Stovall M, et al (Roswell Park Cancer Inst, Buffalo, NY; State Univ of New York, Buffalo; Fred Hutchinson Cancer Research Ctr, Seattle; et al)

Am J Obstet Gynecol 187:1070-1080, 2002 17–6

Background.—Children and adolescents who are successfully treated for cancer may have subsequent adverse reproductive sequelae. The effect of prior treatment for childhood cancer on a woman's pregnancy outcome was investigated.

Methods.—The study group included 1915 women younger than 21 years old at cancer diagnosis who participated in the Childhood Cancer Survivor Study and reported being pregnant. They answered a questionnaire about their pregnancy. Information on their previous cancer treatment was available from medical records. The proximity of the ovaries to the radiation field was also noted. Questionnaires were also sent to siblings of study participants to serve as control answers.

Findings.—Among the 1915 women, 4029 pregnancies were reported: live births, 63%; stillbirths, 1%; miscarriages, 15%; abortions, 17%; unknown, 3%; or in gestation. No significant differences were noted in pregnancy outcome by treatment. The neonates of those treated with pelvic irradiation were more likely to have low birth weight.

Conclusions.—Childhood chemotherapy does not appear to affect subsequent pregnancy of adult survivors. A small but significant adverse effect of prior pelvic irradiation was noted on birth weight.

► The fertility of survivors of childhood cancer has been an important component of late effects studies. The report by Green et al adds important information to this area of survivorship analysis. The study showed a trend toward increased miscarriages among women whose ovaries had been in radiation fields, although this difference did not reach statistical significance. Not surprising was the observation that previous pelvic irradiation was associated with a higher likelihood of a baby weighing less than 2500 g. Interestingly, exposure to most of the chemotherapeutic agents was not associated with adverse pregnancy outcomes, although combinations of pelvic radiation and particular chemotherapy exposures were associated with statistically significant increases in relative risk of low birth weight. The cumulative dose of the chemotherapy agents was also examined and no significant differences were observed in live births, miscarriages, or abortions. However, the details of how the low, medium, and high cumulative dose categories were decided were not included. No information concerning bone marrow transplantation was included. Importantly, the results being reported are from patients under age 21 at the time of their diagnosis who were treated from 1970 to 1986. A lot has changed since then and future information from more modern treatments with detailed information regarding exposures should represent important, future work.

R. J. Arceci, MD, PhD

18 Miscellaneous

Association of Funding and Conclusions in Randomized Drug Trials: A Reflection of Treatment Effect or Adverse Events?

Als-Nielsen B, Chen W, Gluud C, et al (Copenhagen Univ)

JAMA 290:921-928, 2003 18–1

Introduction.—Conclusions in randomized trials have been shown to be more positive toward experimental interventions when funded by for-profit organizations. A meta-analysis was performed in an observational investigation to determine whether the association between funding and conclusions in randomized drug trials reflects the magnitude of the treatment effect or occurrence of side effects.

Methods.—A total of 370 randomized drug trials were included in a meta-analyses from Cochrane reviews selected from the Cochrane Library, May 2001. From a random sample of 167 Cochrane reviews, 25 randomized drug trials were eligible for meta-analyses (evaluated a binary outcome; pooled a minimum of 5 full-paper trials of which at least 1 reported adequate and 1 reported inadequate concealment). The main binary outcome from each meta-analysis was considered the primary outcome for all investigations included in each meta-analysis.

The relationship between funding and conclusions was examined by logistic regression with adjustment for treatment effect, adverse events, and additional confounding factors (methodological quality, control intervention, sample size, publication year, and place of publication). The primary outcome measure was conclusions in trials, classified into whether the experimental drug was recommended as the treatment of choice or not.

Results.—The experimental drug was recommended as the treatment of choice in 16%, 30%, 35%, and 51% of trials funded by nonprofit organizations, trials not reporting funding, trials funded by both nonprofit and for-profit organizations, and trials funded by for-profit organizations, respectively ($P < .001$). Logistic regression analyses showed that funding, treatment effect, and double-blinding were the only significant predictors of conclusions.

Adjusted analyses revealed that trials funded by for-profit organizations were significantly more likely to recommend the experimental drug as the treatment of choice (odds ratio, 5.3; 95% confidence interval, 2.0-14.4) than were trials funded by nonprofit organizations. This relationship did not seem to reflect treatment effect or adverse events.

Conclusion.—Conclusions in trials funded by for-profit organizations may be more positive as a result of biased interpretation of trial findings. Readers need to carefully determine whether conclusions in randomized trials are adequately supported by data.

Factors Associated With Failure to Publish Large Randomized Trials Presented at an Oncology Meeting

Krzyzanowska MK, Pintilie M, Tannock IF (Dana-Farber Cancer Inst, Boston; Univ of Toronto)

JAMA 290:495-501, 2003 18–2

Introduction.—Publication bias refers to the situation in which the results of a study affect the likelihood that it will be published. Given the importance of published trials to treatment decision-making, nonpublication could be an important source of bias in the literature. Factors associated with nonpublication of randomized trials presented at a major oncology meeting were analyzed.

Methods.—The review included 510 abstracts of phase III randomized controlled trials presented at annual meetings of the American Society of Clinical Oncology between 1989 and 1998. All studies had a sample size of at least 200. A literature search was performed to determine whether the studies were published within 5 years after their presentation as well as their time to full publication. If there was no evidence of publication, the authors were contacted. Factors associated with publication and nonpublication were assessed, including the significance of the results, defined as a *P* value of .05 or less for the primary outcome measure; type of presentation; and study sponsorship.

Findings.—Twenty-six percent of the trials were not published within 5 years. The rate of full publication was 81% for studies meeting the criterion for significant results compared with 68% for studies with nonsignificant results. Time to publication was shorter for trials with oral or plenary presentations compared with studies that were not presented. Sponsorship by the pharmaceutical industry was associated with shorter publication times compared with studies sponsored by cooperative groups or those with nonspecified sponsorship. All these factors were independent predictors of publication status on multivariate analysis. When asked why their studies were not published, authors commonly mentioned a lack of resources, such as time or money.

Conclusions.—One fourth of large, phase III, randomized trials presented at a major oncology meeting are still unpublished 5 years later. Nonsignificant results are a key factor in nonpublication, along with type of presentation and study sponsorship. The authors emphasize that nonpublication of clinical trials "breaks the contract" between researchers and their subjects, funders, and ethics boards.

► Will Rogers once said, "All I know is what I read in the papers." I suppose physicians process information from more varied sources, but publications still remain the most reliable source for decision making. These 2 papers (Abstracts 18–1 and 18–2) address different aspects of the same problem: publishing negative results. Negative trials may not provide the opportunity for invited lectures or improve the bottom line for a company, but they are just as important for the patient care as many positive trials.

P. J. Loehrer, Sr, MD

Does Delay in Starting Treatment Affect the Outcomes of Radiotherapy? A Systematic Review

Huang J, Barbera L, Brouwers M, et al (Queen's Cancer Research Inst, Kingston, Ont, Canada; Kingston Regional Cancer Centre, Ont, Canada; McMaster Univ, Hamilton, Ont, Canada)
J Clin Oncol 21:555-563, 2003 18–3

Introduction.—In some publicly funded health care systems, the supply of radiotherapy (RT) has not kept up with increasing demand. This has made it necessary to use waiting lists for RT in several countries, including Canada, Australia, and the United Kingdom. It is not known whether delay adversely impacts the long-term outcome of RT. A literature review was performed to

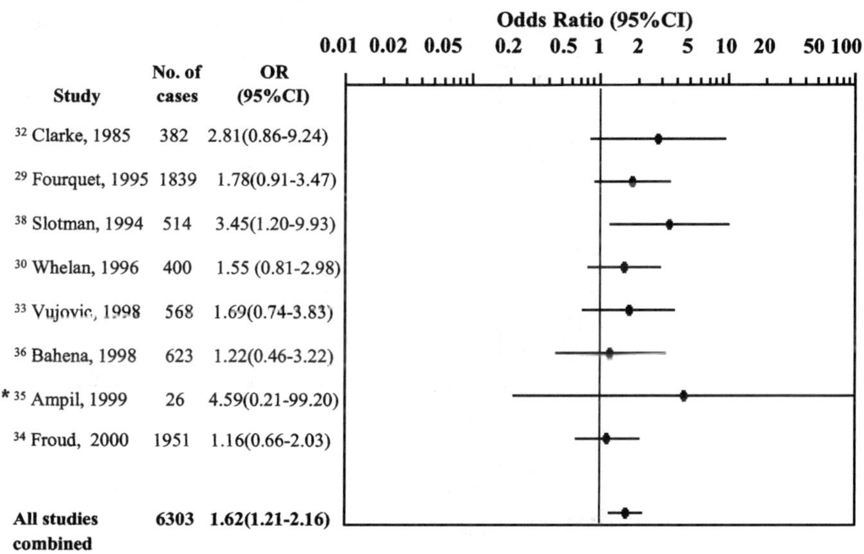

FIGURE 1.—Association between delay in postoperative radiotherapy for breast cancer and local recurrence rates. Local recurrence rates in women treated with postoperative radiotherapy more than 8 weeks after surgery are compared with the rates observed in those women treated within 8 weeks of surgery. Low-quality studies are indicated by an *asterisk*. *Abbreviations: CI*, Confidence interval, *OR*, odds ratio. (Courtesy of Huang J, Barbera L, Brouwers M, et al: Does delay in starting treatment affect the outcomes of radiotherapy? A systematic review. *J Clin Oncol* 21(3):555-563, 2003. Reprinted with permission from the American Society of Clinical Oncology.)

synthesize what is known concerning the relationship between delay in RT and RT outcome.

Methods.—A systematic review of the world literature was performed to identify trials that described the relationship between delay in RT and the probability of local control, metastasis, and/or survival. Searches were conducted using MEDLINE and CANCERLIT databases and appropriate text words or medical subject headings. Trials were classified by clinical and methodologic criteria, and their results were combined by means of a random-effects model.

Results.—Forty-six relevant investigations involving 15,782 patients met minimum methodologic criteria of validity; 42 were retrospective observational trials. Of these, 39 described rates of local recurrence, 21 described rates of distant metastasis, and 19 described survival. The association between delay and the outcome of RT has been examined in diverse situations, most frequently in breast cancer (21 trials) and head and neck cancer (12 trials). Combined analysis revealed that the 5-year local recurrence rate (LRR) was significantly higher among patients treated with adjuvant RT for breast cancer more than 8 weeks after surgery, compared with those treated within 8 weeks of surgery (odds ratio, 1.62; 95% confidence interval, 1.2-2.16) (Figs 1 and 2).

Combined analysis also revealed that the LRR was significantly higher in patients who received postoperative RT for head and neck cancer over 6

Study	No. of cases	OR (95%CI)
[41]Recht, 1991	286	2.61(0.67-10.17)
[40]Buchholz, 1993	100	6.42(0.76-54.26)
[46]Buzdar, 1993	552	1.51(0.49-4.70)
[39]Hartsell , 1995	84	6.83(0.79-59.48)
[42]Leonard, 1995	105	0.49(0.05-4.85)
* [44]Meek, 1996	76	0.65(0.03-16.78)
* [45]McCormick, 1996	139	3.12(0.87-11.22)
[47]Recht, 1996	157	2.99(0.91-9.84)
* [35]Ampil, 1999	21	1.06(0.04-27.30)
* [73]Buchholz, 1999	124	0.11(0.01-2.21)
* [48]Dendale, 2000	283	2.66(1.15-6.18)
All studies combined	**1927**	**2.28 (1.45-3.57)**

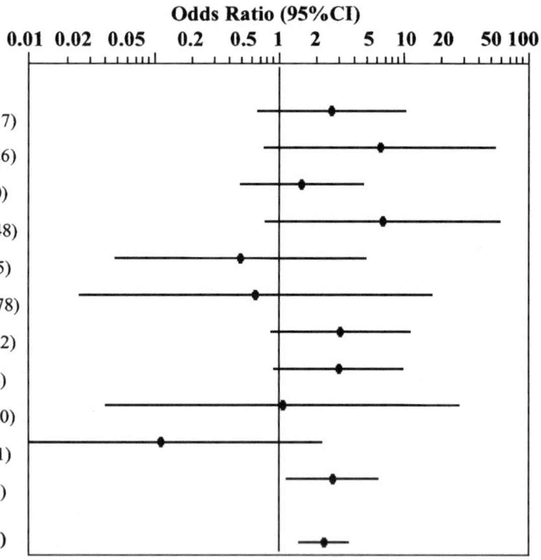

FIGURE 2.—Associations between delay in postoperative radiotherapy and local recurrence rates in studies of the sequencing of adjuvant radiotherapy and chemotherapy for breast cancer. Local recurrence rates in patients who received delayed radiotherapy following initial chemotherapy are compared with the rates observed in those patients who received early radiotherapy by chemotherapy. Low-quality studies are indicated by an *asterisk*. (Courtesy of Huang J, Barbera L, Brouwers M, et al: Does delay in starting treatment affect the outcomes of radiotherapy? A systematic review. *J Clin Oncol* 21(3):555-563, 2003. Reprinted with permission from the American Society of Clinical Oncology.)

weeks after surgery, compared with those treated within 6 weeks of surgery (odds ratio, 2.89; 95% confidence interval, 1.60-5.21). There was little evidence concerning the effect of delay in RT on the risk for metastasis or the probability of long-term survival in any situation.

Conclusion.—Delay in initiation of RT was associated with an increase in LRR in breast cancer and head and neck cancer (greater than 8-week and 6-week delays, respectively). Delays in beginning RT should be as short as reasonably possible.

► In the era of combined modality therapy, there seems to be some controversy as to how to integrate chemotherapy and RT. The basic question is which goes first? If one delays the chemotherapy, there is a concern about the development of metastatic disease that has not been addressed or cannot be well addressed once detection is made. Conversely, if one starts with chemotherapy and then delays RT, there are concerns about local recurrence developing during the period of chemotherapy or shortly thereafter that makes subsequent salvage difficult.

This Canadian study represents a systematic review of the world literature describing any relationship between delay in RT and the probability of local recurrence, metastasis, and survival. The authors were able to find 46 articles that are relevant, of which breast cancer was the more frequently published and some on head and neck cancer.

This article has a lot of data in it, and the data demonstrate reasonably well that for breast cancer, the local recurrence rate is significantly higher in patients treated with adjuvant RT more than 8 weeks after surgery than in those treated earlier. Likewise, in cancer of the head and neck, postoperative RT that begins more than 6 weeks after surgery also is associated with a higher local recurrence rate.

The question is, what does any of this mean? I have always taken the point of view that what is needed is an honest assessment of what the physician thinks the risks are in terms of dissemination versus local recurrence. By that I mean if the surgery was successful in its own right and there are no positive margins, if the patient has positive nodes, dissemination represents the bigger threat. If the nodes are negative, the local recurrence is more likely a bigger issue, especially if there is any question about the adequacy of the margins.

If there is a problem with the surgical resection and the nodes are also positive at the same time, I do not believe it is a question of either/or. In that circumstance, I would prefer to see the patient get chemotherapy and receive local RT to the tumor bed integrated in between cycles of chemotherapy. There may be some cosmetic price with this ping-pong approach, but I think it deals with the patient's disease in the most rational and realistic way in the setting of high risks for both local recurrence and dissemination.

E. Glatstein, MD

Magnetic Resonance Molecular Imaging of the HER-2/*neu* Receptor

Artemov D, Mori N, Ravi R, et al (Johns Hopkins Univ, Baltimore, Md)
Cancer Res 63:2723-2727, 2003 18–4

Introduction.—The HER-2/*neu* receptor belongs to the epidermal growth factor family and is amplified in several cancers. It is being intensely investigated as both a prognostic marker and for treatment, with the use of monoclonal antibodies targeted against the receptor. A novel 2-component gadolinium (Gd)-based magnetic resonance (MR) contrast agent has been developed that can image the HER-2/*neu* receptor. This method was tested in an experimental mouse model of breast carcinoma derived from HER-2/*neu* transgenic mice.

Findings.—Positive T1 contrast in MR images was produced by the specific binding of avidin-Gd complexes to tumor cells prelabeled with an biotinylated anti-HER-2/*neu* antibody. Significant intensity enhancement was seen in HER-2-*neu*-expressing cell lines and in vivo in a breast cancer model. Effective delivery of both components of the cancer to the tumor interstitium was verified by fluorescent analogues of the agents. On the basis of the expression efficiency of the receptor in the tested cells, the estimated MRI detection limit is clearly within the range of 10^6 receptors/cell. This number is within the clinically relevant range of HER-2/*neu* receptor expression, which may surpass 4 million receptors per cell in breast tumors with a HER-2/*neu* histologic score of "3+."

Conclusion.—Potential applications of MRI of the HER-2/*neu* receptor include determination of the HER-2/*neu* status for prognosis and section of tumors appropriate for monoclonal antibody therapy.

► The investigators developed a new gadolinium-based imaging technique for HER-2. This type of functional imaging is receiving tremendous enthusiasm for its ability to predict as well as assess early responses to therapy. In the preclinical studies performed in this trial, the investigators were able to demonstrate that this novel antibody-targeted technique successfully enhanced HER-2 overexpressing tumors both in vitro and in vivo. While the researchers propose that this type of imaging could be useful for the establishment of whether patients' tumors are HER-2 positive, it is feasible that the greatest potential would be in the assessment of the upregulation of HER-2 expression in clinical or experimental models following some type of pharmacologic manipulation. Hence, a HER-2 underexpressing tumor could be treated with an agent developed to increase HER-2 expression and, rather than needing a new biopsy to assess its success, functional imaging with this agent could be used. Other possible uses would need to be explored.

M. S. Gordon, MD

Presurgical Chemotherapy Compared With Immediate Surgery and Adjuvant Chemotherapy for Nonmetastatic Osteosarcoma: Pediatric Oncology Group Study POG-8651

Goorin AM, Schwartzentruber DJ, Devidas M, et al (Dana-Farber Cancer Inst, Boston; Children's Hosp Boston; Harvard Med School, Boston; et al)

J Clin Oncol 21:1574-1580, 2003 18–5

Background.—In patients with nonmetastatic osteosarcoma, adjuvant chemotherapy and surgical resection of the primary tumor have been used successfully for the prevention of disease progression. Presurgical chemotherapy has been recommended for patients with osteosarcoma because several trials that incorporated presurgical chemotherapy resulted in improved outcomes for patients. One possible advantage of presurgical chemotherapy is that it provides immediate treatment of micrometastatic disease and the primary tumor. Other advantages that have been reported are improvement in event-free survival (EFS) and pathologic identification of risk groups. However, a theoretic disadvantage is that it exposes a large tumor burden to marginally effective chemotherapy. The contribution of chemotherapy and surgery timing on the outcome of patients with nonmetastatic osteocarcinoma was examined.

Methods.—This prospective trial was conducted from 1986 to 1993 in patients with nonmetastatic osteosarcoma who were randomly assigned to immediate surgery or to presurgical chemotherapy. With the exception of the timing of surgery (week 0 or week 10), patients received 44 weeks of identical combination chemotherapy that included high-dose methotrexate with leucovorin rescue, doxorubicin, cisplatin, bleomycin, cyclophosphamide, and dactinomycin.

Results.—A total of 106 patients were included in the study, and 6 were subsequently excluded from the analysis. Of the remaining 100 patients, 45 were randomly assigned to chemotherapy and 55 were randomly assigned to immediate surgery. A total of 67 patients were free of disease at the presentation of this study. The projected EFS ± SE was 65% ± 6% at 5 years for presurgical chemotherapy. The incidence of limb salvage was similar for both arms of the study, with 55% for immediate surgery and 50% for presurgical chemotherapy.

Conclusions.—This study found that chemotherapy was successful in both groups and that no advantage was gained from presurgical chemotherapy in terms of EFS.

► Neoadjuvant therapy in the treatment of osteosarcoma had its origin in part because of the need to have time for the preparation of artificial limb prostheses. In addition, there were also theoretical advantages of using presurgical chemotherapy to immediately treat micrometastatic disease and possibly permit safer and more complete tumor resections. Nevertheless, whether presurgical therapy actually improves outcome has not been formally tested. In the study by Goorin et al, patients with nonmetastatic osteosarcoma were randomly assigned to receive presurgical chemotherapy or to go directly to surgery. All patients then received the same intensive postsurgical chemotherapy. With about 50 patients assigned to each arm of the study, the results showed no advantage in EFS for patients who received neoadjuvant therapy. It will be of interest to see whether neoadjuvant therapy continues to be used in future trials. Certainly, one of the advantages of an initial biopsy of the tumor followed by chemotherapy and then definitive surgical resection is the opportunity to study biological markers that might predict outcome and help direct therapy. At this time, the percentage of necrosis following neoadjuvant therapy has been helpful in predicting outcome. This, however, has not been helpful in all patients with a predicted good prognosis and has not led to effective alternative therapies for those patients with a predicted poor prognosis. Unfortunately, while the study by Goorin et al presents important results, it does not help us better utilize pre- and postchemotherapy tumor samples and may make some investigators reconsider the utility of using neoadjuvant therapy in osteosarcoma at all.

R. J. Arceci, MD, PhD

Overweight, Obesity, and Mortality From Cancer in a Prospectively Studied Cohort of U.S. Adults

Calle EE, Rodriguez C, Walker-Thurmond K, et al (American Cancer Society, Atlanta, Ga)

N Engl J Med 348:1625-1638, 2003 18–6

Background.—An increasing number of Americans are overweight or obese, and the health risks from overweight and obesity are frequently topics in the popular media. The relationship between excess body weight and mortality not only from all causes but also from cardiovascular disease are well established. It has been known for some time that excess weight is also a significant factor in death from cancer, but there are only limited data on the magnitude of this relationship, both for all cancers and for cancers at individual sites, and the public health effect of excess weight in regard to total mortality is unclear. Previous studies have consistently shown associations between adiposity and increased risk of cancers of the endometrium, kidney, gallbladder (in women), and colon (particularly in men). The relationships between body mass index (BMI) and the risk of death from cancer at specific sites were determined.

Methods.—This prospective study enrolled more than 900,000 adults (404,576 men and 495,477 women) who were cancer-free at enrollment in 1982. There were 57,145 deaths from cancer during 16 years of follow-up. This study examined the relationship between BMI in 1982 and the risk of death from all cancer and from cancers at individual sites. Multivariate proportional hazards models were used to control for other risk factors. The proportion of all deaths from cancer that was attributable to overweight and obesity in the US population was calculated on the basis of risk estimates from the current study and national estimates of the prevalence of overweight and obesity in the US adult population.

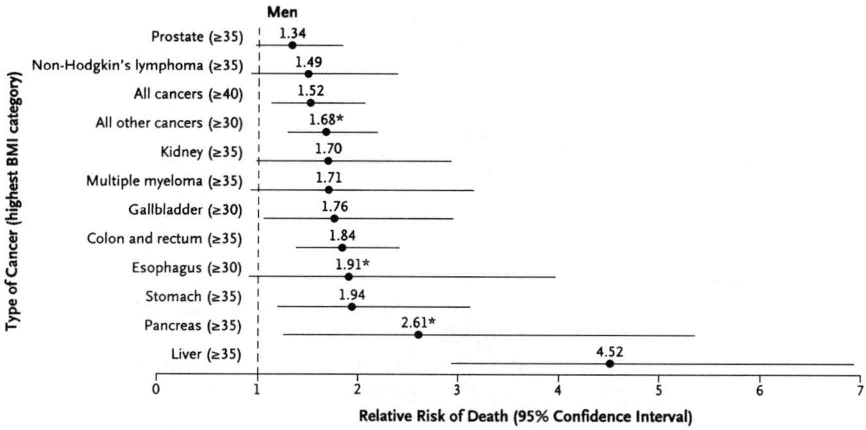

FIGURE 1.—Summary of mortality from cancer according to body mass index for US men in the cancer prevention study II, 1982 through 1998. For each relative risk, the comparison was between men in the highest body mass index (*BMI*) category (indicated in parentheses) and men in the reference category (body mass index, 18.5 to 24.9). Asterisks indicate relative risks for men who never smoked. Results of the linear test for trend were significant ($P \leq .05$) for all cancer sites. (Reprinted by permission of *The New England Journal of Medicine* from Calle EE, Rodriguez C, Walker-Thurmond K, et al: Overweight, obesity, and mortality from cancer in a prospectively studied cohort of U.S. adults. *N Engl J Med* 348:1625-1638, 2003.)

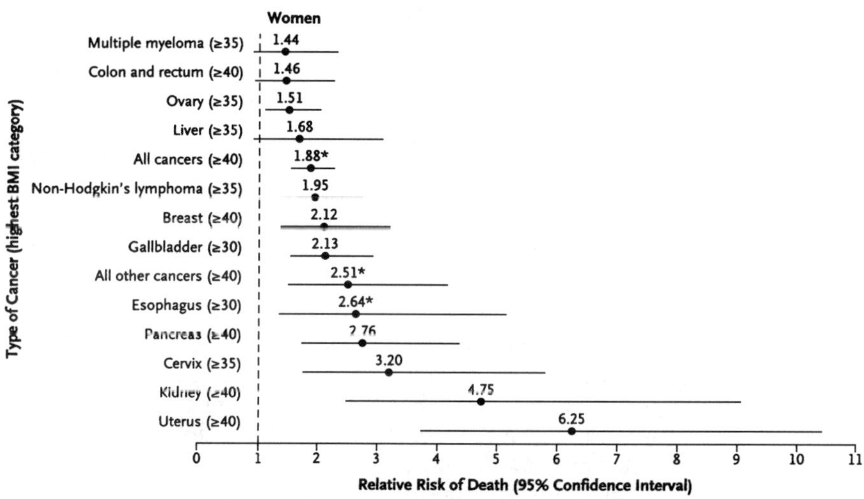

FIGURE 2.—Summary of mortality from cancer according to body mass index for US women in the cancer prevention study II, 1982 through 1998. For each relative risk, the comparison was between women in the highest body mass index (*BMI*) category (indicated in parentheses) and women in the reference category (body mass index, 18.5 to 24.9). Asterisks indicate relative risks for women who never smoked. Results of the linear tests for trend were significant ($P \leq .05$) for all cancer sites. (Reprinted by permission of *The New England Journal of Medicine* from Calle EE, Rodriguez C, Walker-Thurmond K, et al: Overweight, obesity, and mortality from cancer in a prospectively studied cohort of U.S. adults. *N Engl J Med* 348:1625-1638, 2003.)

Results.—The members of this cohort with a BMI of 40 had death rates from all cancers combined that were 52% higher for men and 62% higher for women, than the rates in men and women of normal weight (Fig 1). BMI was also significantly associated in both men and women with higher rates of death from cancer of the esophagus, colon and rectum, liver, gallbladder, pancreas, and kidney. This was also true for death from non-Hodgkin's lymphoma and multiple myeloma. Significant trends of increasing risk with higher BMI values were noted for death from cancers of the stomach and prostate in men and death from cancer of the breast, uterus, cervix, and ovary in women (Fig 2). It was estimated from these findings that current patterns of overweight and obesity in this country are responsible for 14% of all deaths from cancer in men and 20% of cancer deaths in women.

Conclusions.—This prospective study in a large population cohort of adults in the United States found that increased body weight was associated with increased death rates from all cancers combined as well as cancers at multiple specific sites.

► This is an exhaustive study that points again another reason why obesity is bad for you. The findings are even more impressive when the breadth of diversity of malignant diseases is noted even among those patients who are nonsmokers. The preclinical explanation for obesity-related carcinogenesis is largely unknown. One can even take the extreme and ask whether cancer-related cachexia is a natural response to fight cancer. All of this is worth further study, but until then: eat well and exercise.

P. J. Loehrer, Sr, MD

Occupational Risk Factors for Selected Cancers Among African American and White Men in the United States

Briggs NC, Levine RS, Hall I, et al (Meharry Med College, Nashville, Tenn; Ctrs for Disease Control and Prevention, Atlanta, Ga; Univ of Miami, Fla)

Am J Public Health 93:1748-1752, 2003 18–7

Background.—The incidence of cancer among black men in the United States is much higher than in white men. However, cancer incidence is similar among black and white women. This disparity may be attributed in part to the disproportionate exposure of black men to hazardous working conditions. However, there are few data regarding race-specific occupations risk factors for cancer. The published reports have generally been based on data from death certificates and other secondary sources, which has raised questions regarding the validity of these findings because of racial disparities in accuracy. Occupational risks for non-Hodgkin's lymphoma, Hodgkin's disease, and soft tissue sarcoma were evaluated among black and white men.

Methods.—Race-specific multivariate logistic regression analyses were performed with data from a large US population-based case control study. The final study population was composed of 959 cases of non-Hodgkin's lymphoma (66 blacks and 893 whites), 291 cases of Hodgkin's disease (22 blacks and 269 whites), 243 cases of soft tissue sarcoma (38 blacks and 205 whites), and 1620 control subjects (132 blacks and 1488 whites). Interviewers collected data about demographics, medical history, lifestyle, and occupation, including every full-time and part-time job held for at least 1 year since the age of 18 years and all occupational exposures implicated as etiologic determinants for 1 or more of the selected cancers.

Results.—Significant occupational risks were limited to blacks. Chromium was associated with non-Hodgkin's lymphoma, and wood dust was associated with Hodgkin's disease and soft tissue sarcoma.

Conclusions.—Racial disparities may exist in levels of exposure to occupational carcinogens; race-specific occupational risk factors for cancer were evident only among black men.

▶ Numerous cultural and dietary papers have been published about disparity of cancer incidence and mortality rate between black and white populations. This is a nicely written study that illuminates another plausible cause: occupation. Worthy of follow-up.

P. J. Loehrer, Sr, MD

Subject Index

A

B

C

E

G

H

I

J

K

L

M

N

O

Q

R

S

T

U

V

W

Author Index

A

B

C

D

E

F

G

H

I

J

K

L

M

N

O

P

Q

R

S

T

V

W